Emergency Radiology COFFEE Case Book

Case-Oriented Fast Focused Effective Education

Emergency Radiology COFFEE Case Book

Case-Oriented Fast Focused Effective Education

Bharti Khurana MD

Director, Emergency Radiology Fellowship, Brigham and Women's Hospital, and Assistant Professor of Radiology, Harvard Medical School, Boston, MA, USA

Jacob Mandell MD

Staff Radiologist in Musculoskeletal Imaging and Intervention at Brigham and Women's Hospital, and Instructor of Radiology at Harvard Medical School, Boston, MA, USA

Asha Sarma MD

Diagnostic Radiology Chief Resident, Brigham and Women's Hospital and Harvard Medical School, Boston, MA, USA

Stephen Ledbetter MD MPH

Chief of Radiology, Brigham and Women's Faulkner Hospital; former Section Chief of Emergency Radiology, Brigham and Women's Hospital; Assistant Professor of Radiology, Harvard Medical School, Boston, MA, USA

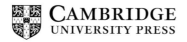

CAMBRIDGE
UNIVERSITY PRESS

CAMBRIDGE
UNIVERSITY PRESS

University Printing House, Cambridge CB2 8BS, United Kingdom

Cambridge University Press is part of the University of Cambridge.

It furthers the University's mission by disseminating knowledge in the pursuit of education, learning and research at the highest international levels of excellence.

www.cambridge.org
Information on this title: www.cambridge.org/9781107690769

First published 2016

Printed in the United Kingdom by Bell and Bain Ltd

A catalog record for this publication is available from the British Library

Library of Congress Cataloging in Publication data
Emergency radiology COFFEE case book : case-oriented fast focused effective education / [edited by]
Bharti Khurana, Jacob Mandell, Asha Sarma, Stephen Ledbetter.
    p. ; cm.
Includes bibliographical references and index.
ISBN 978-1-107-69076-9 (pbk. : alk. paper)
I. Khurana, Bharti, editor.   II. Mandell, Jacob, editor.   III. Sarma, Asha, editor.
IV. Ledbetter, Stephen (M. Stephen), editor.
[DNLM: 1. Emergencies–Case Reports.   2. Radiography–Case Reports.   3. Diagnosis,
Differential–Case Reports. WN 200]
RC78
616.07′572–dc23   2015000788

ISBN 978–1–107-69076-9 Paperback

....

Contents

Contributors

Sona A. Chikarmane MD
Radiology resident, Brigham and Women's Hospital and Harvard Medical School, Boston, MA, USA

Avni Chudgar MD
Radiologist, Brigham and Women's Hospital and Clinical Instructor, Harvard Medical School, Boston, MA, USA

Peter D. Clarke MD
Radiologist, Brigham and Women's Hospital and Assistant Professor, Harvard Medical School, Boston, MA, USA

Naman S. Desai MD
Radiology resident, Brigham and Women's Hospital and Harvard Medical School, Boston, MA, USA

Ritu R. Gill MD
Radiologist, Brigham and Women's Hospital and Assistant Professor, Harvard Medical School, Boston, MA, USA

Asha R. Goud MD
Radiology Fellow, Brigham and Women's Hospital and Harvard Medical School, Boston, MA, USA

Liangge Hsu MD
Radiologist, Brigham and Women's Hospital and Assistant Professor, Harvard Medical School, Boston, MA, USA

Pamela D. Ketwaroo MD
Radiology resident, Brigham and Women's Hospital and Harvard Medical School, Boston, MA, USA

Paryssa V. Khadem MD
Radiology Fellow, Brigham and Women's Hospital and Harvard Medical School, Boston, MA, USA

Bharti Khurana MD
Director, Emergency Radiology Fellowship, Brigham and Women's Hospital, and Assistant Professor of Radiology, Harvard Medical School, Boston, MA, USA

Wendy B. Landman MD
Radiologist, Brigham and Women's Hospital and Clinical Instructor, Harvard Medical School, Boston, MA, USA

Stephen Ledbetter MD MPH
Chief of Radiology, Brigham and Women's Faulkner Hospital; former Section Chief of Emergency Radiology, Brigham and Women's Hospital; Assistant Professor of Radiology, Harvard Medical School, Boston, MA, USA

Jacob Mandell MD

Staff Radiologist in Musculoskeletal Imaging and Intervention at Brigham and Women's Hospital, and Instructor of Radiology at Harvard Medical School, Boston, MA, USA

Asha Sarma MD

Diagnostic Radiology Chief Resident, Brigham and Women's Hospital and Harvard Medical School, Boston, MA, USA

Scott E. Sheehan MD

Radiology resident, Brigham and Women's Hospital and Harvard Medical School, Boston, MA, USA

Daniel A. Souza MD

Radiologist, Brigham and Women's Faulkner Hospital, and Clinical Instructor, Harvard Medical School, Boston, MA, USA

Leticia M. Souza MD

Radiology Fellow, Brigham and Women's Hospital and Harvard Medical School, Boston, MA, USA

David S. Titelbaum MD

Radiologist, Shields Health Care, Brockton, MA, USA

Gregory L. Wrubel MD

Radiology Fellow, Brigham and Women's Hospital and Harvard Medical School, Boston, MA, USA

Preface and acknowledgments

Emergency radiology is a rapidly growing area of clinical practice that focuses primarily on the imaging of the acutely ill, injured, or severely traumatized patient. When organized as a subspecialty service, it aggregates all emergent imaging and realigns the clinical practice of radiology with the principal referring services of emergency medicine and trauma surgery. It requires the rapid application of a diverse body of knowledge across multiple other radiology subspecialties that have been defined historically by organ system or modality divisions. Reliable, timely, and accurate imaging interpretation is vital in emergency radiology. This book's principal aim is to quickly augment this core competency for its reader.

An image-rich, case-based approach to diagnosis, with an emphasis on spectrum of disease and differential considerations has proven a fast and effective educational method that has been popularized in Continuing Medical Education courses over the past decade. We initially coined the acronym Case Oriented Fast Focused Effective Education (COFFEE) to describe this educational approach, which we first began to use in our emergency radiology CME courses in the early 2000s. We have now repurposed the COFFEE acronym for this book.

The book is intended to be a "go to" resource for both radiologists and clinicians during their active clinical work to improve their performance and confidence relative to imaging performed in Emergency Departments. The book is organized by clinical presentation rather than traditional organ system or imaging modality so as to more closely simulate real clinical radiology practice in the Emergency Department setting. Each chapter begins with an index case, presented as an unknown with a standardized format that includes a focused summary of major teaching points, disease variants, clinical and/or imaging management, instructional figures, helpful illustrations, and differential diagnosis. The self-assessment that accompanies each case provides additional learning about the significance of specific clinical and imaging findings with "pearls" of wisdom that often come from seasoned experience.

The editors are indebted to the contributing authors of this text for their expertise and collaboration. This book has been a significant undertaking that has benefitted tremendously from a close working relationship with our inspiring and enthusiastic clinical colleagues in radiology, emergency medicine, and trauma surgery. More broadly, we would also like to thank members of the Department of Radiology at Brigham and Women's Hospital for creating such a rich environment of learning through the sharing of cases and knowledge. Finally, our most heartfelt appreciation goes to each of our families for their patience, encouragement, and support during the many hours it takes to complete work on projects of this nature.

Bharti Khurana
Jacob Mandell
Asha Sarma
Stephen Ledbetter

PART I Non-Traumatic Conditions

SECTION 1 ABDOMEN

Section 1.1 Upper Quadrant and Epigastric Pain

Case 1   44-year-old obese woman presenting with right upper quadrant pain

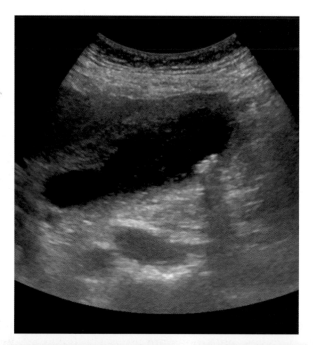

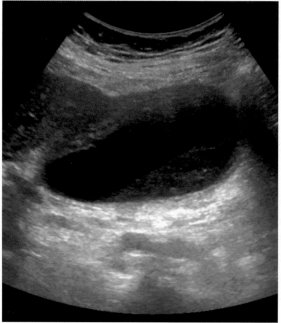
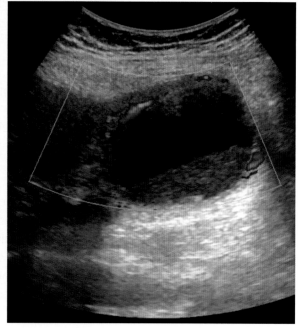

***Diagnosis:*
**Acute
calculous
cholecystitis**

Sagittal grayscale ultrasound images of the gallbladder (left and middle images) show diffuse, asymmetric gallbladder wall thickening (yellow arrows), and a shadowing gallstone (red arrow). There is layering, echogenic sludge (blue arrows). Transverse color Doppler image (right image) shows increased vascular flow within the gallbladder wall, suggestive of acute inflammation. Pain was worsened by compression of the gallbladder by the ultrasound transducer (positive sonographic Murphy sign).

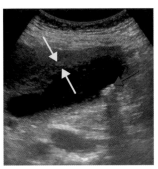 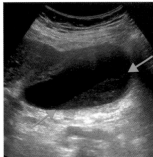 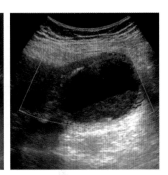

Discussion

Overview of acute cholecystitis

- Acute cholecystitis is defined as acute inflammation of the gallbladder. In 90–95% of cases, gallstones are the cause (acute calculous cholecystitis).
- Acute calculous cholecystitis is thought to result from luminal obstruction by an impacted calculus at the gallbladder neck (infundibulum), which leads to impaired drainage of bile, increased intraluminal pressure, venous congestion, and mural ischemia. This is analogous to the pathophysiology of acute appendicitis.
- Although most patients with cholelithiasis are asymptomatic, gallstones can cause many complications, including biliary colic, acute cholangitis, acute pancreatitis, gallstone ileus, gallbladder-enteric fistula, Mirizzi syndrome, and gallbladder perforation.
- Cholesterol stones are the most common type of gallstones. These are more common in obese, premenopausal female patients (a commonly memorized mnemonic is "forty, fat, female, fertile"). Up to 25% of women over age 50 have gallstones. Pigment stones are less common, and are often associated with hemolytic states (e.g., spherocytosis, prosthetic cardiac valve), cirrhosis, and longstanding bile duct stenosis (e.g., *Clonorchis sinensis* infection).

Imaging of acute cholecystitis

- Ultrasound is the modality of choice for evaluation of the gallbladder and the first line imaging test in the investigation of right upper quadrant (RUQ) pain.
- The sonographic diagnosis of acute cholecystitis is made from a combination of the following findings: sonographic Murphy sign, impacted calculus in the gallbladder neck, distention of the gallbladder (>10 cm in sagittal dimension and >4–5 cm in transverse dimension), gallbladder wall thickening (>3 mm), and the presence of pericholecystic fluid or edema in the surrounding fat or adjacent hepatic parenchyma. In isolation, none of the above listed findings establishes the diagnosis and, conversely, the diagnosis may be made without all of these findings being present.
- In particular, it should be noted that diffuse gallbladder wall thickening is not specific for acute cholecystitis – systemic and local conditions associated with gallbladder wall thickening include gallbladder contraction due to a recent meal, hypoalbuminemia (as in cirrhosis or nephrotic syndrome), acute hepatitis, and gallbladder adenomyomatosis.
- CT is the imaging modality of choice when most complications of cholelithiasis are suspected. Cross-sectional imaging modalities also allow for the detection of hyper-enhancement of the gallbladder wall and pericholecystic tissues, a finding consistent with inflammation.
- MR is most useful when common bile duct pathology is suspected, based on common bile duct dilation seen by other imaging modalities or an obstructive pattern of bilirubin elevation. The advantages of MRI include lack of ionizing radiation and improved detection of choledocholithiasis with MR cholangiopancreatography (MRCP).
- The spectrum of acute cholecystitis ranges from uncomplicated disease to gangrene, necrosis, and perforation of the gallbladder.

Acalculous cholecystitis

- Acalculous cholecystitis is gallbladder inflammation *not* caused by an obstructing stone.
- Establishing the diagnosis of acute acalculous cholecystitis (5–10% of cases) is challenging. This condition is thought to result from gallbladder wall ischemia, and may be suspected in severely ill patients, especially those predisposed by diabetes, sepsis, trauma, major surgery, or AIDS. A nuclear medicine hepatobiliary (HIDA) scan may be necessary for confirmation.

Clinical synopsis   This patient was admitted and underwent laparoscopic cholecystectomy. In some cases, intravenous antibiotics and gallbladder decompression with percutaneous cholecystostomy may be preferred before surgical intervention.

Self-assessment

- *What are the two most specific US findings in acute cholecystitis?*

- *List three common alternative diagnoses associated with diffuse gallbladder wall thickening.*

- *List four common complications of cholelithiasis besides acute cholecystitis.*

- Sonographic Murphy sign
- Impacted gallstone at the gallbladder neck

- Recent meal (gallbladder contraction)
- Cirrhosis (hypoalbuminemia and ascites)
- Acute hepatitis

- Acute pancreatitis
- Acute cholangitis
- Gallstone ileus
- Mirizzi syndrome (obstruction of the common bile duct by an impacted gallstone in the gallbladder neck or cystic duct)

Spectrum of acute cholecystitis

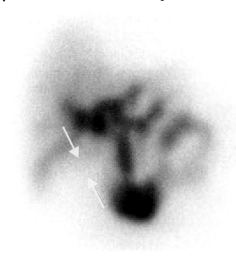

Acute cholecystitis on HIDA scan

Hepatobiliary iminodiacetic acid scintigraphy (HIDA scan) is highly sensitive in detecting cystic duct obstruction, which is the hallmark of acute cholecystitis. Normally, serial images acquired after injection of radiotracer should demonstrate progressive hepatic uptake and subsequent excretion into the biliary system and gallbladder. If the gallbladder is not visualized, cystic duct obstruction is presumed. One-hour delayed static image from a HIDA scan demonstrates absence of gallbladder uptake (yellow arrows). There is normal excretion into the biliary tree and small bowel.

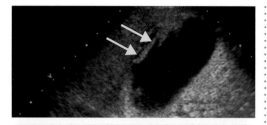

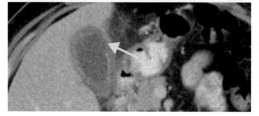

Gangrenous cholecystitis

Gangrenous cholecystitis is a severe form of cholecystitis characterized by mural necrosis. Imaging findings are nonspecific, but include heterogeneous, irregular thickening of the gall-bladder wall, which may demonstrate decreased perfusion (on color Doppler) or reduced enhance-ment (on enhanced CT). Treatment is prompt open cholecystectomy. Ultrasound (top image) demonstrates an irregularly thickened gallbladder wall with projections into the lumen representing desquamating mucosa (arrows). Axial enhanced CT image shows wall thickening with an area of reduced enhancement medially (arrow), with adjacent pericholecystic fat stranding.

Perforated cholecystitis

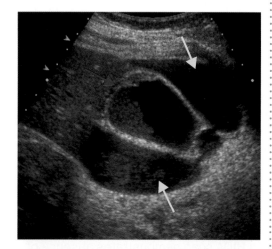

Gallbladder perforation is a rare complication of acute cholecystitis. Spillage of bile into the peritoneal cavity causes chemical, and later, infectious peritonitis. Ultrasound demonstrates a large amount of heterogeneous fluid surrounding the gallbladder (yellow arrows), suggestive of gallbladder perforation and intra-peritoneal spill-age of bile. There is focal thickening and contour irregularity at the gallbladder fundus (red arrow), which is likely the site of rupture.

Emphysematous cholecystitis

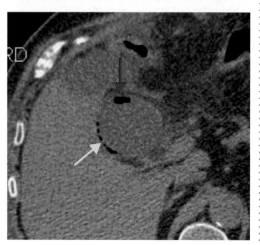

Emphysematous cholecystitis is a rare form of acute cholecystitis that occurs in elderly patients with diabetes or peripheral atherosclerotic dis-ease. CT is the most sensitive and specific imaging modality for identifying gas within the gallbladder lumen or wall, which is produced by gas-forming organisms. Axial unenhanced CT demonstrates gas in the gallbladder wall (yellow arrow) and a small amount of nondependent gas in the gall-bladder fundus (red arrow).

Differential diagnosis of acute cholecystitis

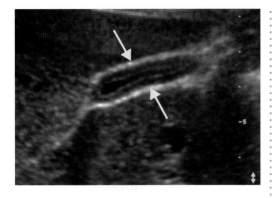

Recent meal (gallbladder contraction)

Eating causes gallbladder contraction and apparent wall thickening; this may result in an erroneous diagnosis of acute cholecystitis upon imaging. Fasting for at least 4–6 hours prior to the examination is recommended for adequate evaluation of the gallbladder. Sagittal ultrasound demonstrates a contracted gallbladder with an apparently thickened wall (arrows).

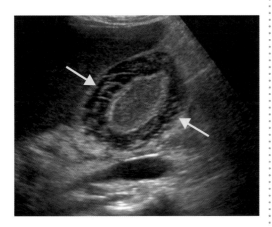

Acute hepatitis

Diffuse gallbladder wall thickening may be due to a systemic process. In particular, viral hepatitis can lead to marked gallbladder wall thickening without cholecystitis. Ultrasound demonstrates marked diffuse hypoechoic gallbadder wall thickening (arrows). The gallbladder is non-distended (in contrast to acute cholecystitis). The gallbladder lumen is filled with mildly echogenic sludge.

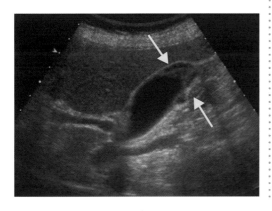

Adenomyomatosis

Adenomyomatosis is a usually asymptomatic finding caused by cholesterol deposition into intramural mucosal diverticula (Rokitansky–Aschoff sinuses). It may be diffuse, circumferential, or focal. Focal adenomyomatosis typically occurs at the gallbladder fundus. Comet-tail artifacts may be seen due to the cholesterol crystals. Sagittal ultrasound image demonstrates focal hypoechoic mural thickening of the gallbladder fundus (arrows).

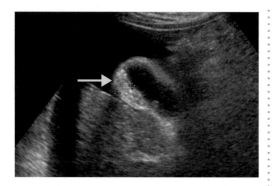

Cirrhosis and ascites

Cirrhosis and other hypoalbuminemic states such as nephrotic syndrome are common causes of diffuse gallbladder wall thickening. Ultrasound demonstrates diffuse gallbladder wall thickening (arrow) associated with moderate ascites. Note that the gallbladder is not distended, which suggests that wall thickening is due to a condition other than acute cholecystitis.

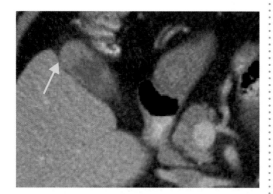

Gallbladder metastasis

Metastases to the gallbladder are rare, and usually are only seen in patients with known widespread metastatic disease. Melanoma is known to metastasize to the gallbladder, as in this patient. Axial enhanced CT images demonstrate an enhancing mural nodule at the gallbladder fundus (arrow). PET/CT performed at later date (not pictured) showed intense FDG uptake at this site and within other organs, highly suspicious for metastases.

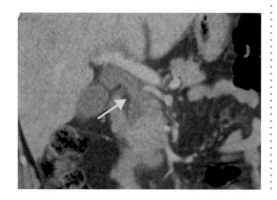

Acute cholangitis

Acute cholangitis is the clinical syndrome of fever, jaundice, and abdominal pain caused by infection in the biliary tract. Coronal contrast-enhanced CT in a patient with fever and jaundice demonstrates wall thickening and hyper-enhancement of the common bile duct (arrow). ERCP later confirmed the presence of mild ductal dilatation and pus within the common bile duct.

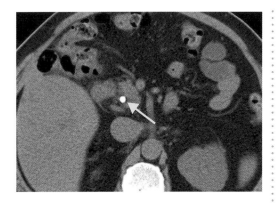

Retained common bile duct stone after cholecystectomy

Approximately 1% of patients undergoing chole-cystectomy experience subsequent choledocho-lithiasis, which may be due to a pre-existing stone and lack of clinical suspicion at time of cholecys-tectomy, or stone migration occurring at the time of cholecystectomy. Axial unenhanced CT in a patient status post recent cholecystectomy dem-onstrates a radiopaque calculus at the distal common bile duct (arrow), consistent with choledocholithiasis.

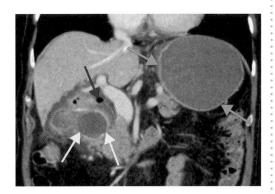

Bouveret syndrome

Bouveret syndrome is gastric outlet obstruction due to impaction of a gallstone within the proximal duodenum. Gallbladder inflammation/adhesions cause a cholecystogastric or cholecystoduodenal fistula to form, which allows a potential large stone to cause obstruction. Coronal enhanced CT dem-onstrates a large radiolucent gallstone (yellow arrows) and adjacent biliary gas (red arrow) suggestive of cholecystoenteric fistula. There is gastric distension (blue arrows).

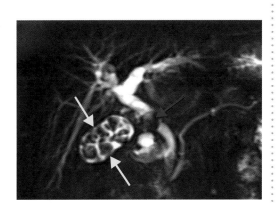

Mirizzi syndrome

Mirizzi syndrome is caused by an impacted gall-stone in the gallbladder neck or cystic duct, which leads to stricture formation in the common hepatic or common bile duct. Thick-slab MRCP image shows multiple gallstones within the gallbladder lumen (yellow arrows). An impacted calculus (red arrow) at the infundibulum causes proximal dilation of the common hepatic duct and mild intrahepatic biliary ductal dilatation.

Further reading

Bennett GL *et al.* CT Findings in Acute Gangrenous Cholecystitis. *AJR* 2002; 178:275–281.

Bortoff GA *et al*. Gallbladder Stones: Imaging and Intervention. *Radiographics* 2000; 20:751–766.

Catalano OA *et al*. MR Imaging of the Gallbladder: A Pictorial Essay. *Radiographics* 2008; 28:135–155.

Grayson DE, Abbott RM, Levy AD *et al*. Emphysematous Infections of the Abdomen and Pelvis: A Pictorial Review. *Radiographics* 2002; 22:543–561.

Lassandro F *et al*. Clinical Observations: Role of Helical CT in Diagnosis of Gallstone Ileus and Related Conditions. *AJR* 2005; 185:1159–1165.

O'Connor OJ, Maher MM. Imaging of Cholecystitis. *AJR* 2011; 196:W367–374.

Shakespear JS *et al*. Pictorial Essay: CT Findings of Acute Cholecystitis and Its Complications. *AJR* 2010; 194:1523–1529.

Case 2   33-year-old woman presenting with acute onset of right upper quadrant pain

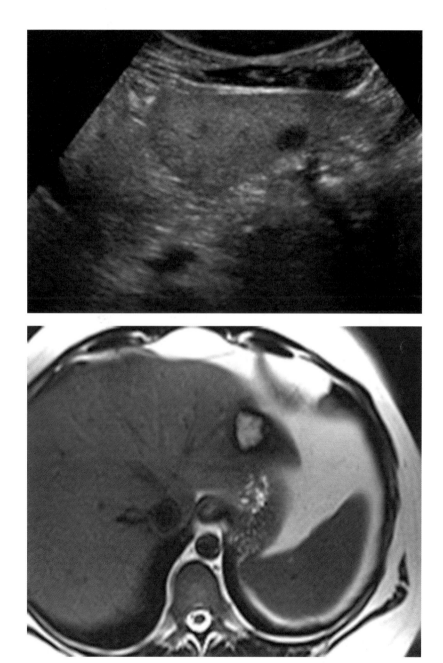

Diagnosis:
Ruptured
hepatic
adenoma

Sagittal US image shows hyperechoic liver, consistent with fat deposition (steatosis), with a subcapsular hypoechoic nodule (yellow arrow) within the left hepatic lobe, nonspecific by imaging. Hepatic adenomas do not have specific sonographic features, and further evaluation is often needed with contrast-enhanced MRI, as was performed in this case.

Subsequently performed axial T2-weighted MRI of the abdomen shows a heterogeneous T2-hyperintense lesion within the left hepatic lobe. The lesion has a peripheral low signal rim (red arrows), demonstrating magnetic susceptibility and suggestive of hemosiderin, consistent with prior hemorrhage. It is important to note that other hypervascular liver lesions such as hepatocellular carcinoma (HCC), angiosarcoma, and hypervascular metastases (e.g., breast, neuroendocrine tumor, kidney, thyroid, and sarcoma) are also associated with increased risk of hemorrhage or hemoperitoneum, particularly when large and/or subcapsular in location.

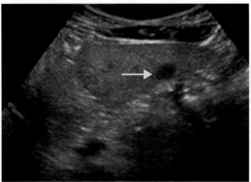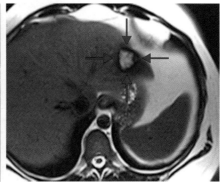

Discussion

Hypervascular liver masses are the most common cause of atraumatic hepatic hemorrhage.

- The most common causes of atraumatic hepatic rupture (hemorrhage) are hypervascular neoplasms such as HCC and hepatic adenoma. Less common causes include focal nodular hyperplasia (FNH), hemangioma, and metastases.
- Hepatocellular adenomas (HA) are rare benign liver tumors of uncertain origin. They are solitary in the majority of cases (70–80%). Histologically, they are characterized by large cords of well-differentiated hepatocytes separated by dilated sinusoids, interspersed with feeding vessels. There is a paucity of connective tissue.
- Development of HA is classically associated with oral contraceptive use but may also be seen in patients with glycogen storage disease, liver adenomatosis, diabetes mellitus, or iron overload, and in males using anabolic steroids.

- Adenomas are prone to spontaneous bleeding.
- Though the normal hepatocytes contained within an HA are capable of producing bile, the absence of bile ductules is a key histologic feature that distinguishes HA from FNH.
- Malignant transformation of an adenoma into hepatocellular carcinoma is rare but has been reported to occur.
- Hepatocellular carcinoma is commonly seen in the setting of cirrhosis or chronic hepatic inflammation due to viral hepatitis or fatty liver disease. Large and peripheral tumors are at higher risk for rupture.

CT is the preferred imaging modality for symptomatic hepatic masses and suspected hemoperitoneum in the acute setting.

- CT is useful for distinguishing lower-attenuation simple ascites from higher-attenuation blood ($\approx$30–45 Hounsfield units). "Sentinel clot," the highest attenuation clotted hematoma, is often adjacent to the site of bleeding, and can be a useful sign to localize the site of extravasation. Lower-attenuation unclotted blood tends to be located farther from the source. Because erythrocytes are denser than plasma and peritoneal fluid, hematocrit levels may form in dependent areas such as the paracolic gutters.
- On contrast-enhanced CT, focal attenuation higher than that of clotted blood (closer to metal or bone) within a mass or clot indicates freely extravasating intravenous contrast, or active bleeding. This finding usually warrants emergent embolization or surgical treatment. To troubleshoot, noncontrast images may be helpful to differentiate actively extravasating contrast from calcification or metal artifact and delayed phase imaging may be helpful to exaggerate the appearance of extravasating contrast.

MRI is superior to CT in definitively characterizing focal liver lesions.

- Ideally, MRI is performed in the stable patient after resolution of hemorrhage. Contrast-enhanced MRI is typically performed with traditional extracellular contrast agents alone, with increasing interest in the use of combined agents. Combined agents contain both traditional extracellular gadolinium preparations that are retained in the intravascular space and "hepatobiliary specific" agents such as gadoxetate disodium (Eovist, Bayer) that are taken up by hepatocytes and excreted in the bile.
- FNH is the prototypical lesion distinguished by uptake and retention of hepatobiliary specific gadolinium contrast.

Clinical synopsis   The patient was admitted and treated with endovascular embolization.

Self-assessment

- *Name three causes of atraumatic hepatic hemorrhage.*

- *What is the utility of the "sentinel clot" sign?*

- *What is the most common lesion associated with spontaneous hepatic rupture?*

- HCC, adenoma, telangiectatic hemangioma.

- To locate the source of bleeding.

- HCC.

Spectrum of hepatic adenoma

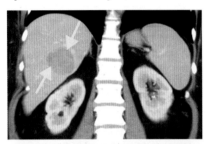
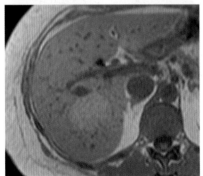
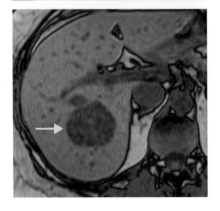

Uncomplicated fat-containing hepatic adenoma

It is rarely possible to make the diagnosis of adenoma from CT alone; however, if a liver mass contains fat or hemorrhage then an adenoma should be considered. Coronal enhanced CT demonstrates a nonspecific, heterogeneous mass (arrows) with slightly lobular contours. Neither hemorrhage nor fat is apparent. In-phase (middle image) and out-of-phase (lower image) axial MR images demonstrate signal loss on the out-of-phase images (arrow), consistent with intracellular lipid. Recently, studies have characterized steatotic (fat-containing) adenomas as the least aggressive subtype, with minimal risk of bleeding and negligible malignant potential. *Case courtesy Cheryl Sadow, MD.*

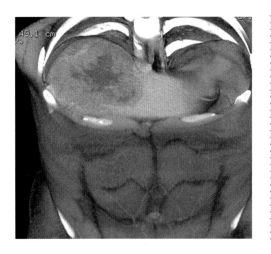

Hepatic adenoma that has undergone malignant transformation into HCC in a male patient with history of anabolic steroid use

Volume-rendered coronal oblique image shows a large, heterogeneous adenoma in the liver dome that has undergone malignant transformation into HCC. This male patient with a non-cirrhotic liver was a weightlifter with a longstanding history of anabolic steroid use. The patient had multiple hypervascular liver lesions. Rupture has been reported in up to 14% of HCCs in Asia and Africa where they are prevalent.

Differential diagnosis of hepatic adenoma

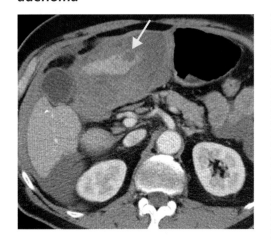

Ruptured hepatocellular carcinoma

Axial contrast-enhanced image demonstrates large hemoperitoneum and a small subcapsular liver lesion in the left lobe, within hepatic segment III (arrow). Hepatic contour irregularity suggests underlying chronic liver disease (cirrhosis). The mass was resected with subsequent pathologic confirmation of a moderately differentiated HCC in the setting of cirrhosis.

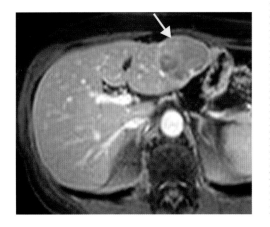

Well-differentiated hepatocellular carcinoma

Adenomas and HCCs are hepatocellular tumors and share similar imaging characteristics. Although best performed with MRI, preoperative differentiation can be difficult, particularly in the absence of clinical correlation. Axial contrast-enhanced T1-weighted MR image obtained in the delayed (equilibrium) phase demonstrates a large, subcapsular lesion in the left hepatic lobe (arrow), with signal intensity lower than the surrounding liver and an enhancing pseudocapsule.

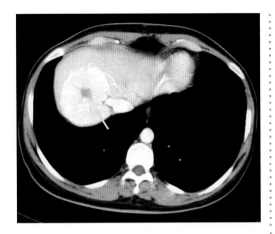

Focal nodular hyperplasia (FNH)

FNH is a benign hepatocellular lesion that is thought to represent focal hyperplastic response to injury due to an underlying vascular malformation. Approximately 20% of patients with FNH have multiple lesions. The female-to-male ratio is 8:1. Axial contrast-enhanced CT image demonstrates a hypervascular, homogeneous lesion with a stellate, hypodense central scar (arrow). There are enlarged feeding vessels.

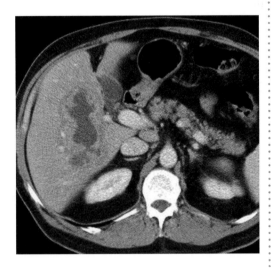

Hepatic abscess

Hepatic abscesses can be classified as pyogenic, amebic, or fungal. They can present as micro-abscesses (<2 cm) or macroabscesses. Although their appearances may be variable, typical large abscesses are irregularly contoured, thick-walled lesions with low attenuation content and occasional rim enhancement. The presence of gas is a relatively uncommon but helpful clue for the diagnosis of infection, which is most commonly polymicrobial.

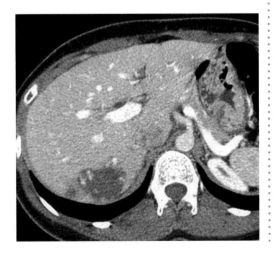

Hemangioma

Hepatic hemangioma is the most common benign tumor of the liver. The classic diagnostic CT appearance is a hypodense lesion with peripheral, globular enhancement with centripetal fill-in pattern, with the attenuation of the enhancing areas identical to that of the aorta and blood pool, such as in this axial enhanced CT.

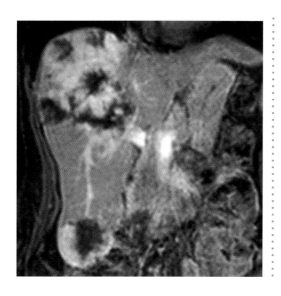

Hepatic hemangiomatosis

Hemangiomas are multiple in 10% of cases (hemangiomatosis). Coronal T1-weighted post-contrast (portal venous phase) MR demonstrates a giant hemangioma (>5 cm) in the right hepatic lobe at the dome and a smaller hemangioma at the caudal tip of the right lobe. In the portal venous phase, the masses demonstrate peripheral, nodular, discontinuous enhancement that progresses centripetally to uniform enhancement in the delayed phases (not pictured). A central area of fixed hypointensity is often seen in giant hemangiomas.

Further reading

Blood in the Belly: CT Findings of Hemoperitoneum. Lubner M, Menias C, Rucker C, *et al. Radiographics* 2007; 27:109–125.

Genetics and Imaging of Hepatocellular Adenomas: 2011 Update. Katabathina VS, Menias CO, Shanbhogue AK, *et al. Radiographics* 2011; 31:1529–1543.

Imaging of Nontraumatic Hemorrhagic Hepatic Lesions. Casillas VJ, Amendola MA, Gascue A, *et al. Radiographics* 2000; 20:367–378.

Hepatic Adenomas: Imaging and Pathologic Findings. Grazioli L, Federle M, Brancatelli G, *et al. Radiographics* 2001; 21:877–894.

Case 3   42-year-old man with acute onset of epigastric pain

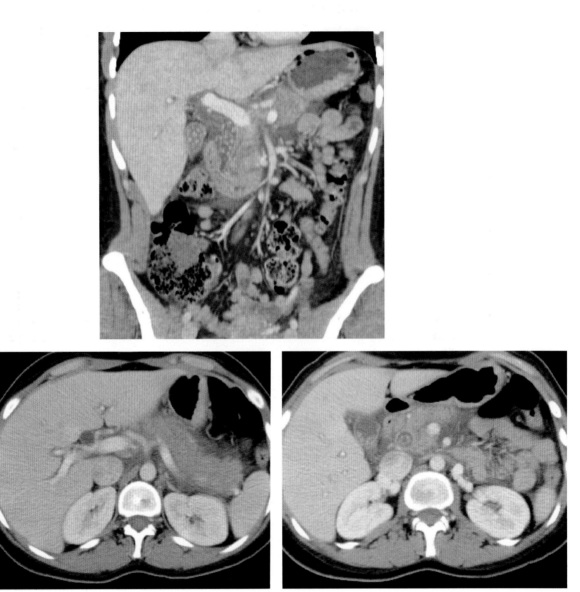

Diagnosis: **Acute gallstone pancreatitis**

Coronal (left image) and axial (middle and right images) contrast-enhanced CT images show diffuse enlargement and hypoattenuation of the pancreas (yellow arrows) with extensive peripancreatic fat stranding and diffuse peri-portal stranding. The common bile duct is distended by numerous calculi (red arrows) and there are innumerable tiny layering gallstones in the gallbladder lumen (blue arrows).

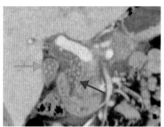 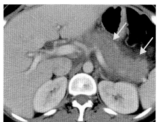 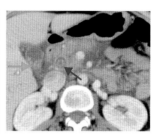

Discussion

Overview of acute pancreatitis

- Acute pancreatitis is an inflammatory process of the pancreas with variable clinical manifestations. Severity ranges from mild abdominal pain to severe life-threatening disease.
- Mortality in severe acute pancreatitis has been reported to be around 10–20%. Severe acute pancreatitis is associated with multi-organ failure and/or local complications such as infected necrosis and abscess formation.
- Treatment is primarily supportive.

Clinical diagnosis of acute pancreatitis

- The clinical diagnosis of acute pancreatitis requires the presence of at least two of the following features: typical abdominal pain (epigastric, radiating to the back), serum amylase and/or lipase activity at least three times the upper limit of normal, and/or characteristic imaging findings of acute pancreatitis.

CT imaging of acute pancreatitis

- Intravenous contrast-enhanced CT is considered to be the imaging modality of choice for diagnosis and staging. It should be reserved for patients who present atypically, those with organ failure or other reliable clinical or biochemical predictors of severe acute pancreatitis, and those who are suspected to have a severe local complication.

- The pancreas can appear normal or enlarged in acute pancreatitis, with or without peripancreatic fat stranding. Local edema may extend along the mesentery, transverse mesocolon, or hepatoduodenal ligament. Peripancreatic fluid collections consist of exudate, fat necrosis, or hemorrhage.
- Contrast-enhanced CT is very specific for the diagnosis of necrosis. Necrosis usually develops between 24 and 48 hours after the onset of acute pancreatitis. Distinction between sterile and infected necrosis is essential, because of differences in natural history, treatment of choice, and prognosis. Unlike patients with sterile necrosis, most patients with infected necrosis require long-term antibiotic therapy and surgical or image-guided intervention. Diagnosis of infected necrosis can be made by image-guided fine-needle aspiration and culture, or on the basis of extraluminal gas bubbles within pancreatic or peripancreatic collections, which are virtually pathognomonic for infection by gas-forming organisms.

Classification of complications of acute pancreatitis

- The revised Atlanta Classification includes specific nomenclature and CT criteria for local pancreatic complications based on location (intra- or peripancreatic), presence and degree of encapsulation, contents (fluid or non-liquid necrotic debris), age, infectious status (sterile or infected), and history of interventional therapy (necrosectomy). Major emphases are on distinguishing necrotizing from non-necrotizing pancreatitis and acute from delayed findings.

Non-necrotizing pancreatitis

- According to the revised Atlanta Classification, an acute peripancreatic fluid collection (APFC) usually develops less than four weeks after the onset of symptoms and is often associated with interstitial edematous (non-necrotizing) pancreatitis (IEP).
- An APFC is of homogeneous fluid density, confined by normal peripancreatic fascial planes, and lacks a definable wall. In contrast, a pseudocyst is typically diagnosed at least four weeks after the onset of symptoms. Like APFC, pseudocysts are of homogeneous fluid density.

Necrotizing pancreatitis

- An acute necrotic collection (ANC) occurs less than four weeks after onset of symptoms in necrotizing pancreatitis. An ANC is an often-heterogeneous fluid collection that may have liquid and non-liquid densities and varying degrees of loculation. It may be intra- or extrapancreatic and lacks a definable wall.

- Walled-off necrosis (WON), on the other hand, generally appears after four weeks. This is an encapsulated, often heterogeneous collection that may be intra- or extrapancreatic.
- Post-necrosectomy pseudocyst is the term used to describe a completely encapsulated homogeneous fluid density collection (round or oval) that is intra- or extrapancreatic and arises following surgical necrosectomy.

MR imaging of acute pancreatitis

- MRI findings are analogous to CT findings, and the same descriptive terminology applies.
- The major role of MR, specifically MRCP, is to identify gallstones (also evaluable by ultrasound in many cases) and main pancreatic duct disconnection.
- MRI is also superior to CT in differentiating pancreatic abscess (collection of infected fluid without solid debris) from infected necrosis (collection of infected fluid with solid debris).
- Early MRCP should be avoided because fluid collections often compress the pancreatic and biliary ducts, obscuring gallstones.

Clinical synopsis The patient was admitted and treated with supportive measures. After the resolution of acute inflammation, ERCP was performed to remove the gallstones.

Self-assessment

- *Cite five local complications arising from acute pancreatitis.*

- Acute fluid collections, pseudocyst, abscess, necrosis, main pancreatic duct disconnection.

- *Cite four late or remote complications of acute pancreatitis.*

- Diabetes, chronic pancreatitis, splenic artery pseudoaneurysm, splenic vein thrombosis.

- *Cite eight causes of acute pancreatitis.*

- Gallstones, alcohol, trauma, drugs, autoimmune disease, hyperlipidemia, viral infection, ERCP.

- *What are the indications for CT in acute pancreatitis?*

- CT may be performed early during the course of acute pancreatitis when the diagnosis is uncertain. More often, it is performed after 72 hours (typically 7–10 days after presentation) for assessment of complications.

Spectrum of acute pancreatitis

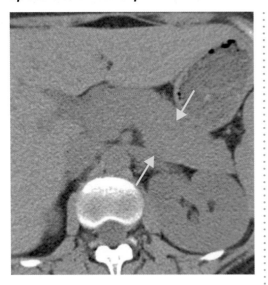

Mild acute pancreatitis

The diagnosis of acute pancreatitis relies primarily on clinical and laboratory findings. In cases of mild (interstitial edematous) pancreatitis, the pancreas may appear normal on CT. This axial unenhanced CT image of a patient with an iodine allergy shows a mildly, diffusely enlarged pancreas (arrows) that appears otherwise unremarkable. Imaging findings of inflammation include diffuse gland enlargement and peripancreatic fat stranding and fluid. It is controversial whether IV contrast should be administered within the first 72 hours of an episode of acute pancreatitis, since complications are almost always absent in this time frame.

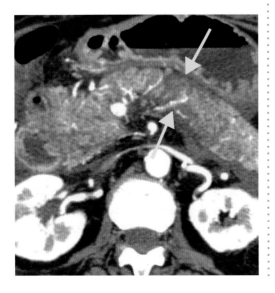

Severe acute pancreatitis

In this case of severe acute pancreatitis complicated by necrosis, as shown by an axial contrast-enhanced CT image, there are scattered areas of parenchymal hypo- and non-enhancement (arrows). There is extensive fat stranding and a significant amount of free fluid surrounding the gland. Approximately 15–20% of cases of acute pancreatitis are complicated by necrosis, which adversely affects prognosis.

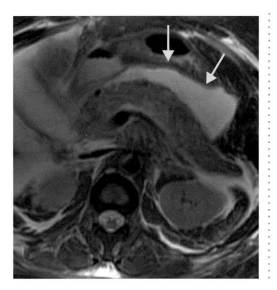

MR imaging of severe acute pancreatitis

MRI is useful in patients with iodine allergies, for characterization of fluid collections, evaluation of an abnormal or disconnected pancreatic duct, and in cases of choledocholithiasis. In this case of severe pancreatitis, an axial T2-weighted MR image demonstrates mild enlargement of the pancreas, which is surrounded by fat stranding and a large homogeneous fluid collection (arrows).

Variants of acute pancreatitis

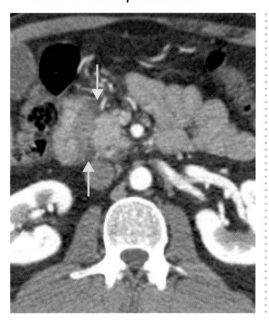

Groove pancreatitis

Groove pancreatitis is a rare type of chronic segmental pancreatitis that is characterized by the formation of fibrosis in the anatomic space between the pancreas, duodenum, and common bile duct – the pancreatico-duodenal groove. In this contrast-enhanced axial CT image, there is ill-defined soft tissue and fat stranding between the pancreatic head and duodenum (arrows). Groove pancreatitis may be caused by disturbance of pancreatic outflow through the accessory pancreatic duct. There are typically several small cystic lesions in the region of the pancreatic head and duodenum (not seen in this case).

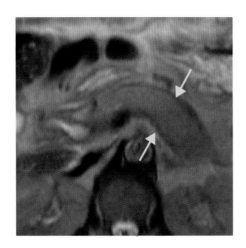

Autoimmune pancreatitis

Autoimmune pancreatitis is a manifestation of systemic IgG4 disease. This systemic, chronic fibro-inflammatory process affects multiple organs, including the pancreas, salivary glands, bile ducts, kidneys, lungs, retroperitoneum, and lymph nodes. Diffuse involvement is the most common pattern, with effacement of the pancreatic contour that causes the pancreas to appear sausage-shaped, as in this T2-weighted MR image. A T2-hypointense halo (arrows) can be seen in 12–40% and is thought to represent inflammatory cell infiltration. Treatment with corticosteroid therapy often results in complete resolution.

Complications of acute pancreatitis

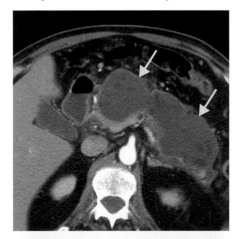

Pancreatic necrosis

Necrosis results from disruption of the pancreatic microcirculation. In severe cases of acute pancreatitis, there is necrosis and liquefaction of the pancreas, as seen in this axial contrast-enhanced CT image. There is complete replacement of the normal parenchyma by an encapsulated, heterogeneous fluid collection containing internal debris (arrows).

Hemorrhagic pancreatitis

The term "hemorrhagic pancreatitis" has been abandoned, since many peripancreatic fluid collections contain blood, and the presence of hemorrhage does not correlate with the severity or extent of necrosis, which has come to be recognized as the key prognostic factor. This axial contrast-enhanced CT image demonstrates heterogeneous, slightly hyperattenuating peripancreatic fluid (arrows) consistent with peripancreatic hemorrhage.

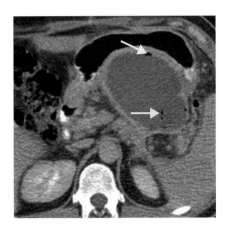

Pancreatic pseudocyst

Pseudocysts are sterile, organized peripancreatic fluid collections that contain pancreatic secretions. They are encapsulated by fibrous walls, which take more than 4 weeks to develop (after the onset of symptoms). Although 40% of pseudocysts resolve spontaneously, persistent enlargement, hemorrhage, and infection may occur. This contrast-enhanced axial CT image shows foci of gas (arrows) within the pseudocyst, raising concern for superinfection by gas-forming organisms.

Differential diagnosis of acute pancreatitis

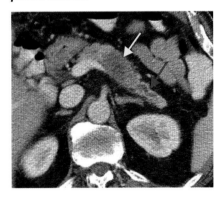

Pancreatic adenocarcinoma

Pancreatic adenocarcinoma is sometimes indistinguishable from focal pancreatitis; however, indirect signs, such as atrophy of the distal gland parenchyma and ductal dilatation, should raise the suspicion for malignancy. In rare cases, acute pancreatitis can be secondary to obstruction by tumor. This axial contrast-enhanced CT image shows an ill-defined, mass-like, hypoenhancing area in the body of the pancreas (yellow arrow) with dilatation of the distal main pancreatic duct (red arrow) and atrophy of the distal gland.

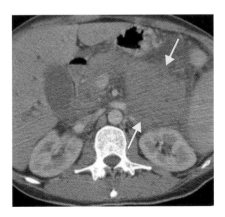

Pancreatic lymphoma

Pancreatic lymphoma is most commonly B-cell non-Hodgkin's lymphoma. Secondary lymphoma, from direct extension of peripancreatic lymphadenopathy, is more common than primary pancreatic lymphoma. Primary pancreatic lymphoma is rare, and is more common in middle-aged men and immunocompromised patients. This axial contrast-enhanced CT image depicts the diffuse form of primary pancreatic lymphoma. There is infiltration of the pancreas with diffuse glandular enlargement (arrows) and effacement of peripancreatic fat. Pancreatic lymphoma may sometimes simulate acute or autoimmune pancreatitis.

Further reading

Balthazar EJ, Robinson DL, Megibow AJ, *et al*. Acute Pancreatitis: Value of CT in Establishing Prognosis. *Radiology* 1990; 174:331–336.

Balthazar EJ. Acute Pancreatitis: Assessment of Severity with Clinical and CT Evaluation. *Radiology* 2002; 223:603–613.

Bollen TL, van Santvoort HC, Besselink MGH, *et al*. Update on Acute Pancreatitis: Ultrasound, Computed Tomography, and Magnetic Resonance Imaging Features. *Semin Ultrasound CT MRI* 2007; 28:371–383.

Bollen TL. Imaging of Acute Pancreatitis: Update of the Revised Atlanta Classification. *Radiol Clin N Am* 2012; 50:429–445.

Casas JD, Diaz R, Valderas G, *et al*. Prognostic Value of CT in the Early Assessment of Patients with Acute Pancreatitis. *AJR* 2004; 182:569–574.

Lecesne R, Taourel P, Bret P, Atri M, *et al*. Acute Pancreatitis: Interobserver Agreement and Correlation of CT and MR Cholangiography with Outcome. *Radiology* 1999; 211:727–735.

Lenhart DK, Balthazar EJ. MDCT of Acute Mild (Nonnecrotizing) Pancreatitis: Abdominal Complications and Fate of Fluid Collections. *AJR* 2008; 190:643–649.

O'Connor OJ, McWilliams S, Maher MM. Imaging of Acute Pancreatitis. *AJR* 2011; 197:W221–W225.

Sahani DV, Kalva SP, Farrell J, *et al*. Autoimmune Pancreatitis: Imaging Features. *Radiology* 2004; 233:345–352.

Whitcomb DC. Acute Pancreatitis. *N Engl J Med* 2006; 354:2142–2150.

Case 4   52-year-old woman status post laparoscopic cholecystectomy
presenting with fever and right upper quadrant pain

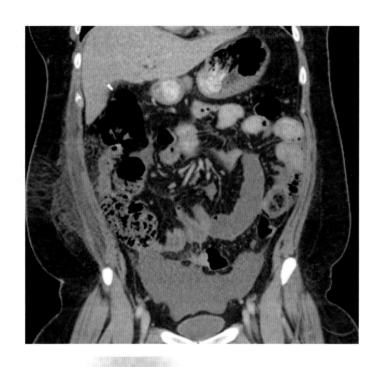

Diagnosis:
Bile leak after laparoscopic cholecystectomy

Coronal enhanced CT (left image) shows a large, low attenuation fluid collection in the pelvis (yellow arrow) and extensive fat stranding along the right paracolic gutter and subcutaneous tissues (red arrows). Note the cholecystectomy clip in the gallbladder fossa (blue arrow). Delayed hepatobiliary scintigraphy (HIDA scan; right image) shows accumulation of the radiotracer in the right lower quadrant (yellow arrow), correlating with the fluid collection on CT and consistent with bile leak.

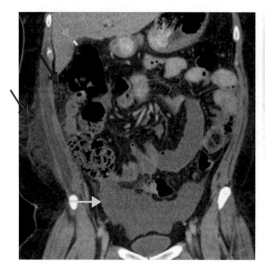 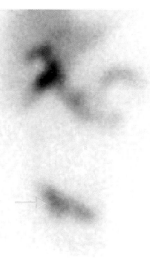

Discussion

Overview of bile leaks

- Bile leaks are one of the most common complications of cholecystectomy, occurring in 0.4% of cases. Both open and laparoscopic procedures can be complicated by bile leaks, typically the result of unrecognized, inadvertent damage to the normal bile duct during surgery.
- In up to 30% of the population, anatomic variation in the relationship of the intrahepatic bile ducts or cystic duct with the common hepatic duct and gallbladder may predispose to bile duct injury during surgery. Other predisposing conditions include intrahepatic position of the gallbladder, adherent gallbladder due to chronic cholecystitis, accessory cystic duct, or ducts of Luschka (accessory ducts that directly drain into the gallbladder lumen).
- Bile leaks at the cystic duct may occur when clips become dislodged or do not encompass the entire duct. Leaks from the surgical bed occur when accessory or anomalous bile ducts have been damaged, or when

the plane of dissection into the liver is too deep, resulting in injury to small biliary radicles.

- Postoperative bile leaks that result in intraperitoneal collections are typically sterile. Usually, they do not produce severe bile peritonitis. In contrast, intraperitoneal collections after acute cholecystitis complicated by gallbladder perforation are usually infected.
- Other common post-cholecystectomy complications include retained calculi, hematomas, hemobilia, abscess, ascending cholangitis, cystic duct or gallbladder remnants, and biliary strictures.

Imaging of suspected bile leak

- CT is the imaging modality of choice to diagnose post-cholecystectomy complications, as it demonstrates the site and morphology of the fluid collection.
- Bile collections are usually close to the site of leakage, but can be remote as in this case. If a fluid collection is identified, further investigation with other imaging studies may be undertaken.
- If a T-tube is present, a cholangiogram may reveal the presence and site of the leak. If not, more invasive examinations such as ERCP, percutaneous cholangiography, or image-guided percutaneous drainage can confirm the diagnosis. These modalities may also provide means for intervention.
- Hepatobiliary scintigraphy (HIDA scan) has the advantage of presenting the physiologic course of biliary excretion and leakage of bile from the biliary tract in real-time. This technique, however, is limited by poor spatial resolution that limits identification of the site of the leak. CT correlation is often required, particularly if the leak is small.
- Gadoxetate disodium (Eovist, Primovist, Bayer HealthCare Pharmaceuticals) enhanced MRI has been described as an alternative approach for the diagnosis of bile leaks. This "hepatocyte-specific" contrast agent is taken up by normal hepatocytes and excreted into the biliary tree, with optimal hepatobiliary visualization 20 minutes after injection. Delayed imaging hours after IV contrast administration may be required for diagnosis.

Clinical synopsis

Percutaneous image-guided drainage was performed to exclude the possibility of superimposed infection. ERCP and papillotomy were used to evaluate for the presence of persistent bile leak and to decrease biliary pressure.

Self-assessment

- *Cite five complications arising from cholecystectomy.*

- *Cite two common anatomic variants that may give rise to post-cholecystectomy complications.*

- *Name three CT findings that suggest superinfection in postoperative fluid collections.*

- Bile leak, hemorrhage, abscess, retained calculi, cystic duct or gallbladder remnants, biliary strictures.

- Low medial insertion of the cystic duct, accessory cystic duct or ducts of Luschka.

- Presence of gas, heterogeneous content, enhancing, thick walls.

Spectrum of bile leak

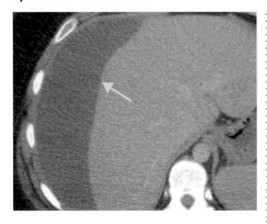

Large postoperative bile leak

Large bile leaks may cause mass effect upon the liver. Even in the absence of specific imaging signs of superimposed infection (such as gas locules), drainage is often indicated to exclude infection in the setting of clinical suspicion. Axial enhanced CT demonstrates a large, crescentic, homogeneous fluid collection (arrow) along the right hepatic lobe, causing moderate mass effect upon the liver.

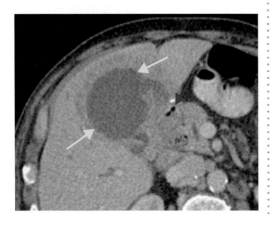

Abscess formation post bile leak

Axial enhanced CT demonstrates an irregularly shaped fluid collection (yellow arrows) in the cholecystectomy bed with an enhancing, thick wall, suspicious for abscess. Note two foci of gas (red arrow) at the periphery of the fluid collection, which may denote infection by gas-forming organisms or communication with bowel. When accessible percutaneously, postoperative abscesses are most often treated with image-guided drainage.

Differential diagnosis of bile leak

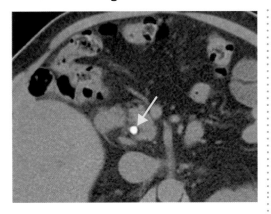

Retained calculi

A retained stone is a biliary tract stone that was not removed at surgery. Postoperative axial non-contrast CT performed for persistent abdominal pain after cholecystectomy demonstrates an impacted, retained gallstone in the common bile duct (arrow). Only a minority of gallstones are visible at CT. In cases of retained calculi, endoscopic removal is recommended.

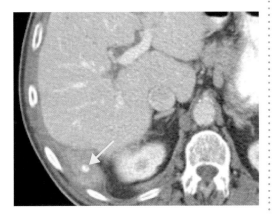

Dropped gallstone

Dropped gallstone is a documented complication of laparoscopic cholecystectomy where a gallstone "drops" from the gallbladder during surgery. Granulomatous reaction or, rarely, abscess formation may result. Axial enhanced CT demonstrates a fusiform soft tissue mass in the hepatorenal fossa, surrounding a dropped gallstone (arrow) in Morison's pouch. There is adjacent inflammatory fat stranding. Dropped gallstones are typically seen in this dependent location.

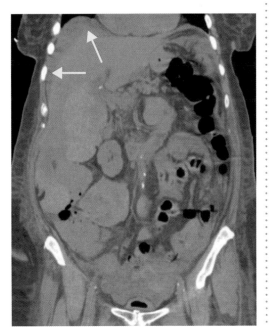

Postoperative hemorrhage

Coronal noncontrast CT performed due to decreasing hematocrit after cholecystectomy demonstrates a large, heterogeneous collection surrounding the liver (arrows), extending along the right paracolic gutter and pooling in the pelvis. There are areas of relative hyperdensity, consistent with hemorrhage. Extensive, diffuse subcutaneous fat stranding indicates generalized edema (anasarca).

Further reading

Hoeffel C, Azizi L, Lewin M, *et al*. Normal and Pathologic Features of the Postoperative Biliary Tract at 3D MR Cholangiopancreatography and MR Imaging. *Radiographics* 2006; 26:1603–1620.

Kapoor V, Baron RL, Peterson MS. Pictorial Essay: Bile Leaks After Surgery. *AJR* 2004; 182:451–458.

O'Connor OJ, O'Neill S, Maher MM. Imaging of Biliary Tract Disease. *AJR* 2011; 197:551–558.

Seale MK, Catalano OA, Saini S, *et al*. Hepatobiliary-specific MR Contrast Agents: Role in Imaging the Liver and Biliary Tree. *Radiographics* 2009; 29:1725–1748.

Yeh BM, Liu PS, Soto JA, *et al*. MR Imaging and CT of the Biliary Tract. *Radiographics* 2009; 29:669–1688.

Case 5   20-year-old man with a history of left flank pain and IV drug abuse

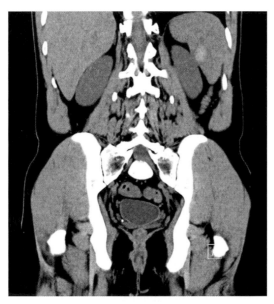

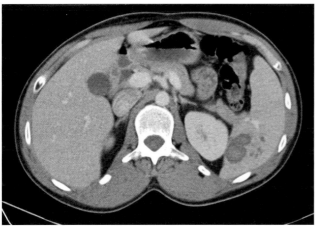
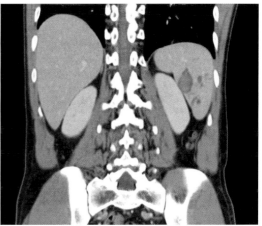

Diagnosis:
Splenic infarction

Initial unenhanced coronal CT (left image) demonstrates a hyperdense lesion (arrow) in the medial spleen, consistent with hemorrhage. Subsequent contrast-enhanced axial (middle image) and coronal (right image) CT images demonstrate a corresponding peripheral, slightly lobular, wedge-shaped, hypoenhancing region (arrows). Multiple smaller, round, hypoenhancing areas are seen adjacent. The splenic capsule remains smooth in contour. Taken together, these findings indicate acute, hemorrhagic splenic infarction.

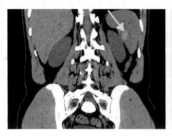 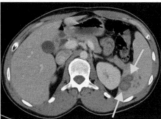 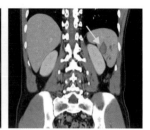

Discussion

Splenic pathology is often clinically unsuspected until diagnosed by imaging.

- The spleen is a vascular organ that is best evaluated with intravenous contrast. Unlike most other solid organs, the normal spleen demonstrates heterogeneous enhancement in the arterial phase; thus, the portal venous or parenchymal phase of contrast is optimal for splenic imaging.
- CT is sensitive for splenic infarction, and is the diagnostic modality of choice when splenic pathology is suspected. In one study, only 18% of 48 patients with CT-demonstrated splenic infarction had corroborating sonographic findings.
- Splenic infarcts may be hemorrhagic because the spleen is inherently vascular.
- Different types of splenic lesions may have similar CT appearances, so a detailed clinical history is essential to differentiate among them. Because patients with splenic infarction may have fever (27%) and leukocytosis (58%), it can be difficult to exclude superimposed infection. Multiplicity of infarcts suggests the possibility of an infectious etiology.

Splenic infarction should be considered in the differential diagnosis of both left upper quadrant and left flank pain.

- 80% of patients with splenic infarction present with either left upper quadrant or left flank pain.

- 70% of patients with splenic infarction have an identifiable predisposing factor. The most common of these is atrial fibrillation, found in about one quarter of patients with splenic infarct. Rapid enlargement of the spleen is another important risk factor for infarction, germane to patients with viral mononucleosis or hematologic disease. Less common causes include hypercoagulable states, hemoglobinopathies such as sickle cell disease, and splenic vein thrombosis secondary to pancreatitis.

Clinical synopsis

This 20-year-old man with a long history of intravenous drug abuse presented with left flank pain. He also had a history of nephrolithiasis, so an unenhanced CT was initially performed to evaluate for renal stones. The diagnosis of hemorrhagic splenic infarction was posited, and more definitely characterized following contrast administration on a subsequent study. Given the patient's history of IV drug abuse, a biopsy was performed and cultures were sent for microbiology. There was no growth and the patient was managed conservatively.

Self-assessment

- *Name three risk factors for splenic infarction.*
  - Atrial fibrillation
  - Splenomegaly (especially when associated with EBV/CMV infection, hematologic malignancy, or sickle cell disease and other hemoglobinopathies)
  - Prosthetic heart valve
  - Endocarditis

- *Name three complications of splenic infarction.*
  - Subcapsular hemorrhage
  - Hemoperitoneum
  - Pseudocyst
  - Abscess

- *What is the treatment for splenic infarction?*
  - Splenic infarction itself usually requires no invasive treatment; however, the finding should prompt evaluation for an underlying condition, which can be appropriately managed upon diagnosis. Because splenic infarction may be a manifestation of a systemic embolic phenomenon, other organs susceptible to infarction (e.g., the kidneys, lungs, and brain) should be carefully evaluated in relevant clinical contexts.

Spectrum of splenic infarction

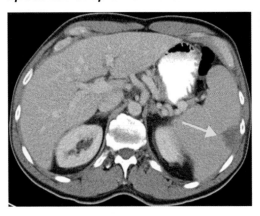

Non-hemorrhagic splenic infarct

The index case demonstrated a hemorrhagic splenic infarct, but splenic infarction may also present without internal hemorrhage. Axial enhanced CT demonstrates a classic wedge-shaped region of hypoattenuation of the peripheral spleen (arrow), consistent with a splenic infarction. No hyperattenuating focus is seen to suggest hemorrhage.

Differential diagnosis of splenic infarction

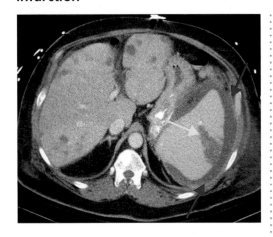

Ruptured spleen / splenic laceration

Splenic laceration as the result of blunt trauma may appear as focal peripheral hypodensity within the splenic parenchyma, simulating infarction. Unlike infarction, however, it is almost always accompanied by subcapsular hematoma or hemoperitoneum. History may be important in establishing the diagnosis. Rarely, delayed rupture may present after an initially normal CT scan. Axial enhanced CT demonstrates a peripheral, wedge-shaped region of low attenuation (yellow arrow) in the spleen. There is an extensive subcapsular hematoma (red arrow).

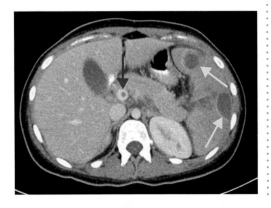

Splenic abscess

Splenic abscesses are usually a complication of systemic infection, and immunodeficiency is an important risk factor. CT is highly sensitive (96%) for splenic abscess. Unlike infarcts, abscesses are typically rounded, with rim enhancement. Treatment with antibiotics alone may be sufficient in patients unable to undergo percutaneous drainage. Axial enhanced CT demonstrates several rounded, peripherally enhancing abscesses (yellow arrows) in the spleen. Note the concomitant portal vein thrombosis, appearing as a filling defect at the portosplenic confluence (red arrow).

Splenic lymphoma

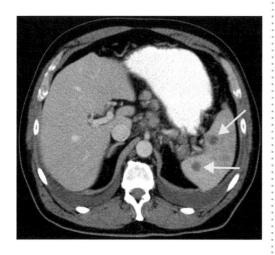

Lymphoma is the most common malignancy involving the spleen, though primary splenic lymphoma is relatively rare. Extranodal lymphoma is usually non-Hodgkin's, and the most common subtypes are Diffuse Large B-Cell Lymphoma (DLBCL) and follicular lymphoma. Diffuse involvement is more common than discrete lesions. Extranodal lymphoma generally portends a worse prognosis. Axial enhanced CT demonstrates several nonspecific round hypoattenuating foci in the spleen (arrows) in a patient with known lymphoma. There are bilateral pleural effusions.

Splenic metastases

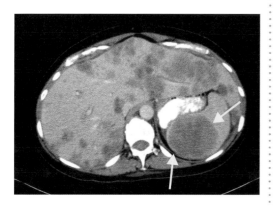

Splenic metastases are most often hematogenous. The most common primary tumors are breast carcinoma, lung carcinoma, and melanoma. Axial enhanced CT in a patient with metastatic cervical cancer demonstrates a large lesion in the posterior spleen (arrows). The splenic mass focally expands the normal contour of the spleen, a finding suspicious for malignancy. There are also numerous hepatic metastases.

Splenic sarcoidosis

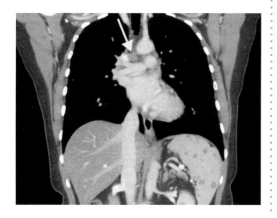

Splenic sarcoidosis should be considered when multiple, hypodense splenic lesions occur with pulmonary manifestations of sarcoidosis. Splenic sarcoidosis is rare in the absence of pulmonary sarcoidosis. An elevated serum acetylcholinesterase (ACE) level supports, but is not necessary for, the diagnosis. Coronal enhanced CT demonstrates numerous nonspecific hypoattenuating foci in the spleen in a patient with known sarcoidosis and mediastinal adenopathy (arrow).

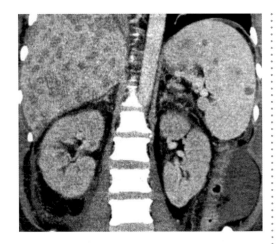

Splenic fungal microabscesses

The most common causal organism of disseminated fungal infection is *Candida albicans*. Hepatosplenic fungal microabscesses are generally multiple, small (<1.5–2 cm), hypodense, and heterogeneously enhancing. Because the condition may be fatal if untreated, diagnosis is critically important, especially in immunocompromised patients. Unfortunately, the systemic inflammatory response to disseminated fungal infection after the immune system starts to recover can also be fatal. The treatment for isolated splenic fungal microabscesses is usually splenectomy, though some patients are managed more conservatively with systemic antifungal therapy. There may be coexistent involvement of the liver, kidneys, gastrointestinal tract, or pleura. Coronal enhanced CT demonstrates innumerable tiny hypoattenuating foci in the liver and spleen.

Splenic cyst

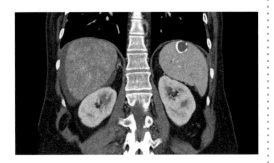

The majority of splenic "cysts" are actually pseudocysts that lack epithelial lining. These are thought to be sequelae of prior trauma or infection. Splenic cysts are usually solitary, asymptomatic, well-circumscribed, simple fluid density lesions that may or may not have peripheral calcification. True cysts and pseudocysts are indistinguishable by imaging. Operative management may be indicated in lesions >5 cm or in patients with symptoms such as early satiety or left upper quadrant pain. Coronal enhanced CT demonstrates a circumscribed fluid attenuation lesion in the superior spleen with smooth peripheral calcification.

Further reading

Antopolsky M., *et al*. Splenic infarction: 10 years of experience. *American Journal of Emergency Medicine*, 27, 262–265 (2009).

Chaing I., *et al*. Splenic abscesses: review of 29 cases. *J Med Sci.*, 19(10), 510–515 (2003).

Chew F., *et al*. Candidal splenic abscesses. *AJR,* 156, 474 (1991).

Geraghty M., *et al*. Large primary splenic cyst: a laparoscopic technique. *Journal of Minimal Access Surgery*, 5(1), 14–16 (2009).

Giovinale M., *et al*. Atypical sarcoidosis: case reports and review of the literature. *European Review for Medical and Pharmacological Sciences*, 13(1), 37–44 (2009).

Gupta P., *et al*. Delayed splenic rupture. *J Surg Radiol.*, 1(2), 110–113 (2010).

Lee W., *et al*. Abdominal manifestations of extranodal lymphoma: spectrum of imaging findings. *AJR,* 191(1), 198–206 (2008).

Moore N., *et al*. Systemic candidiasis. *Radiographics*, 23(5), 1287–1290 (2003).

Nelken N., *et al*. Changing clinical spectrum of splenic abscess: a multicenter study and review of the literature. *American Journal of Surgery*, 154(1), 27–34 (1987).

Nores M., *et al*. The clinical spectrum of splenic infarction. *American Surgeon*, 64(2), 182–188 (1998).

Rabushka L, *et al*. Imaging of the spleen: CT with supplemental MR examination. *Radiographics*, 14(2), 307–332 (1994).

Case 6   78-year-old female with history of chronic obstructive pulmonary disease and lung cancer complaining of right upper quadrant pain for 24 hours

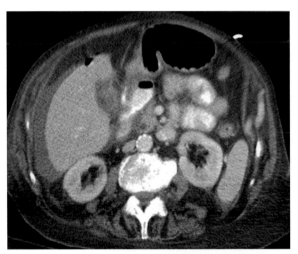
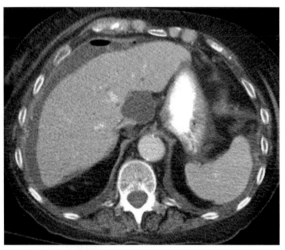
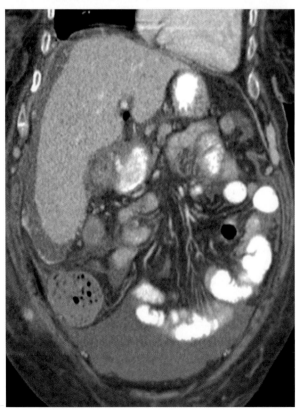

Diagnosis: **Perforated duodenal ulcer**

Axial and coronal oral and intravenous contrast-enhanced CT images show a thickened duodenal wall, with oral contrast extravasating through a wall defect (yellow arrow). There is perihepatic and pelvic ascites (red arrows), with several locules of gas (blue arrows) in the prehepatic space indicating pneumoperitoneum. A focal portocaval fluid collection (green arrow) compresses the inferior vena cava.

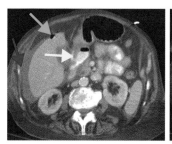 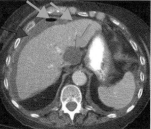 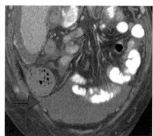

Discussion

Overview of peptic ulcer disease

- The most common cause of nontraumatic gastrointestinal tract perforation is perforated duodenal ulcer.
- The vast majority of duodenal ulcers are related to *Helicobacter pylori* infection, with a markedly reduced incidence in the past decades due to treatment with antibiotics and acid blocker medications. Other risk factors for duodenal ulcer disease include alcohol, smoking, and chronic corticosteroids. Duodenal ulcers and gastric ulcers share risk factors; however, duodenal ulcers are approximately 2–3 times more common than gastric ulcers, and duodenal peptic ulcers are less commonly malignant in comparison to gastric ulcers.
- Duodenal ulcers occur most frequently in the duodenal bulb. Ulcers distal to the duodenal bulb are suspicious for Crohn's disease or Zollinger–Ellison syndrome, and ulcers distal to the ampulla of Vater are very rare but should raise concern for duodenal adenocarcinoma. Secondary inflammation of the duodenum, which may be seen in pancreatitis, tends to be more diffuse than inflammation in primary ulcer disease.
- Complications of untreated duodenal ulcer include bleeding, rupture, and stricture that may lead to gastric outlet obstruction. Perforation of the anterior duodenal wall may lead to peritonitis and pneumoperitoneum, whereas perforation of the posterior wall may lead to catastrophic bleeding from injury to the gastroduodenal artery, which lies posterior to the first portion of the duodenum.

- Treatment of ruptured duodenal ulcer is typically emergent surgery; however, percutaneous drainage may be performed in patients who are poor surgical candidates.

Imaging of peptic ulcer disease

- Uncomplicated duodenal peptic ulcer disease may be difficult to diagnose by CT because mucosal ulcers and wall thickening are most often not apparent. Upper gastrointestinal endoscopy has higher sensitivity for uncomplicated peptic ulcer disease. CT is reserved for evaluation of patients with signs and symptoms of complicated disease.
- CT findings of perforated duodenal ulcer include focal mural thickening, periduodenal fluid, and free peritoneal or retroperitoneal gas (the majority of the duodenum is retroperitoneal—only the proximal segment of the first portion of the duodenum is intraperitoneal). If enteric contrast is administered, there may be free extravasation of contrast through the mural defect, as in the index case; however, this finding is unusual.

Clinical synopsis	The patient was determined to be a high-risk surgical candidate due to her concomitant pulmonary insufficiency. Several image-guided percutaneous periduodenal fluid collection drainages were performed. There was no significant improvement in her tenuous clinical status, and the patient died approximately 10 days later from vancomycin-resistant enterococcus sepsis.

Self-assessment

- *Name three inflammatory processes that can cause duodenal wall thickening.*

  - Peptic ulcer disease, pancreatitis, radiation therapy.

- *What are the CT findings of perforated duodenal ulcer?*

  - Duodenal wall thickening, periduodenal fluid and gas, oral contrast extravasation.

- *Cite three possible complications of untreated duodenal peptic ulcer.*

  - Bleeding, perforation, stricture with gastric outlet obstruction.

Spectrum of duodenal peptic ulcer disease

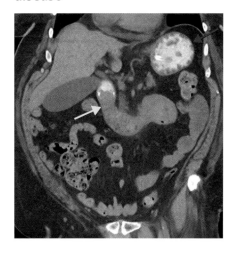

Bleeding duodenal ulcer

Hemorrhage is the most common complication of duodenal ulcers. Coronal enhanced CT demonstrates no passage of oral contrast to the second portion of the duodenum (yellow arrow), and moderate gastric distention (red arrow). These CT findings are nonspecific. Upper endoscopy showed a bleeding ulcer in the first portion of the duodenum with extensive intraluminal hematoma distal to the second portion.

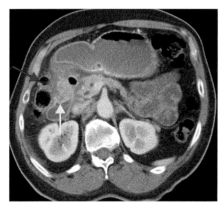

Duodenal ulcer perforation

Perforation is the second most common complication of duodenal ulcers. Acute perforation may also occur with acute or severe systemic stressors, such as burns (Curling's ulcer), intracranial hypertension/trauma (Cushing's ulcer), sepsis, and intensive chemotherapy or radiotherapy. Axial enhanced CT demonstrates marked thickening of the first portion of the duodenum (yellow arrow), associated with free periduodenal fluid and locules of free air (red arrow).

Differential diagnosis of duodenal ulcer disease

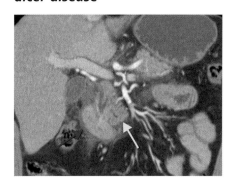

Duodenal inflammation secondary to pancreatitis

Adjacent pancreatitis is the most common cause of secondary duodenal inflammation. Enhanced coronal CT in a patient with epigastric pain and elevated amylase shows an enlarged pancreatic head (yellow arrow), with free peripancreatic fluid and fat stranding, consistent with acute pancreatitis. The adjacent duodenal wall is diffusely thickened (red arrow) with associated periduodenal fluid.

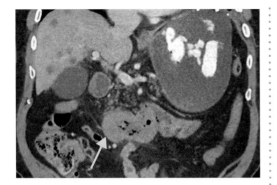

Duodenal metastasis

Metastases may involve the duodenum by local extension (e.g., pancreatic cancer) or hematogenous spread from distant sites (e.g., melanoma). Coronal enhanced CT demonstrates marked wall thickening of the third portion of the duodenum (arrow), with gastric distention. Endoscopic biopsy showed metastasis from lung squamous cell carcinoma.

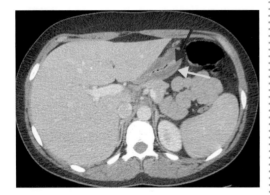

Acute gastritis

This is a very common cause of epigastric pain. Predisposing factors include alcohol, aspirin, NSAIDs, stress, and *H. pylori* infection. The antrum is most commonly affected, but the proximal stomach can also be involved. Gastric carcinoma and MALT lymphoma may complicate *H. pylori* gastritis. Axial enhanced CT image of a patient with epigastric pain shows prominent, hypodense submucosal edema (yellow arrow) and mucosal hyperenhancement (red arrow) of the gastric antrum, which was subsequently confirmed to represent *H. pylori* infection by endoscopic biopsy. Lobulated or polypoid mucosal folds should raise suspicion for malignancy and prompt recommendation for biopsy.

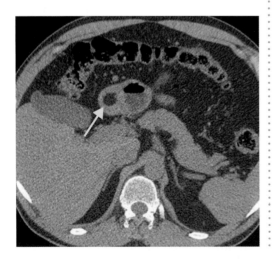

Duodenal lipoma

Lipomas can occur anywhere in the gastrointestinal tract. They are one of the most common benign tumors of the duodenum, often found incidentally. Axial noncontrast CT image shows a well-circumscribed, fat-density lesion in the proximal duodenum (arrow), consistent with lipoma.

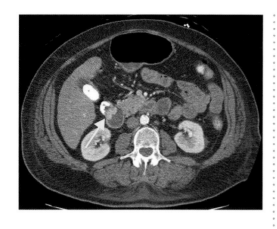

Duodenal GIST

Gastrointestinal stromal tumors (GISTs) are mesenchymal tumors arising from the interstitial cells of Cajal. GISTs most commonly arise from the stomach; however, between 3% and 5% are duodenal in origin. Upper gastrointestinal tract GISTs tend to be benign. Axial enhanced CT shows an exophytic, enhancing, nonobstructing mass in the second part of the duodenum (arrow). Growth is often extraluminal, with internal necrosis and calcification being common features of large tumors. CT findings suggestive of malignant GIST are size >5 cm and central necrosis. The hyper-vascular nature of GISTs renders them susceptible to hemorrhage, a common clinical presentation.

Further reading

Ba-Salamah A, Prokop M, Uffmann M, *et al.* Dedicated Multidetector CT of the Stomach: Spectrum of Diseases. *Radiographics* 2003; 23:625–644.

Burkill GJ, Badran M, Al-Muderis O, *et al.* Malignant Gastrointestinal Stromal Tumor: Distribution, Imaging Features, and Pattern of Metastatic Spread. *Radiology* 2003; 226:527–532.

Hong X, Choi H, Loyer EM, *et al.* Gastrointestinal Stromal Tumor: Role of CT in Diagnosis and in Response Evaluation and Surveillance after Treatment with Imatinib. *Radiographics* 2006; 26:481–495.

Jayaraman MV, Mayo-Smith WW, Movson JS, *et al.* CT of the Duodenum: An Over-looked Segment Gets Its Due. *Radiographics* 2001; 21:S147–S160.

Pearl MS, Hill MC, Zeman RK. CT Findings in Duodenal Diverticulitis. *AJR* 2006; 187:W392–W395.

Section 1.2   Flank Pain

Case 7   55-year-old man with right lower quadrant pain

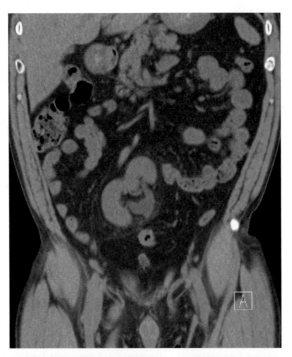

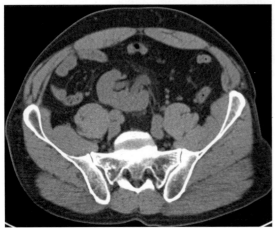

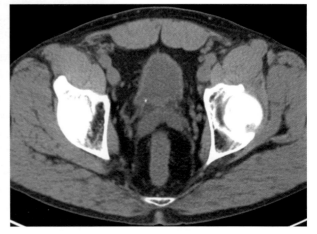

Diagnosis:
Obstructive right ureterovesical junction (UVJ) stone with a pelvic kidney

Coronal (left image) and axial (middle image) unenhanced CT images demonstrate a pelvic right kidney (yellow arrows) with mild hydroureteronephrosis. There is mild perinephric fat stranding, indicating an acute process (red arrow). Axial image through the bladder (right image) demonstrates a punctate, obstructing calcified stone at the right UVJ (blue arrow).

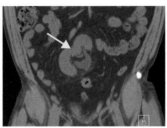 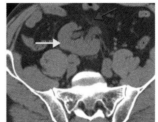 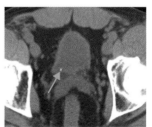

Discussion

Unenhanced CT is highly sensitive (97%) and specific (96%) for the detection of renal and ureteral stones.

- Unenhanced CT is usually the preferred modality for the evaluation of renal and ureteral stone disease because of its ability to resolve between calcified stones, dense non-calcified concretions, and normal renal parenchyma. CT may also detect pathology in other organs that mimics renal colic.
- Initial ultrasound rather than CT may be selected for follow-up in patients with known stone disease or in young patients in whom diagnostic testing without ionizing radiation exposure is desired. However, focused ultrasound for nephroureterolithiasis can be technically challenging and is insensitive for small stones, stones at the ureteropelvic junction (UPJ), and stones in the mid ureter. Estimation of stone size may be inaccurate. Ultrasound is more useful in cases of stones >5 mm and cases with hydroureteronephrosis. In most cases with a negative ultrasound and ongoing concern for stone disease, unenhanced CT is performed. Stones are seen as echogenic foci with posterior acoustic shadowing. Absence of a "ureteral jet" in the bladder on the affected side may be seen with Doppler imaging.
- The most common cause of calcification/calcium density in the renal parenchyma is nephrolithiasis. Medullary nephrocalcinosis and vascular calcification sometimes confound the diagnosis.

Dual-energy CT is an emerging technique that helps distinguish between uric acid and non-uric acid stones.

- Dual energy CT acquires images with two x-ray tubes set 90 degrees apart that simultaneously scan the patient at higher (140 kVp) and lower (80 kVp) energy levels. Because different types of stones have different chemical composition, and hence k-edges, they absorb photons differently at different energy levels. The composition of different stones can be reliably predicted by calculating a ratio of the attenuation at low and high energy levels.
- The distinction between uric acid and non-uric acid stones may be clinically important because some uric acid stones are treated with pharmacologic urine alkalinization rather than invasive procedures.

The most common locations of obstruction by ureteral calculi are in areas of normal ureteral narrowing.

- Special attention should be paid to these areas when evaluating for stones:
  - Ureteropelvic junction (UPJ)
  - Pelvic brim, where the ureter crosses the iliac vessels
  - Ureterovesical junction (UVJ)
- A pelvic venous phlebolith may be differentiated from a ureteral calculus by the "soft tissue rim" sign, which represents the thickened, inflamed ureteral wall around the calcification. If this is present, it is more likely that the calcification represents a ureteral calculus.

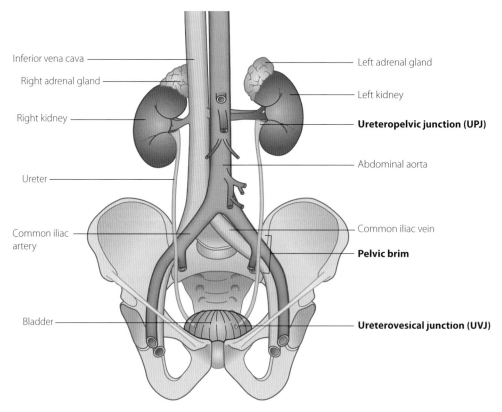

Urosepsis may complicate obstructive uropathy from upper tract stones. Emergent procedures to decompress the collecting system are necessary.

- Ureteral stents or percutaneous nephrostomy tubes temporize until the patient has clinically stabilized.
- Yoshimura *et al.* published that the strongest risk factors for requiring emergent surgical drainage with obstructive calculi were poor performance status (e.g., spinal cord injury), female sex, and age >75.

Clinical synopsis	Because this patient's stone was only 2 mm in diameter, the patient was managed conservatively with fluids and pain control. The stone passed spontaneously, and the patient was discharged from the Emergency Department.

Self-assessment

- *Name two types of kidney stones that are not radiopaque on plain film. Which of these cannot be seen even with CT?*

  - Uric acid stones, matrix stones, and indinavir stones are radiolucent on plain film.
  - Indinavir stones may be radiolucent even on CT. These stones are the crystallized form of the protease inhibitor indinavir, taken by some HIV positive patients on highly active anti-retroviral therapy (HAART).
  - Note that ultrasound can be used to identify both radiolucent and radiopaque stones.

- *What important size threshold helps predict whether renal calculi are likely to pass without intervention?*

  - 80% of stones 4 mm or smaller will pass through the UVJ spontaneously.

- *What important factors affect the sensitivity of ultrasound (but not CT) for the detection of renal calculi?*

  - Size: Calculi <3 mm may not demonstrate posterior acoustic shadowing and therefore may be missed. Very large calculi may also lack posterior acoustic shadowing due to reverberation "filling" the acoustic shadow.
  - Patient body habitus – larger patients have more subcutaneous fat, and lower frequency (lower resolution) probes are required to penetrate through to the kidneys. The resulting images are lower in resolution and contrast.
  - Operator skill.

Spectrum of renal stone disease

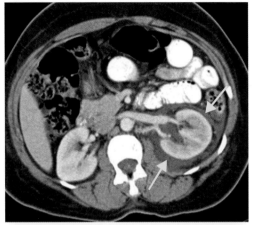

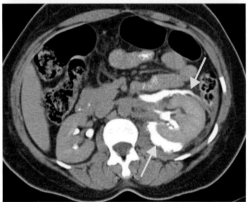

Forniceal rupture

Forniceal (calyceal) rupture results from elevated pressure in the renal collecting system leading to urinary extravasation around the affected kidney. The most common cause is obstructive renal calculi, followed by obstructing malignancy. In this case, there was an obstructing stone in the pelvic ureter (not shown). Portal venous phase axial enhanced CT (upper image) demonstrates mild hydronephrosis, perirenal fat stranding, and low-density fluid (arrows). Post-contrast axial CT obtained ten minutes after administration of IV contrast (in the delayed or excretory phase) shows contrast in the renal collecting system and extravasation into the perirenal space (arrows).

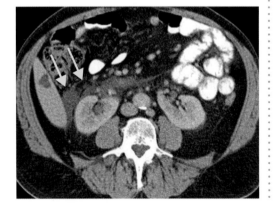

Forniceal rupture in a horseshoe kidney

Horseshoe kidneys span the midline. This results in arrest of metanephric ascension, as the kidneys get caught on the inferior mesenteric artery during their ascent from the pelvis during embryologic development. Though the kidneys are physically connected, the collecting systems are typically separate. In this patient with horseshoe kidney and an obstructing right-sided UVJ stone (not pictured), axial contrast-enhanced CT shows

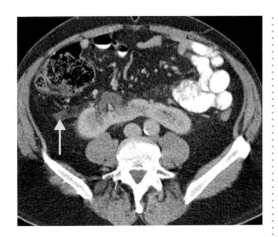

evidence of forniceal rupture involving the right renal moiety. Low density fluid (arrows) around the right moiety of the horseshoe kidney represents extravasated urine.

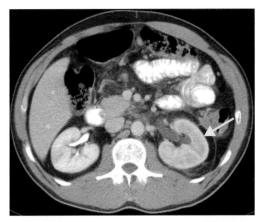

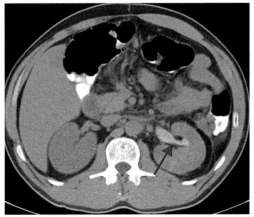

Indinavir stone disease

This HIV positive patient on a HAART regimen including the protease inhibitor indinavir presented with left flank pain. Indinavir stones are radiolucent even on CT. Though no radiopaque stones were seen, obstruction of the left UVJ was suspected by imaging. Initial axial enhanced CT (upper image) demonstrated asymmetric hypo-enhancement of the left kidney (arrow), moderate left hydronephrosis, and no excretion of opacified urine (which is clearly demonstrated on the right). Subsequent axial unenhanced CT performed 24 hours later (lower image) demonstrates faint opacification of the left collecting system (red arrow) and mild persistent left renal enhancement. This markedly delayed excretion of contrast is consistent with distal obstruction.

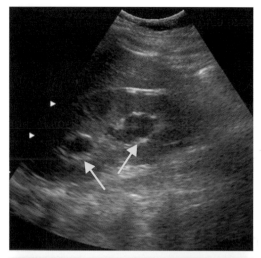

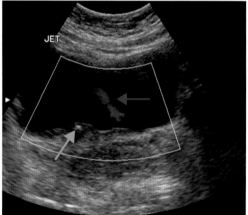

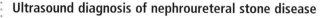

Ultrasound diagnosis of nephroureteral stone disease

Nephroureteral calculi on ultrasound are echogenic, usually demonstrate posterior acoustic shadowing, and tend to be seen in the renal calyces, renal pelvis, UPJ, or UVJ. Sometimes, focal echogenic fat within the renal sinus may result in a false positive. Sagittal grayscale ultrasound of the right kidney (upper image) demonstrates moderate hydronephrosis (yellow arrows). Transverse color Doppler duplex image through the bladder (lower image) demonstrates a normal left ureteral jet (red arrow). An echogenic structure in the expected location of the right UVJ (blue arrow) is highly suggestive of an obstructive right UVJ calculus.

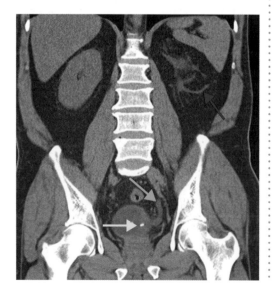

Renal calculus at UVJ

Coronal unenhanced CT demonstrates a calculus at the left UVJ (yellow arrow), with some perirenal fat stranding in the left renal fossa (red arrow) and mild left distal hydroureter (blue arrow).

Differential diagnosis of renal stone disease

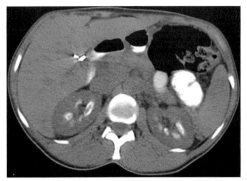

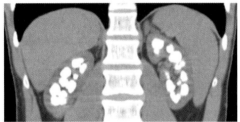

Medullary nephrocalcinosis

Mineralization within the medullary pyramids can be seen in several systemic disorders, including primary hyperparathyroidism, renal tubular acidosis type I, medullary sponge kidney, and long-term furosemide use (particularly in infants). The effect on renal function is variable. Axial unenhanced CT shows a milder case and coronal unenhanced CT represents a more severe case of medullary nephrocalcinosis, characterized by calcification of the renal pyramids. Renal stones are found in the renal collecting system rather than in the renal parenchyma.

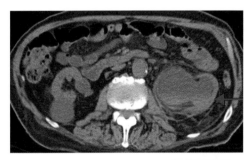

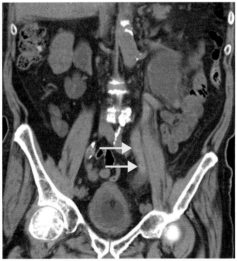

Urothelial carcinoma causing hydronephrosis

Obstructive uropathy and hematuria may herald urothelial malignancy, particularly in the elderly. Hydronephrosis at the time of diagnosis is associated with poorer outcomes in patients with urothelial cancer. If transitional cell carcinoma (TCC) is discovered, screening of the entire urinary tract is mandatory to evaluate for synchronous or metachronous TCC. Any factor resulting in chronic stasis of urine increases the patient's risk of developing upper tract TCC. In this patient, unenhanced axial and coronal CT show severe hydronephrosis and a mix of hemorrhage and hyperdense soft tissue filling the left ureter (yellow arrows). A hematocrit level is seen in the dilated left renal pelvis (red arrow).

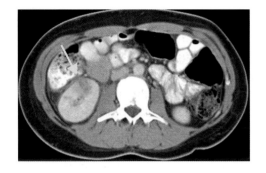

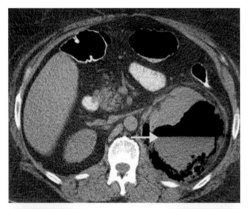

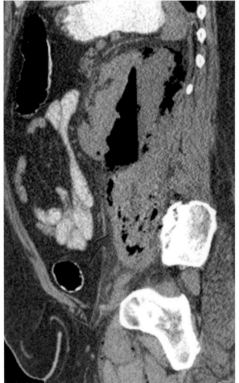

Acute pyelonephritis

Acute pyelonephritis is an affliction with a varying radiological appearance that depends on the degree of severity and presence or absence of complications. This axial enhanced CT in a case of uncomplicated acute pyelonephritis shows an ill-defined area of poor corticomedullary differentiation anteriorly (arrow). Focal hypodensity with bulging of the renal cortex in this area reflects edema and hypoperfusion.

Perinephric abscess

Perinephric abscess may complicate acute pyelonephritis. Less commonly, a perinephric abscess may also develop from a ruptured renal parenchymal abscess or an extrarenal infection such as psoas abscess. In this case, axial and sagittal CT without IV contrast show a complex fluid collection with an air-fluid level (yellow arrow) displacing the left kidney anteriorly. The gas dissects inferiorly into the left iliopsoas muscle (red arrow).

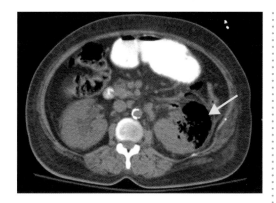

Emphysematous pyelonephritis

Uncomplicated pyelonephritis is a clinical diagnosis that usually does not require imaging; however, imaging is useful for assessing complicated pyelonephritis. The presence of renal parenchymal gas is seen with emphysematous pyelonephritis, which warrants emergent surgical consultation and is often treated with nephrectomy. In this case, axial CT without IV contrast shows extensive gas (arrow) replacing the left renal parenchyma.

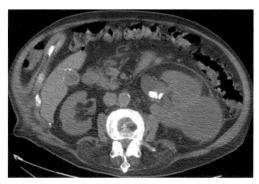

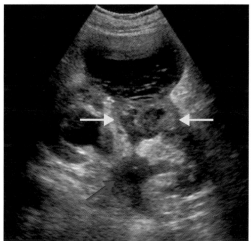

Xanthogranulomatous pyelonephritis (XGP)

XGP is a rare complication of chronic infection, characterized by obstructing staghorn calculi. Causal organisms include *P. mirabilis* and *E. coli*. Over time, the renal parenchyma is replaced and eventually enlarged by fibrofatty tissue. Typical treatment is nephrectomy. Axial unenhanced CT shows enlargement of the left kidney, with replacement of the renal parenchyma with multiple lobular, low attenuation masses (the "bearpaw" sign). Stones are seen in the proximal collecting system. Corresponding ultrasound image demonstrates an enlarged, deformed kidney with a mixed echogenicity mass conforming to the shape of a calyx (yellow arrows) and coexistent upper pole hydronephrosis (red arrow).

Further reading

Eisner B, *et al.* Nephrolithiasis: What Surgeons Need to Know. *AJR* 196: 1274–1278 (2011).

Fowler K, *et al.* US for Detecting Renal Calculi with Nonenhanced CT as a Reference Standard. *Radiology* 222: 109–113 (2002).

Gershman B, *et al.* Causes of Renal Forniceal Rupture. *BJU International* 108: 1909–1912 (2011).

Glodny B, *et al.* Kidney Fusion Anomalies Revisited: Clinical and Radiological Analysis of 209 Cases of Crossed Fused Ectopia and Horseshoe Kidney. *BJU International* 103: 224–235 (2008).

Hidas G, *et al.* Determination of Renal Stone Composition with Dual-Energy CT: In Vivo Analysis and Comparison with X-ray Diffraction. *Radiology* 257(2): 394–401 (2010).

Kawashima A, *et al.* CT of Renal Inflammatory Disease. *Radiographics* 17: 851–866 (1997).

King W, *et al.* Renal Stone Shadowing: An Investigation of Contributing Factors. *Radiology* 154: 191–196 (1985).

Messer J, *et al.* Multi-institutional Validation of the Ability of Preoperative Hydro-nephrosis to Predict Advanced Pathologic Tumor Stage in Upper-tract Urothelial Carcinoma. *Urologic Oncology: Seminars and Original Investigations* 31(6): 904-908 (2013).

Moe O. Kidney Stones: Pathophysiology and Medical Management. *Lancet* 367: 333–344 (2006).

Pickhardt P, *et al.* Infiltrative Renal Lesions: Radiologic–Pathologic Correlation. *Radiographics* 20: 215–243 (2000).

Prando A, *et al.* Urothelial Cancer of the Renal Pelvicaliceal System: Unusual Imaging Manifestations. *Radiographics* 30: 1553–1566 (2010).

Primak A, *et al.* Noninvasive Differentiation of Uric Acid versus Non-Uric Acid Kidney Stones Using Dual-Energy CT. *Acad Radiol* 14: 1441–1447 (2007).

Rao P. Imaging for Kidney Stones. *World J Urol* 22: 323–327 (2004).

Rucker C, *et al.* Mimics of Renal Colic: Alternative Diagnoses at Unenhanced Helical CT. *Radiographics* 24: S11—S33 (2004).

Yoshimura K, *et al.* Emergency Drainage for Urosepsis Associated with Urinary Tract Calculi. *J Urology* 173: 458–462 (2005).

Case 8   67-year-old man with a history of altered mental status, left flank pain, and hypotension, on anticoagulant medications

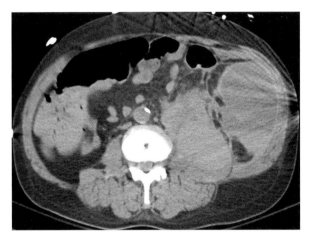
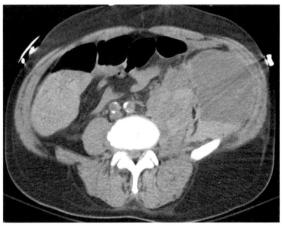
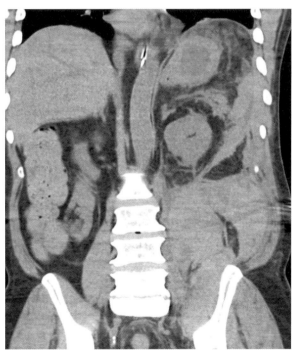

Diagnosis: Axial (left and middle images) and coronal (right image) unenhanced CT
Retroperitoneal images demonstrate a large fluid collection with a hematocrit level (yellow
hematoma arrow). There is hyperdense blood tracking along the posterior pararenal
space (red arrow) and into the left iliopsoas muscle (blue arrow). The IVC is
flattened (green arrow), indicating hypovolemia.

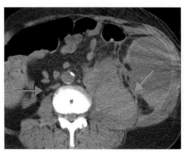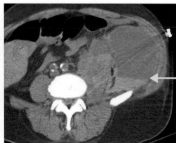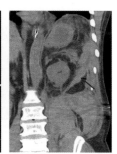

Discussion

Overview of retroperitoneal hematoma (RPH)

- A retroperitoneal hematoma (RPH) is a collection of blood in the
  retroperitoneum. It may be due to trauma, aortic pathology, or coagulopathy.
- In particular, RPH is an important complication of anticoagulation therapy. The
  patient may present with acute anemia or dropping hematocrit, which may or
  may not be accompanied by pain.
- Coagulopathy is often characterized by formation of a "hematocrit level" on
  CT, a term describing the separation of blood into lower-density serous and
  more dependent, higher-density cellular components.
- Physical exam may be misleading since the retroperitoneum cannot be directly
  examined. Thus, imaging is critical to establishing the diagnosis.
- Treatment for bleeding is managed with correction of any coagulopathy,
  intravenous fluids, and administration of blood products if necessary.

If RPH is contiguous with an abdominal aortic aneurysm (AAA), then the diagnosis of aortic rupture should be strongly considered.

- Identifying aortic rupture as the cause of RPH is essential, since aortic rupture
  requires emergent surgery.
- Most patients with atraumatic aortic rupture have an underlying AAA.
- Contiguity of RPH with the aortic wall over a distance of >3 cm is both a
  sensitive and specific sign for ruptured AAA.

- Identification of a site of active extravasation of IV contrast can help to differentiate ruptured AAA from RPH due to coagulopathy. In ruptured AAA, active extravasation is contiguous with the aorta, whereas in RPH, the site of active extravasation is typically noncontiguous. Unless the patient has a known AAA, however, CT for suspected RPH is generally performed without intravenous contrast.

Clinical synopsis

This patient was initially evaluated at an outside hospital, and given left thigh erythema and positive d-dimer, the diagnosis of deep vein thrombosis was presumed despite negative lower extremity ultrasound. Elevated creatine kinase and acute renal failure raised concern for rhabdomyolysis. He was treated with therapeutic doses of low molecular weight heparin (LMWH), after which he developed altered mental status and hypovolemic shock. Renal failure caused delayed drug clearance and prolonged effect of LMWH. The patient's hematocrit dropped to 16%, but his condition improved with reversal of anticoagulation, aggressive fluid resuscitation, and transfusion.

Self-assessment

- *Name three predisposing factors to spontaneous RPH.*

  - Therapeutic anticoagulation or antiplatelet therapy (aspirin, warfarin, heparin, LMWH, clopidogrel, etc.)
  - Inherited or acquired coagulopathy (e.g., coagulation factor deficiency or inhibitor)
  - Thrombocytopenia or platelet dysfunction
  - Chronic renal failure or chronic liver disease, which can lead to platelet abnormalities and secondary factor deficiencies, respectively

- *Name two physical exam signs that may be seen with RPH. What do they represent?*

  - Cullen's sign (periumbilical ecchymosis) was originally described in ruptured ectopic pregnancy, but it can also signify RPH or hemoperitoneum from other causes. The etiology is thought to be blood tracking along the ligamentum teres.
  - Grey–Turner sign (flank ecchymosis) was originally described in hemorrhagic pancreatitis, but may also be seen with RPH from other causes or hemoperitoneum. This sign is thought to be due to blood collecting in the pararenal space along the

posterior abdominal wall musculature, resulting in bilateral flank hematomas (particularly if the patient is supine).

- *What is the typical density of hemo-peritoneum? What factors may lower the density to render it less conspicuous?*

- Clotted blood typically attenuates between 40 and 50 Hounsfield units (HU), which is hyperattenuating relative to simple fluid. Hemoperitoneum is less dense in the setting of anemia (due to lower RBC content) and peritonitis (due to hemolysis and dilution by transudative ascites).

Spectrum of retroperitoneal hematoma

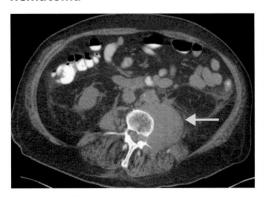

Psoas hematoma

The psoas (or iliopsoas) muscle is not an uncommon site for bleeding. Over time, secondary infection may occur, which may require percutaneous drainage. Axial CT with enteric contrast demonstrates expansion and hyperattenuation of the left psoas muscle (arrow) with haziness and stranding in the adjacent fat.

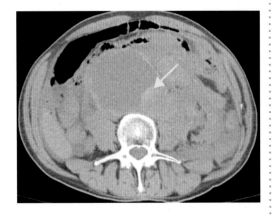

Ruptured AAA with RPH

As previously discussed, it is critical to identify rupture of AAA as the cause of a retroperitoneal hematoma to triage the patient appropriately. The most important finding of ruptured AAA is contiguity of an aortic aneurysm with the hematoma. There may also be a high-attenuation crescent-shaped mural thrombus, interruption of mural calcification, and a periluminal "halo". Axial unenhanced CT shows a large AAA with high-attenuation mural thrombus (arrow), mural irregularity, and adjacent RPH.

Differential diagnosis of retroperitoneal hematoma

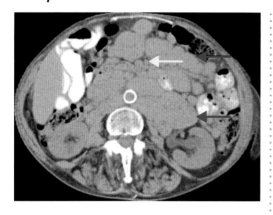

Retroperitoneal malignancy

Lymphadenopathy is the most common retroperitoneal mass and may be due to either lymphoma (as in this case) or metastatic disease. Retroperitoneal metastases are seen in testicular, prostate, renal, urothelial, colon, adrenal, and ovarian cancers. Axial CT with oral contrast only in a patient with lymphoma demonstrates extensive, bulky retroperitoneal and mesenteric lymphadenopathy with "sandwiching" of mesenteric vessels (yellow arrow) between layers of lymph nodes (red arrows), typical for lymphoma.

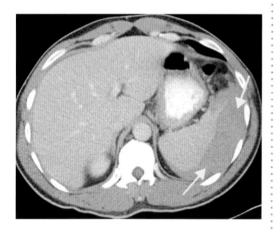

Perisplenic hematoma

The spleen is the abdominal organ most commonly injured by blunt trauma. Contrast-enhanced CT is sensitive for splenic injury. If an adjacent focus of high attenuation is identified on routine portal venous phase images, then delayed images (~5 minutes after contrast administration) should be used to differentiate between active extravasation (extraluminal contrast will remain or increase) and pseudoaneurysm (extraluminal contrast will not persist). Axial CT demonstrates a perisplenic hematoma (arrows) exerting moderate mass effect on the splenic parenchyma, uncomplicated by active extravasation.

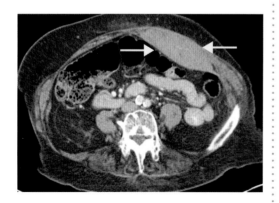

Rectus sheath hematoma

Rectus sheath hematoma is characterized by accumulation of blood within the fascia of the rectus sheath of the anterior abdominal wall, usually due to injury of the epigastric vessels or spontaneous hemorrhage in the setting of coagulopathy or anticoagulation. Because of investment by fascia, it is unusual for a rectus sheath hematoma to cross the midline. The most common clinical presentations are abdominal pain, abdominal mass, and cough. Rectus sheath hematoma is more common in women, presumably due to the protective effect of greater muscle bulk in men. In hemodynamically stable patients with unchanging hematoma, treatment is usually nonsurgical. Enhanced axial CT demonstrates high attenuation and enlargement of the left rectus abdominis muscle (arrows).

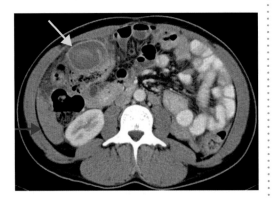

Omental hematoma

Omental hematoma is a very rare entity that usually occurs with trauma. Other causes include neoplasm, varices, and omental torsion with infarction. If the patient is hemodynamically unstable, treatment is resection of the involved omentum. Axial enhanced CT demonstrates a mixed-attenuation mass with surrounding fat stranding centered within the omentum in the right anterior hemiabdomen (yellow arrow). A small amount of hemoperitoneum is also present in the right paracolic gutter (red arrow).

Extraperitoneal/prevesical hematoma compressing the urinary bladder

Extraperitoneal hemorrhage may compress adjacent structures in the pelvis. In the case of bladder compression, acute hydronephrosis may develop. Axial unenhanced CT demonstrates two large hematomas with hematocrit gradients causing significant mass effect on the urinary bladder, as evidenced by displacement of a Foley catheter balloon posteriorly (arrow).

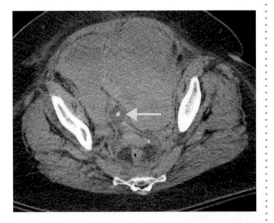

Hemoperitoneum

Hemoperitoneum, or blood within the peritoneal cavity, manifests on CT imaging as hyperdense fluid unbounded by the retroperitoneal fascial planes, distinguishing it from RPH. Axial enhanced CT demonstrates hyperdense blood (arrows) within the pelvis.

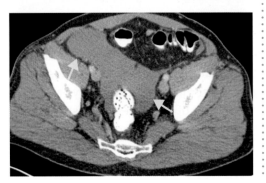

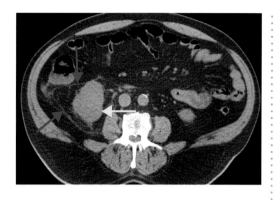

Hemorrhagic renal neoplasm

Renal neoplasm is the most common cause of spontaneous perirenal hemorrhage. Of all renal neoplasms, angiomyolipomas are the most likely to hemorrhage, especially when larger than 4 cm. Renal cell carcinoma is the second most common hemorrhagic renal neoplasm. Axial unenhanced CT in a patient with renal cell carcinoma demonstrates an exophytic solid renal mass (yellow arrow) with high density fat stranding along Gerota's fascia and the lateral conal fascia due to hemorrhage (red arrows).

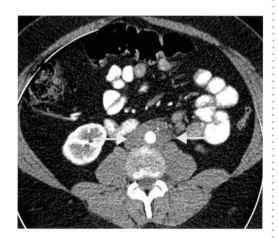

Retroperitoneal fibrosis

Retroperitoneal fibrosis is a poorly understood inflammatory process that may be benign or malignant and either primary (idiopathic) or secondary to autoimmune disease, prior radiation, or medications such as methysergide. Biopsy remains the gold standard for diagnosis, although certain imaging clues can be helpful. CT findings of benign retroperitoneal fibrosis include periaortic soft tissue that does not anteriorly displace the inferior vena cava and aorta, which differentiates it from malignant retroperitoneal fibrosis, lymphoma, and hematoma. There may also be medial displacement of the middle 1/3 of the ureters. MRI appearance is variable, but T1 hypointense, T2 intermediate, variably enhancing retroperitoneal soft tissue is typical. Treatment includes corticosteroids, immunosuppressants, and treatment of underlying causes. Axial enhanced CT demonstrates soft tissue (arrows) that extends almost circumferentially around, but does not significantly anteriorly displace, the aorta. *Case courtesy Amin Chaoui, MD.*

Further reading

Cherry WB, *et al.* Rectus Sheath Hematoma: Review of 126 Cases at a Single Institution. *Medicine* 85(2):105–110 (2006).

Chopra S. *Radcases: Genitourinary Imaging*. Thieme Medical Publishers, New York: 2012.

Chung K. Cullen and Grey Turner Signs in Idiopathic Perirenal Hemorrhage. *CMAJ* 183(16):E1221 (2011).

Cronin C, *et al.* Retroperitoneal Fibrosis: A Review of Clinical Features and Imaging Findings. *AJR* 191:423–431 (2008).

Ernst C. Abdominal Aortic Aneurysm. *NEJM* 328(16):1167-1172 (1993).

Federle M, *et al.* CT Criteria for Differentiating Abdominal Hemorrhage: Anticoagulation or Aortic Aneurysm Rupture? *AJR* 188:1324–1330 (2007).

Levine C, *et al.* Low Attenuation of Acute Traumatic Hemoperitoneum on CT Scans. *AJR* 166:1089–1093 (1996).

Ohno T, *et al.* Idiopathic Omental Bleeding: Report of a Case. *Surg Today* 35:493–495 (2005).

Siegel C, *et al.* Abdominal Aortic Aneurysm Morphology: CT Features in Patients with Ruptured and Nonruptured Aneurysms. *AJR* 163:1123–1129 (1994).

Sunga K, *et al.* Spontaneous Retroperitoneal Hematoma: Etiology, Characteristics, Management, and Outcome. *J Emerg Med* 43(2):e157–161 (August 2012).

Van Dyke J, *et al.* Review of Iliopsoas Anatomy and Pathology. *Radiographics* 7(1): 53–84 (1987).

Zhang J, *et al.* Etiology of Spontaneous Perirenal Hemorrhage: A Meta-analysis. *The Journal of Urology* 167(4):1593–1596 (2002).

Case 9   48-year-old woman with hypotension and acute right flank pain. No history of anticoagulation

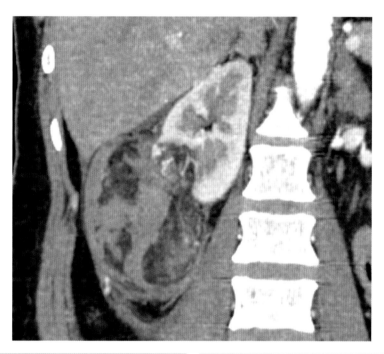

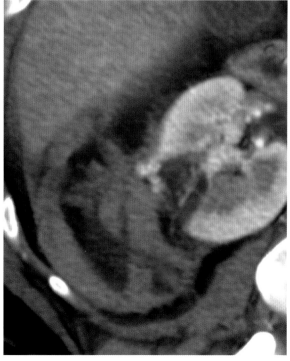

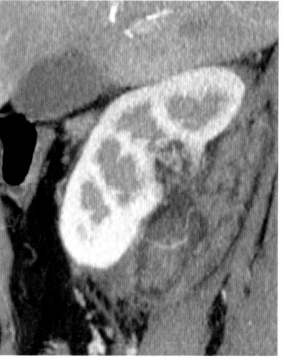

Diagnosis:
Hematoma secondary to a bleeding renal angiomyolipoma

Coronal (left image), axial (middle image), and sagittal (right image) contrast-enhanced CT images demonstrate retroperitoneal hemorrhage surrounding an exophytic, fat-containing, hypervascular right renal mass (yellow arrows). Prominent intratumoral vessels are noted within the lesion (red arrows). Despite predominantly exophytic location, the lesion definitively arises from the renal cortex in the posterior interpolar region, as indicated by the cortical defect (blue arrow).

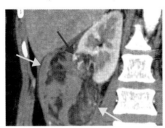 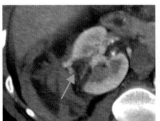 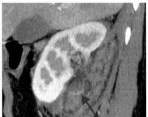

Discussion

Angiomyolipoma and risk of hemorrhage

- As the name implies, angiomyolipoma (AML) is a benign renal tumor comprised of vascular, smooth muscle, and fatty elements.
- Isolated or sporadic AMLs account for the vast majority of cases, in which tumors are typically unilateral and occur in middle-aged women. Up to 80% of patients with tuberous sclerosis have multiple, bilateral AMLs.
- Although they are usually an incidental finding, AMLs may present in the acute setting with hemorrhage, especially if they grow larger than 4 cm. It is thought that abnormal intratumoral vessels are prone to microaneurysm formation and, hence, hemorrhage.
- Clinical presentation of a bleeding AML includes hypotension, decreasing hematocrit, flank pain, and/or hematuria.

Imaging of AML

- The diagnosis of AML relies on identification of intratumoral macroscopic (gross) fat, which is characterized by negative density on CT (typically <-20 HU), or intratumoral fat signal (saturation on fat-suppressed images) on MRI. Overwhelmingly, AML is a diagnosis made by radiologists.
- Imaging diagnosis may be difficult in lipid-poor AMLs (4% of all AMLs). The finding of a small, hyperdense renal mass on CT should raise the suspicion of lipid-poor AML, particularly in a young female patient. Biopsy can be used to make the diagnosis and avoid unnecessary surgery.

- On MR imaging, an AML is seen as a mass that contains focal macroscopic fat signal. Intra-lesional fat signal will follow retroperitoneal or mesenteric fat on all pulse sequences, with the fat-suppressed sequences most helpful. Note that in- and out-of-phase imaging, which is used to evaluate for the presence of water and fat in the same voxel, is not helpful to detect macroscopic fat.
- In extremely rare instances, renal cell carcinomas (RCCs) can contain macroscopic intratumoral fat, which may be secondary to lipid-producing necrosis within a large RCC, intratumoral bone metaplasia with fatty marrow elements (usually associated with calcification), or entrapment of perirenal or sinus fat. Unlike a rare fat-containing RCC, AML should not have any calcification.

Clinical synopsis	This patient was admitted and treated with aggressive fluid resuscitation. After CT diagnosis, she was referred to interventional radiology, where she had an uneventful endovascular embolization. Following the procedure she was asymptomatic and hemodynamically stable, and she was discharged the following day.

Self-assessment

- *Name two factors that predispose to hemorrhage in renal AMLs.*

  - Large size (typically larger than 4 cm in diameter)
  - Prominent microaneurysms
  - Presence of symptoms (which may reflect interval growth)

- *What are the diagnostic criteria for renal AML?*

  - An AML is diagnosed by the presence of macroscopic fat.
  - A renal mass containing fat (<-20 HU) on CT is considered virtually pathognomonic for AML.
  - Ultrasound is not reliable for the diagnosis of macroscopic fat, as the finding of a hyperechoic renal mass is nonspecific. A small RCC may also present as a hyperechoic mass; however, a small hyperechoic renal mass is much more likely to represent an AML.
  - On MRI, the mass should contain internal signal that is similar to the surrounding retroperitoneal fat. Fat-suppression techniques are particularly useful. Note that in- and out-of-phase imaging is not helpful, as this imaging technique detects intracytoplasmic lipid (e.g., to diagnose

• *What is the differential diagnosis for macroscopic fat-containing renal tumors?*

an adrenal lipoma or hepatic steatosis) rather than macroscopic fat.

• Angiomyolipoma
• Lipoma (unusual and does not differ in appearance from AML with predominant adipose component)
• Retroperitoneal liposarcoma (typically lacks the renal cortical defect or indentation in the renal parenchyma seen in exophytic AMLs, and does not feature enlarged vessels arising from the kidney)
• Wilms tumor (rare)
• Renal cell carcinoma (very rare)

Spectrum of renal angiomyolipoma

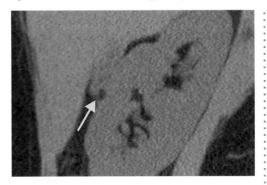

Small angiomyolipoma

A small (<4 cm), asymptomatic fat-containing renal mass is considered nearly pathognomonic for AML. Sagittal noncontrast CT demonstrates a subcentimeter fat-containing lesion (arrow) arising from the renal cortex.

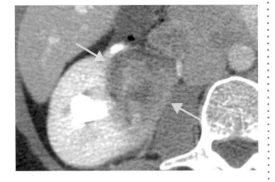

Renal sinus angiomyolipoma

When an AML arises in the region of the renal sinus, it can be difficult to determine with certainty whether the fat is intralesional or related to the renal sinus. Axial enhanced CT demonstrates a heterogeneous, hypervascular renal mass (arrows) abutting the sinus. Although foci of macroscopic fat were seen on the noncontrast CT (not shown), biopsy was performed to confirm that the fat was arising from the tumor rather than the adjacent sinus fat.

Differential diagnosis of renal angiomyolipoma

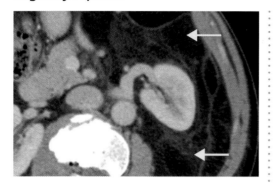

Retroperitoneal liposarcoma

Liposarcoma is a malignant sarcoma that usually contains fat. Axial enhanced CT shows a large, fatty mass (arrows) encasing the kidney and featuring several septations. There is no cortical defect to suggest that the lesion is arising from the renal parenchyma. Intratumoral vessels are also notably absent, which distinguishes this lesion from a large AML.

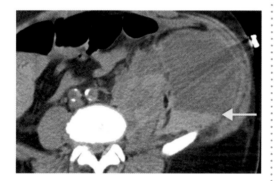

Retroperitoneal hematoma

An idiopathic retroperitoneal hematoma can appear similar to a hemorrhagic AML; however, an idiopathic hematoma will not contain fat. Axial unenhanced CT demonstrates a large left retroperitoneal fluid collection with a hematocrit level posteriorly (arrow). There is expansion of the left psoas, consistent with intramuscular hematoma formation. In contrast to a hemorrhagic AML, there is no fatty component.

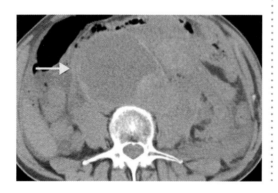

Ruptured abdominal aortic aneurysm

Axial unenhanced CT demonstrates a large abdominal aortic aneurysm (arrow) with mural irregularity, adjacent retroperitoneal hematoma and hemoperitoneum. Contiguity of the retroperitoneal hematoma with the abdominal aneurysm is considered a specific sign of ruptured abdominal aortic aneurysm.

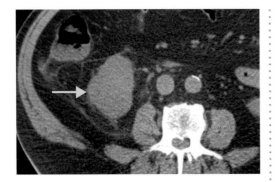

Hemorrhagic renal cell carcinoma

Of all renal neoplasms, AMLs are the most likely to hemorrhage, especially when larger than 4 cm, as shown in the index case. Renal cell carcinoma is the second most common hemorrhagic renal neoplasm. Unenhanced CT in a patient with renal cell carcinoma demonstrates an exophytic solid renal mass (arrow) with high-attenuation fat stranding along Gerota's fascia and lateral conal fascia due to hemorrhage.

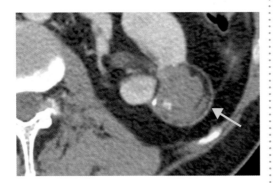

Pseudo renal AML sign after percutaneous thermal ablation

After percutaneous ablation of renal cell carcinoma, the ablation zone forms a pseudocapsule that may contain fat, soft tissue, and punctate calcifications. The presence of fat in the ablation zone may simulate an AML on imaging, although calcification is not typical for an AML. Enhanced CT in a patient post-ablation demonstrates an exophytic, heterogeneous, fat-containing mass (arrow) with a pseudocapsule containing punctate calcification.

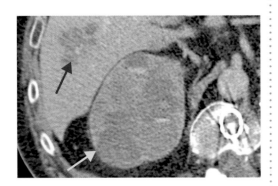

Hemorrhagic adrenal metastasis

An adrenal metastasis may hemorrhage. In contrast to a hemorrhagic renal AML, a hemorrhagic adrenal metastasis will be located in the adrenal gland, and macroscopic fat would be unusual. Enhanced CT shows a heterogeneous right retroperitoneal mass (yellow arrow), which was shown to be superior to the kidney on the coronal images (not shown). Note the irregular hepatic metastasis (red arrow).

Further reading

Beer, *et al*. Comparison of 16-MDCT and MRI for Characterization of Kidney Lesions. *AJR* 186:1639–1650 (2006)

Bosniak, *et al*. CT Diagnosis of Renal Angiomyolipoma: The Importance of Detecting Small Amounts of Fat. *AJR* 151:497–501 (1988)

Hélénon, *et al*. Renal Cell Carcinoma Containing Fat: Demonstration with CT. *Radiology* 188:429–430 (1993)

Hélénon, *et al*. Unusual Fat-containing Tumors of the Kidney: A Diagnostic Dilemma. *Radiographics* 17:129–144 (1997)

Israel, *et al*. CT Differentiation of Large Exophytic Renal Angiomyolipomas and Perirenal Liposarcomas. *AJR* 179:769–773 (2002)

Kim, *et al*. Renal Angiomyolipoma with Minimal Fat: Differentiation from Other Neoplasms at Double-Echo Chemical Shift FLASH MR Imaging. *Radiology* 239:174–180 (2006)

Logue, *et al*. Angiomyolipomas in Tuberous Sclerosis. *Radiographics* 23:241–246 (2003)

Muttarak, *et al*. Renal Angiomyolipoma with Bleeding. *Biomed Imaging Interv* 3(4):1–4 (2007)

Prasad, *et al*. Benign Renal Neoplasms in Adults: Cross-Sectional Imaging Findings. *AJR* 190:158–164 (2008)

Silverman, *et al*. Hyperattenuating Renal Masses: Etiologies, Pathogenesis, and Imaging Evaluation. *Radiographics* 27:1131–1143 (2007)

Yamakado, *et al*. Renal Angiomyolipoma: Relationships between Tumor Size, Aneurysm Formation, and Rupture. *Radiology* 225:78–82 (2002)

Zagoria, *et al*. *Genitourinary Imaging: Case Review Series 2nd Edition*. Mosby-Elsevier Publishers, 2006.

Section 1.3   Lower Quadrant Pain

Case 10   23-year-old man with right lower quadrant pain

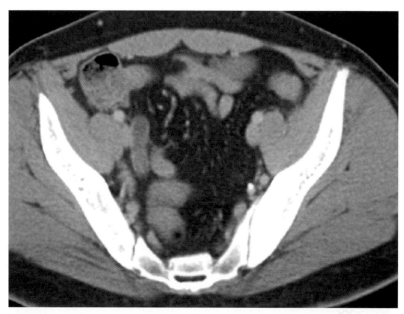

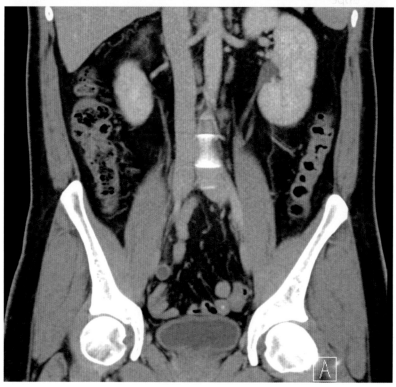

Diagnosis:
Appendicitis

Axial (left image) and coronal (right image) contrast-enhanced CT images show a dilated appendix with mild associated fat-stranding (arrows).

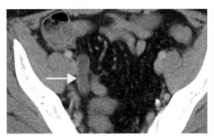 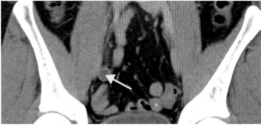

Discussion

Overview of appendicitis

- Although appendicitis is one of the most common causes of an acute abdomen, clinical diagnosis can be difficult due to the varied presentation and large number of clinical mimics. CT plays a crucial role in diagnosing appendicitis, with an accuracy of 98%.
- Appendicitis is thought to be caused by luminal obstruction by an appendicolith (as shown below) or lymphoid hyperplasia, which subsequently causes venous congestion and mural ischemia. The ischemic appendix becomes a nidus for bacterial translocation and inflammation.

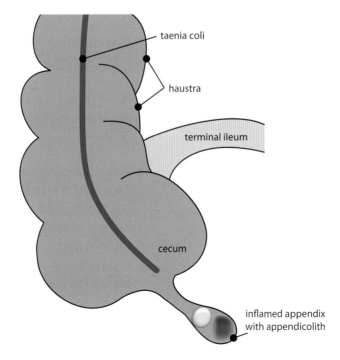

The CT diagnosis of appendicitis depends on both direct and indirect imaging characteristics.

- Direct signs are due to intrinsic abnormalities of the appendix:
  - **Distended appendix**: It is uncommon for the appendix to measure less than 6 mm in a case of appendicitis, although an enlarged appendix in isolation may be a normal variant.
  - **Wall thickening** or **hyperemia** (hyperemia can only be seen on scans with intravenous contrast).
  - **Appendicolith**, which can also be seen in a normal appendix.
- Indirect imaging signs are due to adjacent inflammation:
  - Periappendiceal **fat stranding**
  - **Wall thickening** of **adjacent organs**, such as the base of the cecum
  - **Ileus** or **hydroureter** (due to adjacent inflammation)
- When evaluating for suspected acute appendicitis, it's essential to look for potential clinical mimics *not* related to the appendix, such as pyelonephritis, nephrolithiasis, psoas abscess, and pelvic pathology, all of which can be evaluated by CT.

Clinical synopsis	This patient, a 23-year-old male with early appendicitis, was treated with emergent appendectomy and was discharged without complication the following day.

Self-assessment

- *Describe what "complicated" appendicitis means.*

  - "Complicated appendicitis" implies gangrene, necrosis, perforation, or abscess formation.

- *Name three appendiceal neoplasms that may mimic acute appendicitis.*

  - Appendiceal carcinoma, appendiceal carcinoid, adenocarcinoma metastatic to the appendix.

- *What is secondary appendicitis?*

  - Secondary appendicitis is inflammation of the appendix due to inflammation of the surrounding structures, and is one of the most common causes of false positive CT for appendicitis. Crohn's disease, cecal diverticulitis, enteritis, and pancreatitis may cause adjacent inflammation of the appendix.

- *What is the eponym for appendicitis in the inguinal canal?*

  - Appendicitis in the inguinal canal is known as Amyand's hernia.

Spectrum of appendicitis

The spectrum of appendicitis ranges from tip appendicitis to inflammation of the entire appendix. Advanced appendicitis may rupture, potentially resulting in abscess formation.

Tip appendicitis

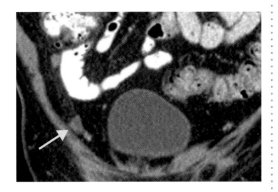

The earliest form of appendicitis can be difficult to detect by CT unless the entire course of the appendix is carefully followed. Occasionally, the entire appendix is normal except for the most distal tip, which is mildly dilated (arrow). The more proximal appendix (inferior to the arrow) is decompressed.

Perforated appendictis

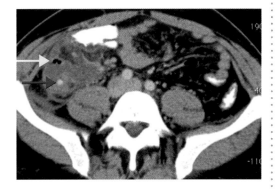

Note the tiny foci of extraluminal air (yellow arrow) signifying that the appendix has ruptured. An appendicolith (red arrow) is also seen.

Periappendicular abscess

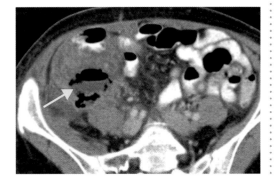

A large periappendiceal fluid collection with gas-fluid levels implies abscess formation. Antibiotic therapy and percutaneous drainage are often the initial steps in treatment. After the infection is treated adequately, elective appendectomy can be considered. Axial enhanced CT demonstrates a large right lower quadrant abscess (arrow) containing gas and fluid.

Appendicitis in pregnancy

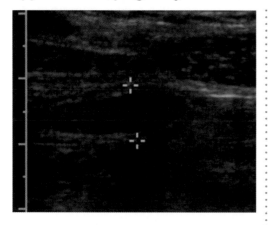

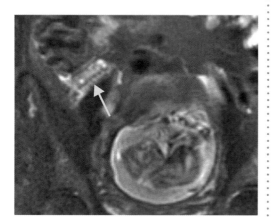

Imaging of appendicitis in pregnancy

Ultrasound with graded compression is the initial imaging technique for suspected acute appendicitis in pregnancy. Visualization of a blind-ending tubular structure in the right lower quadrant dilated to greater than 6 mm is suggestive of appendicitis.

MRI provides excellent soft-tissue contrast and does not expose the patient to radiation. The MR diagnosis of appendicitis relies on the same size criteria established for CT and ultrasound (6 mm). T2-weighted fat-saturation sequences are most useful for the detection of periappendiceal inflammation and edema. Gadolinium-based contrast agents are generally avoided for this indication in pregnant patients.

Top image: Right lower quadrant ultrasound shows a dilated, tubular blind-ending structure (calipers) suggesting acute appendicitis.

Bottom image: Coronal T2-weighted MR with fat suppression in a pregnant patient shows a dilated, hyperintense structure (arrow) in the right lower quadrant reflecting acute appendicitis. A singleton gestation is noted.

Differential diagnosis of appendicitis

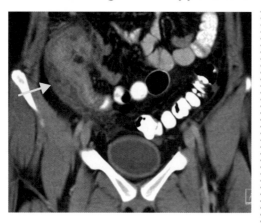

Terminal ileitis

Inflammation of the terminal ileum, most commonly due to Crohn's disease, can spread to the appendix and mimic acute appendicitis. Making the distinction between appendicitis and terminal ileitis is essential, as appendicitis is treated surgically and terminal ileitis is treated medically. If surgery is performed in Crohn's disease, there may be prolonged healing time and potential for complications. Coronal enhanced CT shows extensive wall thickening of the distal ileum with adjacent fat stranding (arrow).

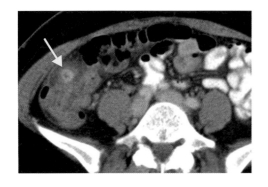

Cecal diverticulitis

Acute inflammation of a bowel diverticulum most commonly occurs in the sigmoid colon. However, cecal diverticulitis can mimic acute appendicitis, and may even involve the appendix with secondary inflammation. A hyperemic cecal diverticulum (arrow) is the epicenter of inflammation in this case of diverticulitis. Diverticulitis is discussed in case 13.

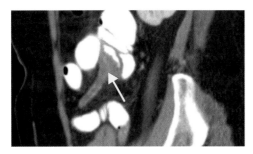

Cecal carcinoma

Cecal carcinoma may cause obstruction of the appendix. Sagittal CT image demonstrates circumferential cecal base thickening (arrow) leading to appendiceal obstruction.

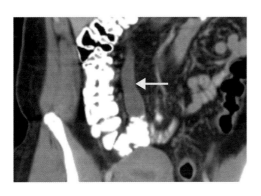

Appendiceal mucocele

The term *mucocele* describes a mucus-containing dilated structure. Appendiceal mucocele may be benign due to cystadenoma or malignant due to mucinous cystadenocarcinoma. In contrast to appendicitis, there is rarely surrounding inflammation. If malignant, there is a propensity for rupture into the peritoneal cavity, causing pseudomyxoma peritonei. Mucoceles are treated surgically. Coronal enhanced CT shows a dilated appendiceal mucocele (arrow) without surrounding inflammatory change.

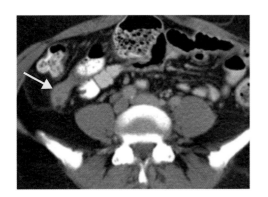

Appendiceal neoplasm

Appendiceal carcinoids are rare tumors of neural crest origin that can occur in any age group. Generally, carcinoids of the appendix have a benign clinical course and do not metastasize. Small tumors less than 2 cm in size can be treated with simple appendectomy. Right hemicolectomy is performed for less commonly encountered advanced disease. Other appendiceal neoplasms include primary and metastatic adenocarcinoma. Axial enhanced CT demonstrates nonspecific mural thickening of the appendix (arrow).

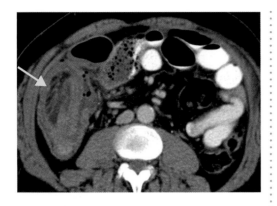

Ileocolic intussusception

Telescoping of the bowel can be idiopathic or due to a lead point mass. In an adult with a history of malignancy, intussusception is concerning for an intraluminal lead point mass. In children, lymphoid hyperplasia is the most common lead point mass. A short-segment intussusception may be treated conservatively, while obstructing intussusceptions are resected. Axial CT demonstrates a classic "targetoid" appearance of intussusception (arrow).

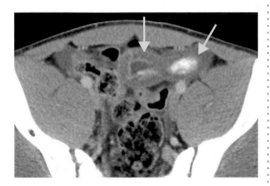

Meckel's diverticulitis

Meckel's diverticulum, a blind-ending ileal diverticulum that is a remnant of the omphalomesenteric duct, may become obstructed and inflamed. Meckel's diverticula are present in 2% of the population, are 2 feet from the ileocecal valve, usually 2 inches long, and usually become symptomatic before age 2. In children, they typically cause bleeding, and in adults they may cause diverticulitis or obstruction. Axial enhanced CT demonstrates a large blind-ending structure (arrows) in the mid and left pelvis with mural thickening.

Further reading

Long, S.S. *et al.* Imaging strategies for right lower quadrant pain in pregnancy. *AJR: American Journal of Roentgenology* 196, 4–12(2011).

Raja, A.S. *et al.* Negative appendectomy rate in the era of CT: an 18-year perspective. *Radiology* 256, 460(2010).

Rybkin, A.V. & Thoeni, R.F. Current concepts in imaging of appendicitis. *Radiologic Clinics of North America* 45, 411–442, vii(2007).

Silva, A.C. *et al.* Spectrum of normal and abnormal CT appearances of the ileocecal valve and cecum with endoscopic and surgical correlation. *Radiographics: A Review Publication of the Radiological Society of North America, Inc* 27, 1039–1054(2007).

Whitley, S. *et al.* The appendix on CT. *Clinical Radiology* 64, 190–199(2009).

Case 11   26-year-old man presenting with diffuse abdominal pain and diarrhea for several weeks

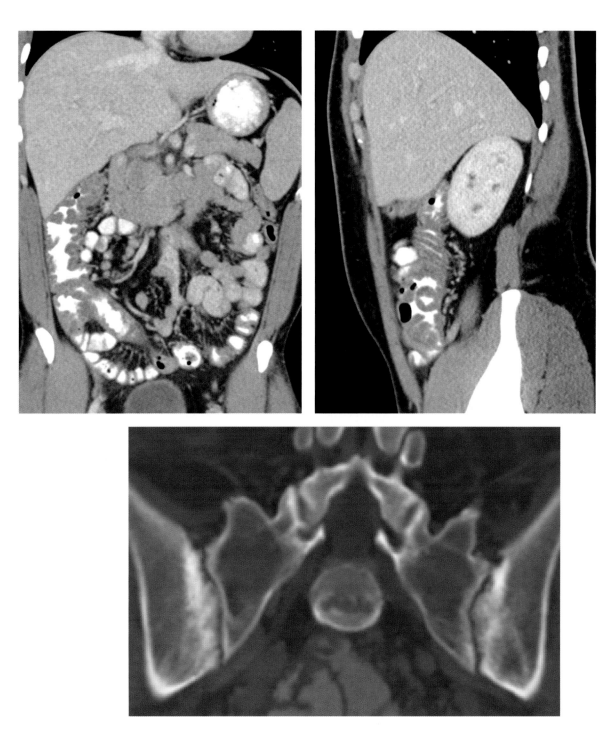

***Diagnosis:*
**Crohn's
disease
(acute flare)**

Coronal (left image) and sagittal (middle image) CT images with oral and intravenous contrast show a long segment of mural thickening (yellow arrows) involving the distal ileum, cecum, and ascending colon, associated with subtle pericolonic fat stranding, representing ileocolitis. Coronal CT in bone window (right image) of the same patient demonstrates symmetrical sclerosis at the iliac aspect of the sacroiliac joints (red arrows), consistent with sacroiliitis.

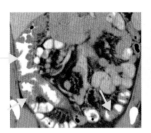 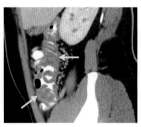 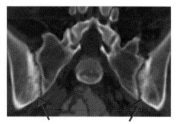

Discussion

Overview of Crohn's disease

- Crohn's disease is a chronic, relapsing granulomatous inflammatory disorder affecting the gastrointestinal tract. Many cases of Crohn's disease are first diagnosed during the workup for acute right lower quadrant pain in the Emergency Department.
- Crohn's disease can involve any segment of the gastrointestinal tract, from the oral mucosa to the anus. The terminal ileum is almost always involved. The involved portions of bowel are characteristically discontinuous in location (e.g., there may be simultaneous involvement of the terminal ileum and anus without any abnormality of intervening bowel segments, a distribution described as "skip lesions"). The affected bowel features ulcerations, full-thickness mural inflammation, and formation of noncaseating granulomas.
- Crohn's disease is most commonly diagnosed in adolescence through the third decade, although onset in late adulthood has also been reported. Patients usually present with chronic diarrhea, abdominal pain, weight loss, and fever.
- Skip lesions and transmural involvement are characteristic of Crohn's disease. In contrast, ulcerative colitis (UC) tends to feature continuous, superficial (mucosal) inflammation. The rectum is almost always involved in UC, with extension proximally.

Imaging of Crohn's disease

- CT is the primary imaging modality for the evaluation of acute right lower quadrant pain due to quick examination time with single-breath-hold scanning and near-universal availability.

- Mesenteric hyperemia leads to many of the CT findings of Crohn's disease. Transversely oriented engorged vessels perpendicular to the longitudinal axis of the involved bowel loop produce the characteristic "comb" sign. Intramural fat and mesenteric fibro-fatty infiltration (called "creeping fat" by pathologists) are indicative of chronic involvement.
- The most common cross-sectional imaging findings during an acute flare include:
  - Wall thickening (>4 mm)
  - Mesenteric vascular engorgement, submucosal and mesenteric edema, and mucosal hyperenhancement
  - Transmural ulceration and fistula formation
  - Enlarged mesenteric lymph nodes
- MR enterography is a highly accurate, dynamic imaging technique that spares the generally young population of patients with inflammatory bowel disease from ionizing radiation exposure.

Abdominal complications and management of Crohn's disease

- There is a high incidence of abdominal complications of Crohn's disease, including bowel stricture, fistula (to other bowel segments, urinary bladder, skin, or perianal tissue), and abscess.
- Differentiation between an acute flare and chronic stenosis is critical, since management differs substantially. An acute flare is usually treated with anti-inflammatory drugs, while a chronic stenosis may require surgery. The absence of acute inflammatory changes and the presence of fibrotic stenoses suggests chronic disease.

Extra-intestinal manifestation of Crohn's disease

- Extra-intestinal inflammatory processes are seen in up to 25% of patients with Crohn's disease and may involve the musculoskeletal, ocular, and mucocutaneous systems. Musculoskeletal involvement includes an inflammatory arthropathy, which characteristically affects the sacroiliac joints (as shown in this case), although any joint may be involved. Ocular manifestations include uveitis. Mucocutaneous findings include erythema nodosum and pyoderma gangrenosum involving the lower extremities, and aphthous ulcers involving the mucous membranes.

Clinical synopsis This patient underwent colonoscopy with biopsy revealing a granulomatous inflammatory process, consistent with Crohn's disease. Appropriate medical treatment was started.

Self-assessment

- *What are the main differences between Crohn's disease and ulcerative colitis?*

- Crohn's disease is a transmural process, most often involving the small bowel with skip lesions. Ulcerative colitis is characterized by superficial inflammation extending proximally from the rectum in a continuous manner.

- *List three imaging findings of an acute flare of Crohn's disease.*

- Bowel wall thickening (>4 mm) with submucosal edema and mucosal hyperenhancement
- Transmucosal ulceration
- Mesenteric engorgement, which may manifest as the "comb" sign
- Mesenteric adenopathy

- *List three common complications of Crohn's disease.*

- Stricture, sinus, fistula, and abscess formation

CT and MR enterography in evaluation of Crohn's disease

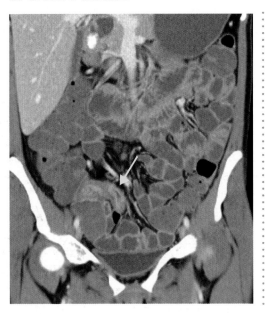

CT enterography

CT enterography allows good visualization of both the small bowel lumen and wall. Dilute barium (which attenuates similarly to fluid) is administered, allowing for better evaluation of the bowel wall compared to standard positive oral contrast. Similar to standard CT, CT enterography may also be used to detect associated pathologic findings such as lymphadenopathy, fistula and sinus formation, abscesses, and abnormal fold patterns. Coronal CT enterography in a patient with known Crohn's disease demonstrates mucosal hyperenhancement and submucosal edema of the distal ileum (arrow), consistent with acute flare.

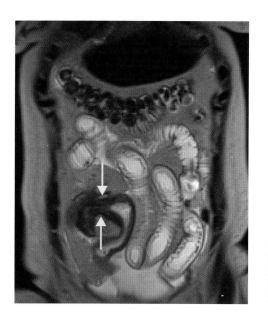

MR enterography

MR offers the advantages of dynamic imaging without ionizing radiation. Similar to CT enterography, MR enterography allows for the evaluation of bowel lumen diameter, bowel wall thickening, patterns of enhancement, and extra-intestinal findings. Focal or multifocal bowel wall thickening are findings suggestive of acute flare, while stenoses or low signal intensity of the bowel wall are seen in chronic disease. Coronal T2-weighted MR demonstrates hypointense wall thickening and narrowing of the distal ileum (arrows), consistent with fibrosis characteristic of chronic disease.

Spectrum of Crohn's disease

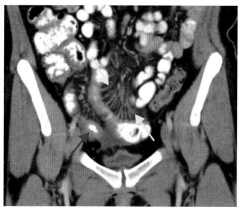

"Comb" sign

The "comb" sign signifies mesenteric vascular engorgement and is seen as multiple parallel vessels on the mesenteric side of the ileum, resembling the teeth of a comb. Coronal enhanced CT demonstrates the comb sign with multiple parallel engorged mesenteric vessels (yellow arrows). Note the thickened distal ileal small bowel loops in the right lower quadrant (red arrow).

Abscess

The transmural nature of the inflammatory process in Crohn's disease and the presence of deep bowel wall ulcers predispose patients to develop abdominal abscesses. Coronal enhanced CT demonstrates a large, peripherally enhancing fluid collection (yellow arrow) in the pelvis, which contains a few small peripheral foci of gas (red arrow). There is an adjacent inflamed loop of bowel (blue arrow) possibly adherent to the abscess.

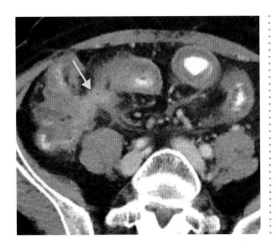

Fistula

Deep transmural ulcers may ultimately communicate with an adjacent epithelial surface and become fistulas. If the inflammatory process forms a blind-ending tract, it is then called a sinus. On CT, fistulas present as enhancing soft tissue tracts. Oral contrast can sometimes be seen within the lumen of the fistula. On MR, fistulas typically manifest as T2-hyperintense tracts. Axial enhanced CT demonstrates a fistulous tract between the distal ileum and the cecum (arrow).

Differential diagnosis of Crohn's disease

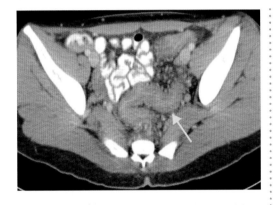

Ulcerative colitis

It is often possible to differentiate between Crohn's disease and ulcerative colitis (UC) on imaging. The hallmark of UC is continuous involvement, extending from the rectum proximally, without skip lesions. Ulcerative colitis involvement is limited to the mucosa and is not transmural. Strictures and fistulas are not typically seen in UC. In this case of ulcerative colitis, axial enhanced CT demonstrates thickening of the rectosigmoid colon (arrow).

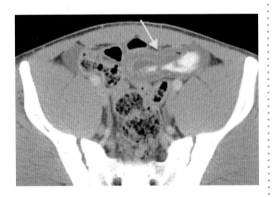

Meckel's diverticulitis

Meckel's diverticulum is due to incomplete obliteration of the omphalomesenteric duct and is located on the antimesenteric side of the ileum, approximately 100 cm from the ileocecal valve. Gastrointestinal bleeding (due to ectopic gastric mucosa) is the most common presentation in children; however, intestinal obstruction or diverticulitis may occur in adults. Axial CT demonstrates a thickened, blind-ending structure (arrow) consistent with Meckel's diverticulitis.

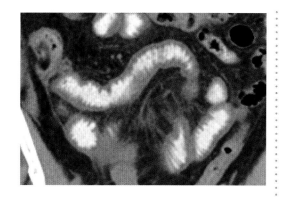

Infectious enterocolitis

Infection of the distal ileum and cecum may be caused by a number of organisms, including *Yersinia enterocolitica*, *Campylobacter jejuni*, and *Salmonella enteritidis*, and have nonspecific imaging features. Clinical presentation and imaging findings may be similar to Crohn's disease, including wall thickening and enhancement of the distal ileum and cecum. Coronal CT in this case of proven *Salmonella* enteritis demonstrates diffuse ileal wall thickening.

Radiation enteritis

Radiation enteritis can affect any segment of the bowel in the radiation field, potentially leading to stenosis, sinus, or fistula formation. Axial contrast-enhanced CT demonstrates nonspecific small bowel wall thickening in the mid-pelvis in this patient who received prior radiation therapy for colon cancer.

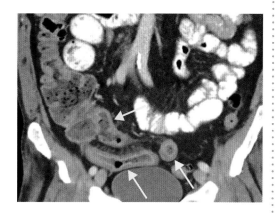

Graft-versus-host disease

Graft-versus-host disease is the most common gastrointestinal complication following allogenic stem cell transplantation, accompanying or preceding hepatic or skin manifestations. Biopsy may be necessary for diagnosis since many of these patients are immunosuppressed and susceptible to infectious enteritis. Coronal enhanced CT demonstrates diffuse mural thickening (arrows) of the small bowel and cecum in the pelvis and right hemiabdomen.

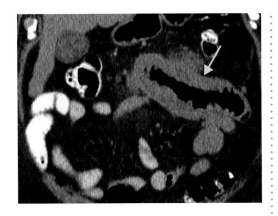

Small bowel lymphoma

The distal ileum is the most common site of primary gastrointestinal lymphoma. A characteristic imaging finding of lymphoma is aneurysmal dilatation of the bowel. Gradual narrowing of the bowel lumen due to circumferential wall thickening, typically without obstruction, can also be seen. Lymphoma of the terminal ileum may also lead to intussusception. Associated bulky mesenteric adenopathy is common. Coronal CT demonstrates segmental wall thickening and "aneurysmal dilatation" of a loop of bowel (arrow).

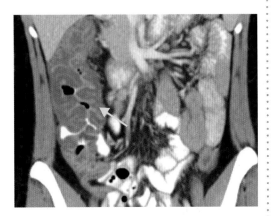

Typhlitis

Also known as neutropenic colitis, typhlitis is seen in the context of neutropenia and can rapidly progress to perforation due to a combination of infection, ischemia, and hemorrhage. It classically involves the right colon. CT findings include circumferential wall thickening with areas of low attenuation secondary to edema or necrosis, and mesenteric fat stranding. Coronal enhanced CT demonstrates marked wall thickening of the cecum (arrow).

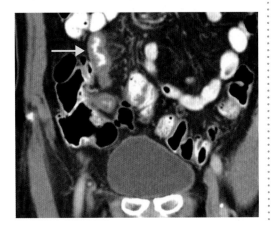

Chemotherapy-related enteritis

Patients undergoing chemotherapy may be susceptible to enteritis, independent of functional immune status. Coronal enhanced CT demonstrates wall thickening and mild associated mesenteric stranding of the distal ileum (arrow) in this patient receiving treatment for colon cancer with irinotecan, 5-FU, and leucovorin.

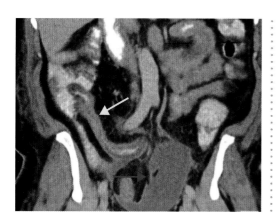

Cocaine-induced vasculitis

Cocaine-induced vasculitis may lead to bowel ischemia and rupture. Imaging findings may mimic Crohn's disease in a young patient presenting with abdominal pain. Coronal enhanced CT demonstrates wall thickening of multiple small bowel loops, including the distal ileum (yellow arrow). A large fluid collection in the lower pelvis (red arrow) resulted from small bowel rupture secondary to this ischemic process.

Further reading

Furukawa A, Saotome T, Yamasaki M, *et al*. Cross-Sectional Imaging in Crohn Disease. *Radiographics* 2004; 24:689–702.

He JD, Liu YL, Wang ZF, *et al*. Colonoscopy in the Diagnosis of Intestinal Graft versus Host Disease and Cytomegalovirus Enteritis following Allogeneic Haematopoietic Stem Cell Transplantation. *Chin Med J* 2008; 121:1285–1289.

Horton KM, Corl FM, Fishman EK. CT Evaluation of the Colon: Inflammatory Disease. *Radiographics* 2000; 20:399–418.

Purysko AS, Remer HM, LeãoFilho HM, *et al*. Beyond Appendicitis: Common and Uncommon Gastrointestinal Causes of Right Lower Quadrant Abdominal Pain at Multidetector CT. *Radiographics* 2011; 31(4);927–947.

Tolan DJM, Greenhalgh R, Zealley IA, *et al*. MR Enterographic Manifestations of Small Bowel Crohn Disease. *Radiographics* 2010; 30:567–584.

Wittenberg J, Harisinghami MG, Jhaveri K, *et al*. Algorithmic Approach to CT Diagnosis of the Abnormal Bowel Wall. *Radiographics* 2002; 22:1093–1109.

Case 12   68-year-old man with left lower quadrant pain and hypotension

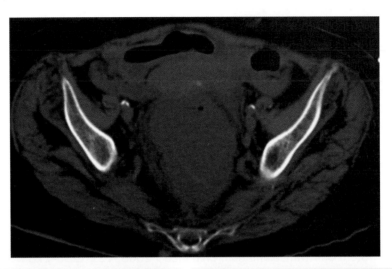

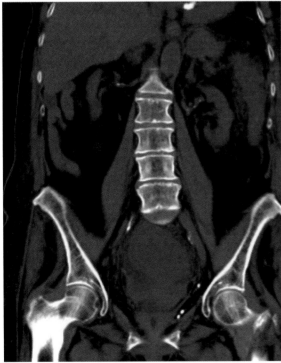

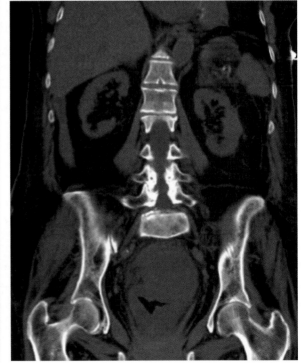

Diagnosis:
Pseudomem-
branous
colitis with
hemorrhage
into bowel
lumen

Axial (left image) and coronal (middle and right images) noncontrast CT images show a markedly thickened sigmoid colon (arrows), with distension of the lumen with high-attenuation fluid, representing intraluminal hemorrhage.

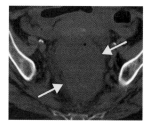 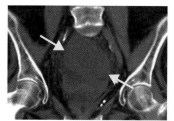 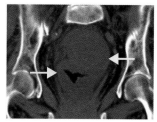

Discussion

Overview and imaging of colitis

- Inflammation of the colon is a common cause of abdominal pain.
- Several unrelated disease processes of infectious, ischemic, or inflammatory etiology can lead to a similar CT appearance of colonic wall thickening. Secondary imaging findings and clinical reasoning are often needed to narrow the differential diagnosis.
- The hallmark CT imaging feature of colitis is bowel wall thickening, and most often, a final diagnosis requires a colonoscopic biopsy. However, there are several other findings that can help narrow the differential diagnosis.
  - For instance, in addition to evaluating the degree of colonic wall thickening, what is the pattern of involvement of the colon and the small bowel? Is there ascites? Is there an associated fluid collection? Is there atherosclerotic disease or thrombosis affecting the vasculature?
- Incidental colonic wall thickening mimicking colitis can be found in greater than 10% of abdominopelvic CT scans.
  - Some authors recommend that any patient with colonic thickening seen on CT receive a follow-up colonoscopy to evaluate for diseases that would require ongoing management, such as colon carcinoma or inflammatory bowel disease.

Clinical
synopsis

This patient, a 68-year-old male with hemorrhagic pseudomembranous colitis and hypotension, was admitted directly to the ICU for stabilization of blood pressure. He required emergent colectomy, and ultimately was discharged to a nursing home after a protracted hospital stay.

Self-assessment

- *Name three radiographic features that favor pseudomembranous colitis over other forms of colitis.*

- Ascites
- Pancolitis (as opposed to partial involvement of the colon)
- Colonic wall thickening >1 cm

- *Name two antibiotics that do not pre-dispose to pseudomembranous colitis.*

- Vancomycin and linezolid (both can be used to treat pseudomembranous colitis).

Etiology of colitis

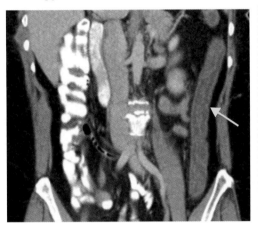

Infectious colitis

Several organisms cause colitis. Yersinia, salmonella, and tuberculosis tend to affect the right colon. Tuberculosis attacks the ileocecal valve with a desmoplastic reaction that may mimic Crohn's disease. Imaging features are often nonspecific. In general, bacterial colitis features pericolonic stranding and ascites; however, stool studies or biopsy are necessary for a definitive diagnosis. Coronal CT demonstrates nonspecific thickening of the left colon (arrow) in this case of infectious colitis.

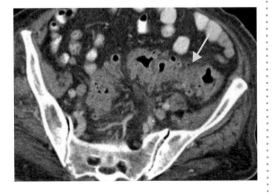

Pseudomembranous colitis

Most commonly associated with recent antibiotic use causing alteration of colonic bacterial flora, *C. difficile* colitis can range from mild diarrhea to life-threatening disease. Typically the rectosig-moid colon is involved, as in this axial enhanced CT (arrow), and stool cultures are positive for *C. difficile* toxin. The "accordion" sign indicates severe colonic edema. Colonic thickening can appear as "thumbprinting" in the transverse colon.

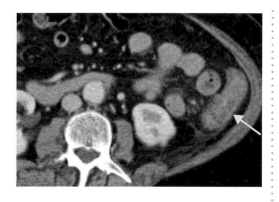

Ischemic colitis

Seen most commonly in elderly patients with vascular disease, ischemic colitis may be due to acute arterial embolism, chronic arterial stenosis, venous occlusive disease, or low-flow states such as congestive heart failure (CHF). Imaging findings are nonspecific and most commonly include wall thickening, as seen on this axial enhanced CT (arrow). Careful evaluation of the vasculature may be helpful. Fulminant cases may cause pneumatosis and bowel necrosis.

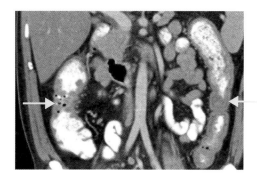

Ulcerative colitis

Ulcerative colitis begins in the rectum and spreads proximally in a continuous manner. Ulcerative colitis does not extend beyond the cecum; however, spread of inflammatory debris into the terminal ileum can cause a "backwash" ileitis that mimics Crohn's disease. There is a greatly increased risk of colon cancer and primary sclerosing cholangitis. Coronal enhanced CT demonstrates mural thickening of the entire visualized colon (arrows).

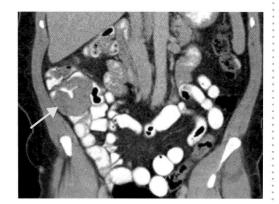

Typhlitis

Neutropenic enterocolitis is a right-sided colitis seen in immunocompromised patients. Broad-spectrum antibacterial and antifungal treatment is indicated as infection can progress to abscess formation, pneumatosis, and sepsis. Imaging findings are similar to other forms of infectious colitis, although findings are generally confined to the right colon. Coronal enhanced CT demonstrates focal mural thickening of the right colon (arrow).

Differential diagnosis of colitis

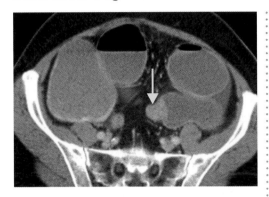

Colon cancer

Although the typical imaging appearance of colon cancer is a concentric, shouldering mass, colon cancer may mimic colitis with diffuse colonic wall thickening. Therefore, it is generally recommended that all patients with bowel wall thickening seen on CT receive a follow-up colonoscopy. Axial enhanced CT in a patient with colon cancer demonstrates focal thickening of the sigmoid (arrow) causing large bowel obstruction.

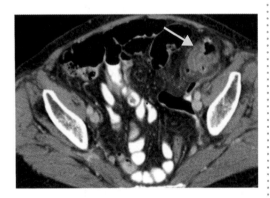

Diverticulitis

Diverticulitis, or acute inflammation of a colonic diverticulum, also causes colonic wall thickening, as demonstrated on this axial enhanced CT (arrow). A culprit diverticulum is often identified as the epicenter of the inflammation. Diverticulitis is overwhelmingly left-sided. Uncomplicated diverticulitis is treated with antibiotics. Percutaneous abscess drainage or surgery may be required in complicated cases.

Further reading

Eskaros, S. *et al.*, 2009. Correlation of incidental colorectal wall thickening at CT compared to colonoscopy. *Emergency radiology*, 16(6), pp.473–476.

Macari, M., Balthazar, E.J. & Megibow, A.J., 1999. The accordion sign at CT: a nonspecific finding in patients with colonic edema. *Radiology*, 211(3), pp.743–746.

Moraitis, D. *et al.*, 2006. Colonic wall thickening on computed tomography scan and clinical correlation. Does it suggest the presence of an underlying neoplasia? *The American surgeon*, 72(3), pp.269–271.

Taourel, P. *et al.*, 2008. Imaging of ischemic colitis. *Radiologic clinics of North America*, 46(5), pp.909–924, vi.

Thoeni, R.F. & Cello, J.P., 2006. CT imaging of colitis. *Radiology*, 240(3), pp.623–638.

Wiesner, W. *et al.*, 2003. CT of acute bowel ischemia. *Radiology*, 226, p.635.

Wolff, J.H. *et al.*, 2008. Clinical significance of colonoscopic findings associated with colonic thickening on computed tomography: is colonoscopy warranted when thickening is detected? *Journal of clinical gastroenterology*, 42(5), pp.472–475.

Case 13 68-year-old man with left lower quadrant pain

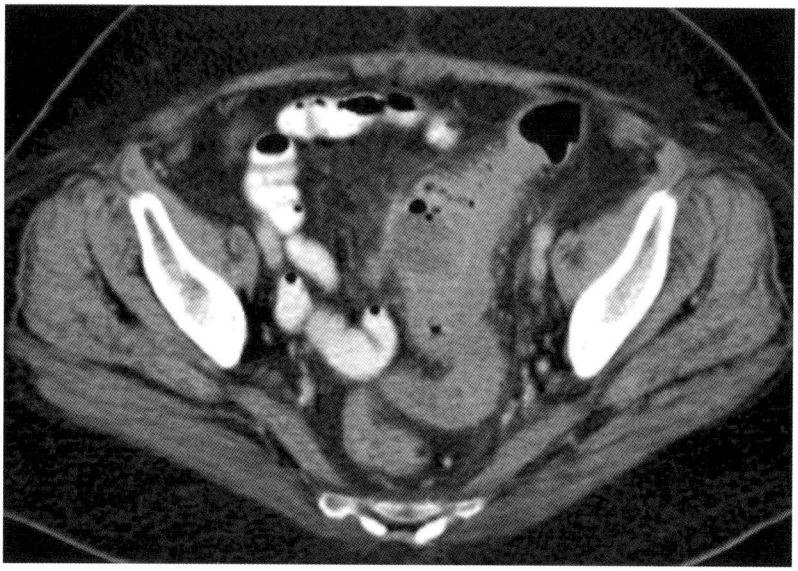

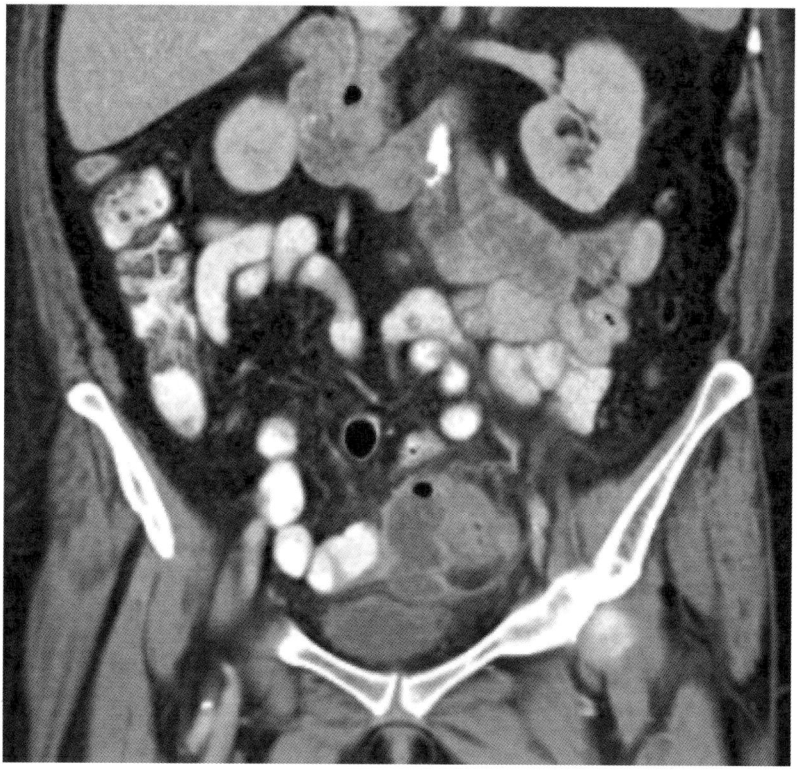

Diagnosis:
Diverticulitis
with abscess

Axial (left image) and coronal (right image) contrast-enhanced CT shows thickening of the sigmoid colon, with pericolonic fat stranding. A focal fluid collection (arrows) containing foci of gas adjacent to the colon is consistent with an abscess.

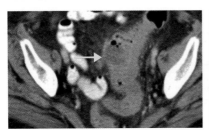 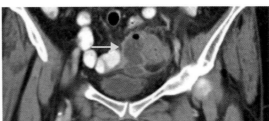

Discussion

Diverticulitis is the acute inflammation and infection of a colonic diverticulum.

- Diverticulosis, the asymptomatic disease of multiple colonic diverticula, is a Western disease thought to be due to low-fiber diet, with increasing prevalence with age.
- Nearly all diverticula are located in the left colon, but occasionally the rare right-sided diverticula can become inflamed and mimic other more common causes of right lower quadrant pain.

CT is the primary modality for imaging acute diverticulitis and plays a central role in triage.

- In addition to confirming the presence and severity of diverticulitis, CT can evaluate for potential complications.

Diverticulitis can be characterized as uncomplicated or complicated.

- Uncomplicated diverticulitis implies that the bowel lumen is intact, and features two primary CT findings:
  - Colonic wall thickening (greater than 3 mm is abnormal)
  - Pericolonic fat stranding. Often, a diverticulum will be identified as the epicenter of the inflammation.
- Diverticulitis can become complicated when one or more associated findings are present in addition to the colonic wall thickening and pericolonic fat stranding:
  - Abscess
  - Extraluminal air, which would signify perforation or microperforation
  - Bowel obstruction
  - Fistula, with colovesicular being the most common
  - Mesenteric vein thrombosis

The difficulty in distinguishing acute diverticulitis from malignancy is a longstanding clinical problem.

- After an initial episode of acute diverticulitis, follow up with either colonoscopy or CT colonography is recommended to evaluate the extent of diverticular disease, and to exclude colon cancer.

Clinical synopsis

This patient, a 68-year-old male with diverticulitis and a small intramural abscess, was admitted and treated initially with intravenous ceftriaxone. He was discharged on a 7-day course of oral antibiotics and did well after this episode.

Self-assessment

- *What is the treatment for uncompli-cated diverticulitis? How would the treatment change for a diverticular abscess?*

- Treatment of uncomplicated diverticulitis is conservative with intravenous antibiotics.
- The presence of an abscess may necessitate percutaneous drainage.

- *Name three indications for surgical treatment (colectomy) for diverticulitis.*

- Two prior episodes of diverticulitis treated conservatively.
- A first episode of colitis in an immunocompromised patient.
- Fistula.

- *If a case of presumed diverticulitis featured prominent lymph nodes adjacent to the thickened colonic segment, what is the most likely alternative diagnosis?*

- Colon cancer.

Spectrum of diverticulitis

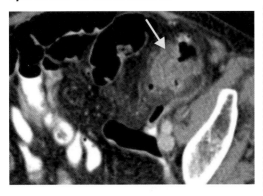

Early diverticulitis

Colonic wall thickening (typically greater than 3 mm) with mild pericolonic fat stranding suggests early diverticulitis. A culprit diverticulum is often apparent. Often, colonic muscular hypertrophy due to chronic diverticular disease may simulate very early diverticulitis before pericolonic fat stranding has developed. Axial enhanced CT shows mild focal colonic wall thickening and pericolonic fat stranding (arrow).

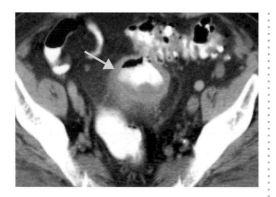

Giant diverticulitis

"Giant diverticula" may arise by a ball-valve mechanism or represent slowly expanding chronic abscesses. This axial enhanced CT demonstrates a diverticulum in the mid-pelvis (arrow) that is larger in diameter than the sigmoid colon from which it arises, with wall thickening and fat stranding.

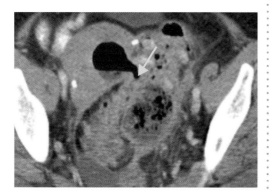

Diverticulitis with colouterine fistula

Severe cases of diverticulitis can cause complications, including fistulization between bowel and other hollow organs. The most common colonic fistula is a colovesical fistula between the colon and the urinary bladder, which is usually evidenced by air within the bladder. This axial enhanced CT demonstrates a fistula (arrow) between the colon and the uterus.

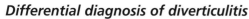

Differential diagnosis of diverticulitis

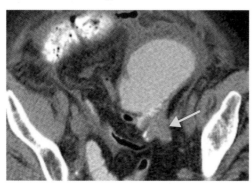

Colon cancer

Colon cancer is the most important differential consideration when the primary concern is diverticulitis. Features that suggest colon cancer are a concentric "shouldering" mass and pericolonic lymphadenopathy. However, there is a great deal of overlap of the imaging findings. Axial enhanced CT in this patient with colon cancer demonstrates sigmoid thickening with pericolonic stranding (arrow) and proximal dilation of the sigmoid colon.

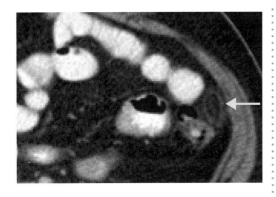

Epiploic appendagitis

Caused by acute torsion of a normal fatty appendage arising from the colon, epiploic appendagitis is a relatively common clinical mimic of diverticulitis. Epiploic appendagitis almost always occurs on the left, most commonly arising from the sigmoid. On CT imaging, epiploic appendagitis appears as an oval fat-attenuation lesion abutting the colonic wall with adjacent fat stranding, as seen in this enhanced axial CT (arrow). Treatment is with anti-inflammatory medication.

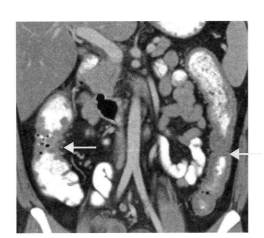

Colitis

Colitis is inflammation of the colon, which may be vascular, ischemic, inflammatory, or infectious. Colonic wall thickening is the hallmark imaging finding of colitis. Coronal enhanced CT demonstrates typical findings of ulcerative colitis with bowel wall thickening involving the entire colon (arrows).

Further reading

Ambrosetti, P., 2008. Acute diverticulitis of the left colon: value of the initial CT and timing of elective colectomy. *Journal of gastrointestinal surgery: official journal of the Society for Surgery of the Alimentary Tract*, 12(8), pp.1318–1320.

Buckley, O. *et al.*, 2004. Computed tomography in the imaging of colonic diverticulitis. *Clinical radiology*, 59(11), pp.977–983.

DeStigter, K.K. & Keating, D.P., 2009. Imaging update: acute colonic diverticulitis. *Clinics in colon and rectal surgery*, 22(3), p.147.

Hjern, F. *et al.*, 2007. CT colonography versus colonoscopy in the follow-up of patients after diverticulitis – a prospective, comparative study. *Clinical radiology*, 62(7), pp.645–650.

Praveen, B.V. *et al.*, 2007. Giant colonic diverticulum: an unusual abdominal lump. *Journal of surgical education,* 64, pp.97–100.

Thoeni, R.F. & Cello, J.P., 2006. CT imaging of colitis. *Radiology*, 240(3), pp.623–638.

Touzios, J.G. & Dozois, E.J., 2009. Diverticulosis and acute diverticulitis. *Gastroenterology clinics of North America*, 38(3), pp.513–525.

Case 14   17-year-old boy with right lower quadrant and suprapubic pain

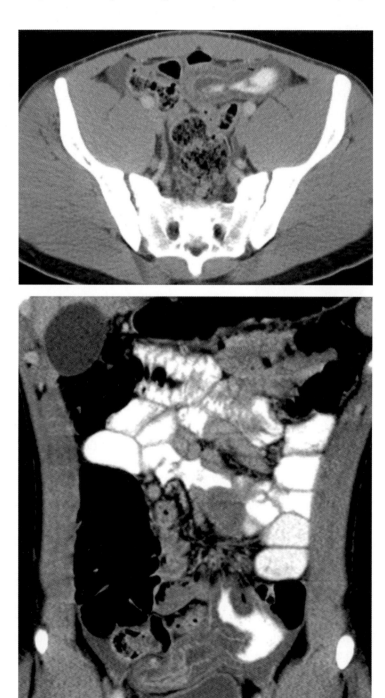

Diagnosis: **Meckel's diverticulitis**	Axial (left image) and coronal (right image) contrast-enhanced CT images show a large, blind-ending tubular structure to the left of midline with thickened walls (arrows). There is some enteric contrast material within this structure, as seen on the axial image.

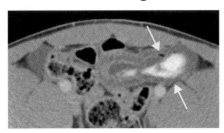 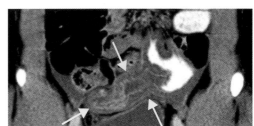

Discussion

Overview of Meckel's diverticulitis

- Meckel's diverticulitis is acute inflammation of a Meckel's diverticulum.
- Meckel's diverticulum is seen in 2% of the population and is the most common congenital gastrointestinal anomaly.
- A Meckel's diverticulum is the result of incomplete regression of the omphalomesenteric (vitelline) duct, which connects the intestine to the yolk sac via the umbilicus in early embryological life. There is a spectrum of anomalies due to incomplete atrophy of the omphalomesenteric duct, with the most rare and dramatic being an umbilicoileal fistula due to complete patency of the duct, which causes fecal drainage from the umbilicus in the neonatal period.
- Meckel's diverticulum is found on the antimesenteric aspect of the distal ileum, usually within 100 cm of the ileocecal valve.
- Although there are many exceptions in real life, the "rule of twos" is often taught: Meckel's are present in 2% of the population, are 2 feet from the ileocecal valve, usually 2 inches long, and usually become symptomatic before age 2.

Complications of Meckel's diverticulum

- While most Meckel's diverticula are asymptomatic, between 4% and 40% of patients will experience a complication during their lifetime, including gastrointestinal hemorrhage, bowel obstruction, or diverticulitis (as in this case).
- There can be ectopic gastric or pancreatic mucosa within the Meckel's diverticulum, which predisposes to complications. Most cases of symptomatic Meckel's diverticulitis occur in the pediatric population, where gastrointestinal hemorrhage is by far the most common complication.
- A Meckel's diverticulum may invaginate or invert into the small intestinal lumen, thereby serving as a lead point for ileocolic intussusception and small bowel obstruction (inverted Meckel's diverticulum).

Clinical synopsis   This patient, a 17-year-old male with Meckel's diverticulitis, underwent laparotomy. An 8 cm inflamed Meckel's diverticulum was found approximately 200 cm from the ileocecal valve. The patient recovered uneventfully after surgery.

Self-assessment

- *What is the eponym for a Meckel's diverticulum trapped within an inguinal hernia?*

- Meckel's diverticulum within an inguinal hernia is called a Littre hernia.

- *What are the histologic layers of a Meckel's diverticulum? How commonly is ectopic mucosa seen?*

- A Meckel's diverticulum is a true diverticulum, containing all the layers of the intestinal wall. Additionally, heterotopic mucosa is seen in 50% of resected Meckel's, more commonly gastric than pancreatic.

- *Describe the nuclear medicine test used to test for Meckel's diverticulum.*

- Tc-99m pertechnetate scintigraphy is used to evaluate gastrointestinal bleeding in a child for whom there is a high suspicion for a bleeding Meckel's diverticulum. Ectopic gastric mucosa and resultant peptic ulceration cause the bleeding. There is pertechnetate uptake only within gastric mucosa.

Differential diagnosis of Meckel's diverticulitis

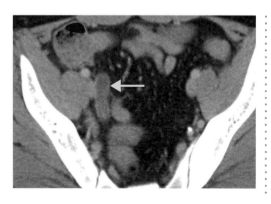

Appendicitis

Appendicitis is acute inflammation and infection of the appendix. Since appendicitis is so common, even experienced radiologists have mistaken cases of Meckel's diverticulitis for appendicitis. Complicating matters further, the appendix can become secondarily inflamed in Meckel's diverticulitis. Axial CT demonstrates a dilated, tubular, fluid-filled structure (arrows) in the right lower quadrant representing early appendicitis.

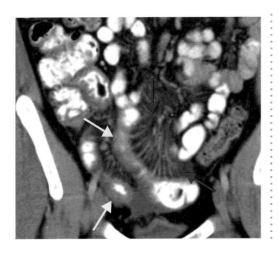

Crohn's disease

Crohn's disease is an idiopathic gastrointestinal inflammatory condition with a propensity for affecting the terminal ileum. In patients with Crohn's disease, the inflammation may spread to adjacent Meckel's diverticula and can result in diverticulitis and possibly perforation or fistula formation. Coronal enhanced CT demonstrates mural thickening of the distal ileum (yellow arrows), with associated mesenteric vascular engorgement (representing the "comb" sign; red arrows).

Further reading

Bennett, G. L., Birnbaum, B. A., & Balthazar, E. J. (2004). CT of Meckel's diverticulitis in 11 patients. *AJR: American Journal of Roentgenology*, 182(3), 625.

Elsayes, K. M., Menias, C. O., Harvin, H. J., & Francis, I. R. (2007). Imaging manifestations of Meckel's diverticulum. *AJR: American Journal of Roentgenology*, 189(1), 81–88.

Levy, A. D. & Hobbs, C. M. (2004). From the archives of the AFIP. Meckel diverticulum: radiologic features with pathologic correlation. *Radiographics: A Review Publication of the Radiological Society of North America, Inc.*, 24(2), 565–587.

Case 15   44-year-old male presenting with left lower quadrant pain

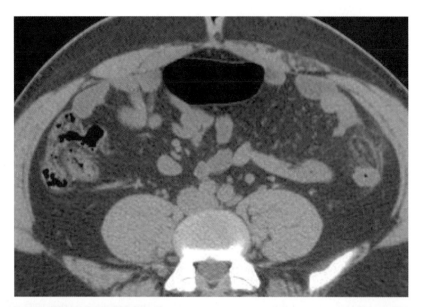

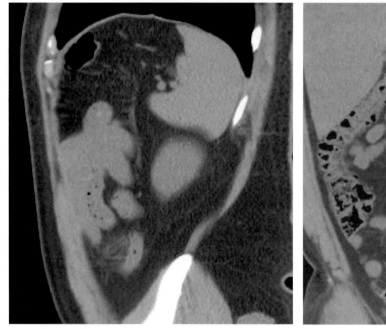

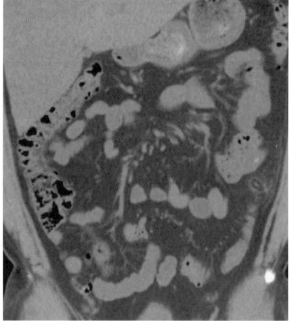

Diagnosis: Axial (left image), sagittal (middle image), and coronal (right image) enhanced
Epiploic CT images of the abdomen and pelvis demonstrate a fat-density oval structure
appendagitis (yellow arrows) arising from the left colon. A central hyperdense focus (red
arrows) represents a thrombosed vein. There is a small amount of peripheral
mesenteric stranding.

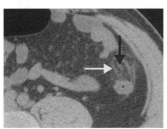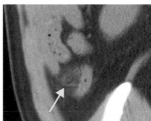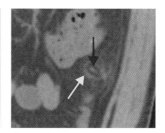

Discussion

Overview of epiploic appendagitis

- Epiploic appendages are small, fat-containing peritoneal outpouchings that
  arise from the serosal surface of the colon. Each epiploic appendage is
  connected to the colon by a vascular stalk, containing paired arterioles and a
  single vein.
- Acute epiploic appendagitis is inflammation of an epiploic appendage, most
  commonly due to torsion that leads to central venous thrombosis and
  consequent ischemia.
- Acute epiploic appendagitis is typically a self-limited condition and treatment
  is anti-inflammatory medications.
- Acute epiploic appendagitis is more commonly adjacent to the left colon than
  to the cecum and right colon. There, the appendages are more numerous and
  longer, and thus, more prone to torsion. Less frequently, epiploic appendagitis
  may occur adjacent to the right colon and cecum.

Imaging of epiploic appendagitis

- The CT appearance of acute epiploic appendagitis is characteristic and usually
  diagnostic. A typical appearance is a fat-density pericolic oval structure with
  surrounding inflammatory fat stranding. A central hyperattenuating focus
  representing the thrombosed vein is often present (the "central dot" sign),
  although epiploic appendagitis may still be diagnosed in the absence of this
  feature. The adjacent colon is usually normal, but mild reactive wall thickening
  may be seen.

Imaging and clinical differential diagnosis of epiploic appendagitis

- Several conditions may mimic acute epiploic appendagitis, both clinically and on imaging, including omental infarction, mesenteric panniculitis, diverticulitis, and fat-containing tumor. When epiploic appendagitis involves the cecum, the condition may be mistaken for acute appendicitis. The distinction between epiploic appendagitis and other mimickers is crucial because epiploic appendagitis is a self-limited condition, whereas other conditions may require more definitive therapy. An adjacent inflammatory process may cause secondary inflammation of one or more epiploic appendages.

Clinical synopsis The patient was diagnosed with acute epiploic appendagitis and was discharged home with pain medication only. She had improvement of her symptoms within a few days.

Self-assessment

- *What is acute epiploic appendagitis and how is it treated?*

  - Epiploic appendagitis is ischemia or inflammation of an epiploic appendage. It is typically self-limited and is treated with pain management only.

- *What is secondary epiploic appendagitis?*

  - Secondary epiploic appendagitis is inflammation of an epiploic appendage from an adjacent inflammatory process, such as colitis, diverticulitis, or appendicitis. It is important to recognize the culprit primary inflammatory process in such cases to direct appropriate treatment.

- *What are the mechanisms leading to primary and secondary epiploic appendagitis?*

  - Primary epiploic appendagitis is caused by spontaneous torsion of the pedicle of the appendage leading to ischemia. Secondary epiploic appendagitis is a result of adjacent inflammation.

Spectrum of epiploic appendagitis

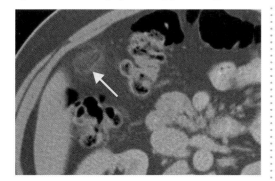

Epiploic appendagitis of the right colon

Inflammation of the epiploic appendages of the right colon is relatively uncommon as the append-ages in this location are less numerous and shorter than those associated with the left colon. Axial unenhanced CT image demonstrates an oval fat density structure adjacent to the ascending colon (arrow), with a small amount of peripheral stranding. A central hyperdense thrombosed vessel is present.

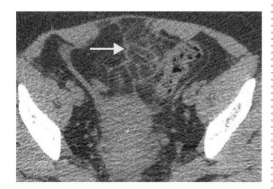

Severe epiploic appendagitis

Axial unenhanced CT image of the pelvis demon-strates severe fat stranding and a moderate amount of free fluid surrounding an epiploic appendage adjacent to the sigmoid colon (arrow). Also note the central hyperdensity consistent with the thrombosed vein. The main differential diag-nosis in this case was omental infarction; how-ever, the typical location of the epiploic appendage led to the diagnosis of acute epiploic appendagitis.

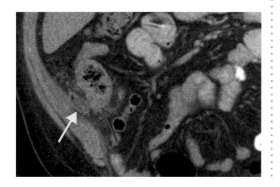

Secondary epiploic appendagitis

Coronal enhanced CT demonstrates an inflamed epiploic appendage (yellow arrow) adjacent to a thickened cecum (red arrow), raising suspicion for colitis with secondary epiploic appendagitis. The patient was treated with antibiotics and pain management.

Differential diagnosis of epiploic appendagitis

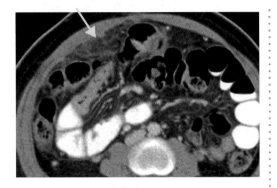

Omental infarction

Omental infarction may be caused by vascular torsion or venous thrombosis. Omental infarction can be primary (precipitated by coughing, straining, or overheating) or secondary, where a vascular insult is caused by surgery, hernia, or adhesion. Axial enhanced CT demonstrates stranding of the anterior omental fat (arrow), with adjacent engorged vessels. The patient had recently undergone a Whipple procedure.

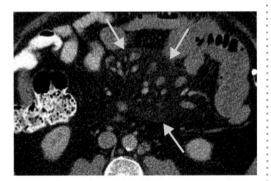

Mesenteric panniculitis

Mesenteric panniculitis is a subtype of sclerosing mesenteritis in which chronic inflammation of the mesenteric fat predominates. It is a self-limited, usually idiopathic condition characterized by variable degrees of mesenteric fat inflammation, necrosis, and fibrosis. Axial enhanced CT demonstrates a typical appearance with a circumscribed region of hazy mesenteric stranding at the root of the small-bowel mesentery with a peripheral pseudocapsule (arrows).

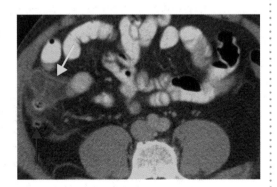

Cecal diverticulitis

As with epiploic appendagitis, diverticulitis is also less common on the right. Axial enhanced CT demonstrates a geographic region of cecal wall thickening and adjacent fat stranding (yellow arrow) centered upon a diverticulum. The visualized appendix (red arrow) appears normal. The characteristic imaging findings of appendagitis (e.g., well-defined, fat-containing structure with a central thrombosed vein) are not present.

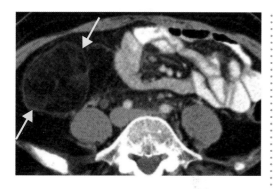

Liposarcoma

Liposarcoma is the second most common soft-tissue sarcoma. Well-differentiated liposarcoma usually appears as a circumscribed, largely lipomatous mass, usually containing enhancing septa or soft tissue components. The most common sites are the retroperitoneum and the thigh. Axial enhanced CT demonstrates a well-circumscribed, fat-attenuating mass (arrows) containing wispy internal septations. The mass abuts the right psoas muscle.

Further reading

Kamaya A, Federle MP, Desser TS. Imaging Manifestations of Abdominal Fat Necrosis and Its Mimics. *Radiographics* 2011; 31: 2021–2034.

Purysko AS, Remer HM, LeãoFilho HM, *et al*. Beyond Appendicitis: Common and Uncommon Gastrointestinal Causes of Right Lower Quadrant Abdominal Pain at Multidetector CT. *Radiographics* 2011; 31(4): 927–947.

Singh AK, Gervais DA, Hahn PF, *et al*. Acute Epiploic Appendagitis and Its Mimics. *Radiographics* 2005; 25: 1521–1534.

Section 1.4 Generalized Abdominal Pain

Case 16   74-year-old woman with a history of metastatic ovarian cancer presenting with abdominal pain, nausea, and vomiting

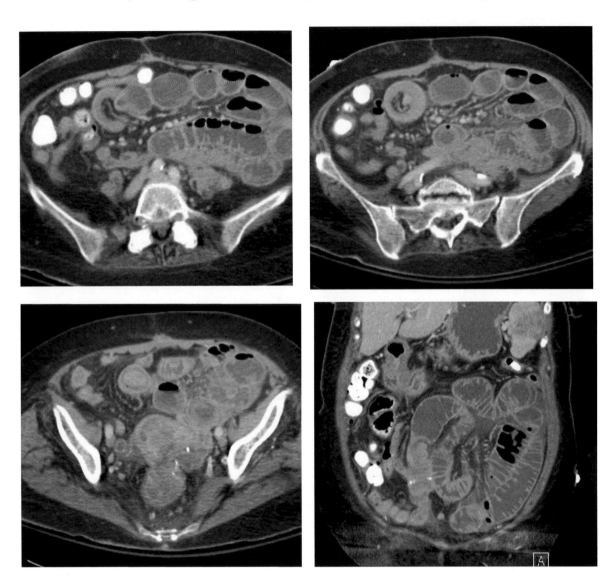

Diagnosis:
Small bowel obstruction (secondary to intussusception from metastatic ovarian cancer)

Axial (first three images at left) and coronal (last image at right) contrast-enhanced CT images show invagination of a bowel loop with its mesenteric fold (intussusceptum, yellow arrows in first two images) into the lumen of a contiguous portion of bowel (intussuscipiens). A soft tissue mass (red arrows in final two images) acts as the lead point. Proximally, obstructed small bowel is dilated and fluid-filled (blue arrows), while distally, the small bowel is decompressed (green arrow).

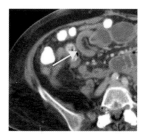 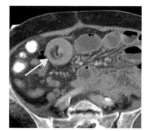 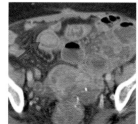 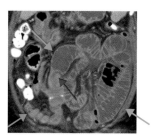

Discussion

Role of imaging in suspected small bowel obstruction

- Small bowel obstruction (SBO) accounts for 12–16% of surgical admissions for acute abdominal pain.
- Nausea and vomiting are typical clinical symptoms. Clinical exam and labs are often insufficient for differentiating simple obstruction from strangulated bowel.

CT is the primary modality for imaging suspected acute SBO and answers the following questions:

- Is there a mechanical obstruction? Mechanical obstruction is characterized by proximally dilated small bowel loops (>2.5 cm between the outer walls) with distal loops that are normal in caliber or decompressed.
- How severe is the obstruction, if present?
  - Mild (low grade): 25–50% discrepancy between proximal and distal small bowel caliber.
  - Moderate (intermediate grade): >50% discrepancy, with residual gas or contrast in distal small bowel.
  - Severe (high grade): >50% discrepancy, with completely collapsed distal small bowel and colon that do not contain residual gas, stool, or contrast.
- Where is the obstruction located? Multiplanar reformats are helpful for determining the site and level of the obstruction. The site of obstruction, or "transition point," is where the caliber change occurs. Two transition points are present in "closed loop" obstruction, which is a surgical emergency.

- What is the cause of the obstruction? The transition point should be carefully inspected to help determine the etiology of the obstruction. The most common cause of SBO is adhesions, which are generally invisible or detectable only by inference on CT. Bowel loops obstructed by adhesions may be abnormally angulated or appear tethered to the abdominal wall or other structures.
  - Other common causes include hernias, Crohn's disease, and neoplasms.
  - Less common causes include intussusception, gallstones, hematomas, tuberculosis, radiation enteritis or fibrosis, endometriosis, and foreign bodies.
- Is strangulation present? Signs of bowel ischemia include decreased bowel wall enhancement, wall thickening, mesenteric fluid/congestion, and ascites.
- Does the patient require emergency surgery? Is there a closed loop obstruction or evidence of strangulation/ischemia?

Clinical synopsis   The patient was deemed a poor surgical candidate due to comorbidities and was treated with a gastrostomy tube for palliative decompression.

Self-assessment

- *What is the "small bowel feces" sign?*

  - The small bowel feces sign is heterogeneous particulate-type material in dilated small bowel that appears similar to mixed solid and gas-containing stool. This sign by itself is neither sensitive nor specific for SBO, and may be simulated by undigested vegetable matter or reflux across an incompetent ileocecal valve; however, in the presence of a SBO, the small bowel feces sign produced by localized stagnation can often help locate the transition zone.

- *Name four signs of a closed loop obstruction.*

  - "U" or "C"-shaped configuration
  - Radial distribution of mesenteric vessels
  - "Beak" sign at the ends of the involved loop
  - Triangular shape
  - "Whirl" sign of the mesenteric vessels
  - Collapsed adjacent loops on either side of the dilated bowel segment
  - Two transition points

Spectrum of small bowel obstruction

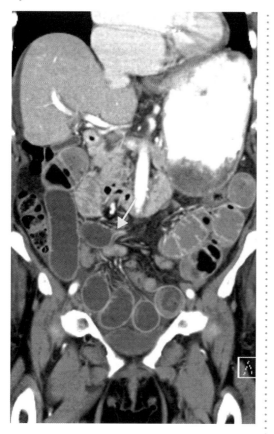

Adhesions

Adhesions are the most common cause of small bowel obstruction, accounting for >70% of cases. Most occur in patients who have had prior abdominal surgery. Rarely, adhesions are the result of prior inflammatory or infectious peritonitis, or are congenital. Adhesive bands are not typically seen – thus, adhesions are generally a diagnosis of exclusion. CT findings include abrupt change in small bowel caliber without mass, inflammation, or bowel wall thickening. Coronal CT with intravenous and oral contrast shows multiple loops of dilated small bowel, with a caliber change (arrow) to distally decompressed small bowel (not pictured). The stomach is also dilated. Multiplanar reformatted images are often important in identifying the transition point.

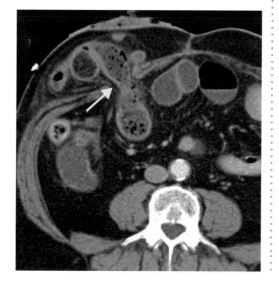

External hernia

Hernias may be the second most common cause of SBO (~10%). Increasingly common elective hernia repair has decreased the occurrence of SBO from abdominal wall hernias. External hernias result from prolapse of intestinal loops through defects in the abdominal or pelvic walls and are often palpable on clinical exam. Incarcerated bowel is irreducible, while strangulated bowel shows signs of ischemia. Axial CT with intravenous and oral contrast shows narrowing of a loop of small bowel (arrow) as it enters a parastomal hernia sac. The small bowel feces sign is present.

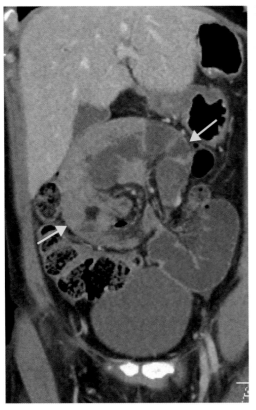

Internal hernia

Internal hernias result from transit of small bowel loops through normal or abnormal peritoneal or mesenteric apertures within the confines of the abdominal cavity. Internal hernias are rare, accounting for less than 6% of all SBO; however, incidence is increasing due to rising numbers of Roux-en-Y gastric bypass and liver transplantation procedures. In patients who have undergone these procedures, internal hernias have been implicated in >50% of SBO. There are several types of internal hernia including paraduodenal, pericecal, foramen of Winslow, transmesenteric/transmeso-colic, intersigmoid, and retro-anastomotic. This patient had an incarcerated, right-sided paraduodenal hernia. Coronal IV contrast-enhanced CT demonstrates typical imaging features such as small bowel obstruction, apparent encapsulation of distended, abnormally located small bowel loops (arrows), abnormal appearance of mesenteric vessels (engorgement, crowding, twisting, stretching), and displacement of other bowel segments.

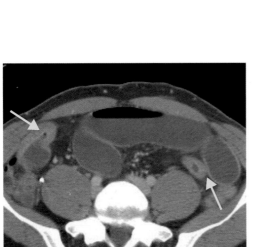

Crohn's disease

SBO is common in various stages of Crohn's disease. Narrowing may follow transmural inflammation. Long-standing disease can result in cicatricial stenosis. Complications of prior surgery, including adhesions, strictures, and incisional hernias, can also cause SBO. Axial IV contrast-enhanced CT shows dilated small bowel loops with areas of narrowing, wall-thickening, and mucosal hyperemia (arrows) representing skip lesions in a patient with an acute flare of Crohn's disease.

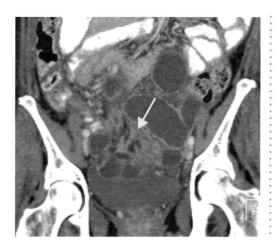

Neoplasia

Neoplasms produce approximately 10–15% of all SBO. Primary small bowel tumors are rare, accounting for <2% of gastrointestinal malignancies. The majority of cases are caused by metastatic disease, typically peritoneal carcinomatosis, as in this case. Coronal IV and oral contrast-enhanced CT shows tethering of loops of small bowel in the pelvis (arrow) due to ovarian cancer-related carcinomatosis. The more proximal small bowel is dilated.

Differential diagnosis of small bowel obstruction

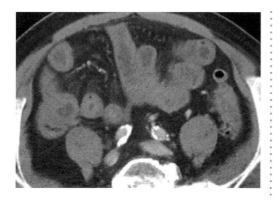

Enteritis

As demonstrated here by axial IV contrast-enhanced CT, infectious or inflammatory enteritis may be characterized by mildly dilated, fluid-filled loops of small bowel with no transition point. There may be bowel wall thickening, as in this case.

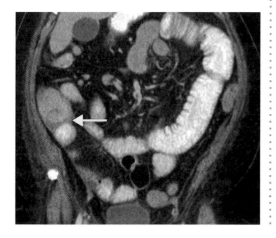

Ileus

Differentiating adynamic ileus and mechanical SBO in the post-operative period can be difficult on clinical grounds. Plain radiographs may be helpful but are often nonspecific. CT may help differentiate between the two entities. The findings in this case are typical for postoperative adynamic ileus. Coronal IV and oral contrast-enhanced CT shows diffuse dilatation of the small bowel without a transition point. The colon (arrow) is also mildly distended and contains oral contrast.

Further reading

Balthazar, E. *et al*. Closed-Loop and Strangulating Intestinal Obstruction: CT signs. *Radiology*. 185:769–775 (1992).

Boudiaf, M. *et al*. CT Evaluation of Small Bowel Obstruction. *Radiographics*. 21:613–624 (2001).

Ha, H. *et al*. Differentiation of Simple and Strangulated Small-Bowel Obstruction: Usefulness of Known CT Criteria. *Radiology*. 204:507–512 (1997).

Kim, Y. *et al*. Adult Intestinal Intussusception: CT Appearances and Identification of a Causative Lead Point. *Radiographics*. 26: 733-734 (2006).

Maglinte, D. *et al*. Radiology of Small Bowel Obstruction: Contemporary Approach and Controversies. *Abdominal Imaging*. 30:160–178 (2005).

Martin, L. *et al*. Review of Internal Hernias: Radiographic and Clinical Findings. *American Journal of Roentgenology*. 186:707–717 (2006).

Nicolaou, S. *et al*. Imaging of Acute Small-Bowel Obstruction. *American Journal of Roentgenology*. 185:1036–1044 (2005).

Taourel, P. *et al*. Value of CT in the Diagnosis and Management of Patients with Suspected Acute Small-Bowel Obstruction. *American Journal of Roentgenology*. 165:1187–1192 (1995).

Case 17   61-year-old woman with a history of Roux-en-Y gastric bypass four years prior presented with progressive abdominal pain, nausea, and small volume emesis

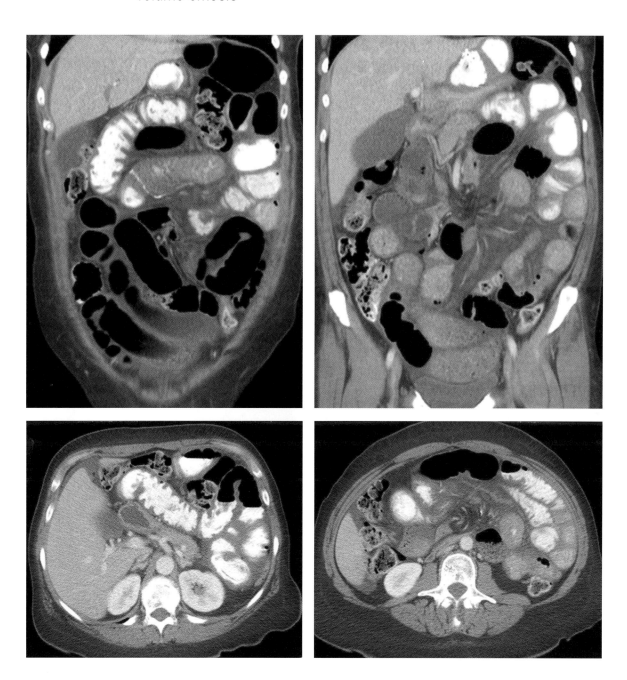

Diagnosis:
Strangulated internal hernia through a Petersen defect in a patient with a history of Roux-en-Y gastric bypass

Coronal (left images) and axial (right images) CT images with oral and IV contrast show multiple dilated loops of small bowel with wall-thickening, gas–fluid levels, and free fluid, worrisome for strangulated small bowel obstruction (SBO). Internal hernia is suggested by the location of the jejunojejunal anastomosis to the right of midline (yellow arrow) and "swirling" of vessels at the root of the mesentery (red arrows). A loop of jejunum with mural thickening (blue arrow) passes posterior to the Roux limb (green arrow). Along with clustered dilated loops in the left upper quadrant, this finding suggests that internally herniated bowel has passed from right to left via a surgically created retro-Roux or "Petersen" defect posterior to the Roux limb and inferior to the transverse colon. There is trace free fluid in the subhepatic space (white arrow).

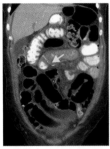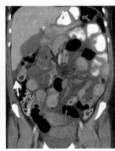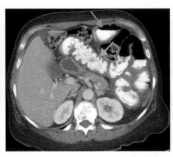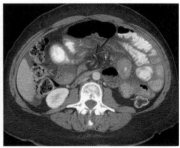

Discussion

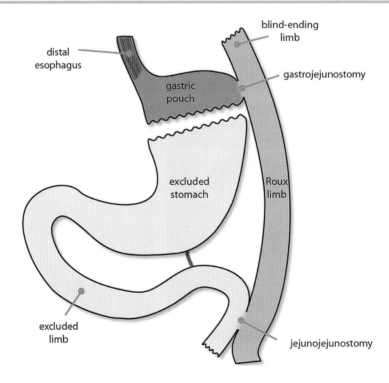

Normal post-Roux-en-Y anatomy (illustration on preceding page): in Roux-en-Y gastric bypass, the stomach is bisected, with a small portion of proximal stomach (gastric pouch) anastomosed to a proximally blind ending jejunal loop (Roux limb). This anastomosis is termed the gastrojejunostomy. So that biliary secretions retain a route of egress into the small bowel, the distal "excluded" stomach and duodenum (excluded or pancreatico-biliary limb) are anastomosed to the Roux limb more distally at the jejunojejunostomy. The jejunojejunostomy is typically located in the left hemiabdomen. Distal to the jejunojejunostomy, the Roux limb is in contiguity with the remainder of the bowel (common limb).

Internal hernias are increasing in incidence as Roux-en-Y gastric bypass (RYGB) and orthotopic liver transplantation (OLT) become more common.

- In both surgeries, the "Roux limb" may be placed either anteriorly (antecolic) or posteriorly (retrocolic) to the transverse colon. In the retrocolic approach, the Roux limb is passed through a surgically created defect in the transverse mesocolon. The retrocolic approach allows for a much shorter Roux limb.
- Rapid weight loss from gastric bypass is thought to increase the size of the surgical defect in the fatty transverse mesocolon, predisposing gastric bypass patients with retrocolic Roux limbs to transmesocolic internal hernia.
- Post-surgical internal hernias may be transmesocolic, through a mesenteric "Petersen" defect posterior to the Roux limb, or through a mesenteric defect created for the jejunojejunal anastomosis.
- When incarcerated or strangulated, internal hernias are a surgical emergency.
- Patients typically present with symptoms of SBO – nausea, vomiting, and abdominal pain that may be postprandial. In patients with RYGB, vomiting is less common, as the volume of secretions in the gastric pouch is low relative to the volume in a normal stomach.

Internal hernias can be difficult to diagnose on imaging.

- Diagnosing the type of internal hernia can be difficult, and is less important than alerting the surgeon that one is present.
- The most sensitive and specific CT finding for internal hernia is the "swirled mesentery" sign, which describes rotation of vessels at the mesenteric root. One study showed that swirling of >90 degrees from anatomic position was highly associated with internal hernia, and that in all patients with swirling of >270 degrees, internal hernia was confirmed intraoperatively.
- Other CT signs of internal hernia include:
  - The "hurricane eye" sign: similar in principle to the "swirled mesentery" sign, but more distal, with loops of bowel swirling around mesenteric fat rather than vessels in the mesenteric root.

- Small bowel (other than duodenum) posterior to the superior mesenteric artery.
- Although this may vary with surgical technique, the jejunojejunal anastomosis is usually placed on the left; right-sided position should raise concern for internal hernia.

Internal hernias after Roux-en-Y gastric bypass. TM: transmesocolic; SB: defect for small bowel anastomosis; RR: retro-Roux or Petersen defect; P: gastric pouch; J: Roux jejunal limb.

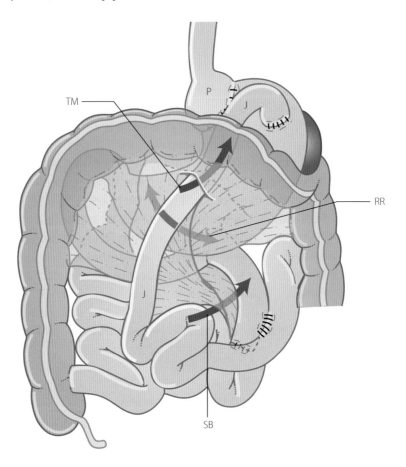

Small bowel obstruction in all patients with a history of RYGB or OLT should raise high suspicion for internal hernia.

- In these populations, over 50% of SBO are due to internal hernia.
- Internal hernia after RYGB nearly always occurs at least 30 days after the initial surgery. If SBO occurs within the first 30 days after surgery, adhesions are a more likely cause.

Internal hernias may occur in the absence of surgery.

- The most common type of non-surgical internal hernia is paraduodenal (53%), which is congenital and more commonly to the left.
- 35% of transmesenteric and transmesocolic internal hernias occur in children. The likely etiology in children is a developmental insult, while surgery, trauma, and inflammation are common predisposing factors in adults.

Clinical synopsis	Given suspicion for ischemia, the patient underwent emergent exploratory laparotomy with reduction of the internal hernia. The bowel was initially felt to be ischemic but viable, so no bowel was resected. The post-operative course was complicated by abdominal compartment syndrome. Upon re-exploration 2 days after the initial hernia reduction, 150 cm of infarcted, necrotic common limb distal to the jejunojejunostomy was resected.

Self-assessment

- *Name three CT signs of small bowel strangulation, a complication of internal hernia.*
  - Bowel mucosal non-enhancement.
  - Free fluid.
  - Pneumatosis intestinalis (gas within the wall of the bowel, particularly on the dependent side, as it may be difficult to differentiate intraluminal from intramural gas on the non-dependent side).
  - "Target" sign – circumferentially thickened loops of small bowel with alternating high and low attenuation from submucosal edema and adjacent mesenteric vascular engorgement.

- *Are internal hernias more common in patients who have had open or laparoscopic RYGB? Why?*
  - Laparoscopic
  - It has been speculated that patients who have undergone open RYGB have more post-operative adhesions, which have a protective effect: by tethering small bowel loops, adhesions may prevent herniation through abnormal apertures.

- *Name three types of internal hernia that may occur in adult patients without a history of surgery.*
  - Paraduodenal hernia

- Foramen of Winslow hernia:
  - Loops of small bowel cluster between the posterior wall of stomach and the pancreas in the lesser sac, which may result in mass effect on the stomach and gastric outlet obstruction.
- Pericecal hernia:
  - Small bowel loops are found lateral to the cecum and ascending colon.

Spectrum of internal hernia

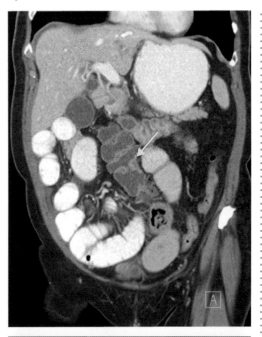

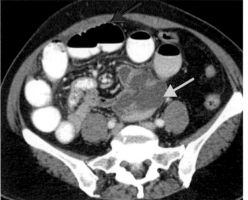

Transmesenteric internal hernia

In adults, transmesenteric hernias usually occur as sequelae of surgery, trauma, or inflammation. The mesenteric defect is not visible, so secondary findings, such as clustering of small bowel loops, are critical for diagnosis. Coronal and axial IV and oral contrast-enhanced CT show multiple distended loops of small bowel with gas–fluid levels, consistent with SBO. The right colon is medially displaced (yellow arrows). Normal intervening omental fat is absent between the abnormal bowel loops and the anterior abdominal wall (red arrow). These imaging findings could represent transmesenteric or pericecal internal hernia. The final diagnosis was established during surgical exploration.

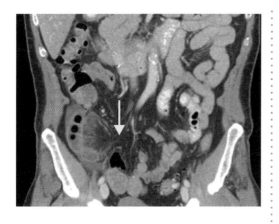

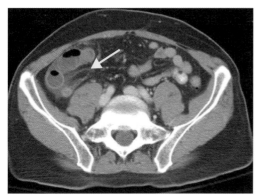

Transomental hernia

Transomental hernia may occur in the postsurgical setting or may be related to a congenital defect in the omentum. Tethering of the mesentery as it passes through an omental defect in the right lower quadrant is evident on these IV and oral contrast-enhanced coronal and axial CT images (arrows). Abnormal, mildly distended loops of small bowel with gas–fluid levels in the right lower quadrant are surrounded by a small amount of free fluid.

Post-RYGB left paraduodenal internal hernia

Paraduodenal hernias are three times more common on the left than on the right. They are the only internal hernia with a sex predilection – the male to female ratio is 3:1. Paraduodenal recesses may be postsurgical or may be congenital. Congenital defects predispose to recurrent hernia. As demonstrated by this axial IV contrast-enhanced CT image, left paraduodenal hernias are characterized by a left upper quadrant, retrogastric, sac-like cluster of small bowel loops (arrow).

Other complications of RYGB

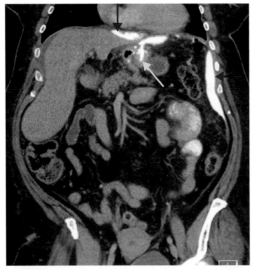

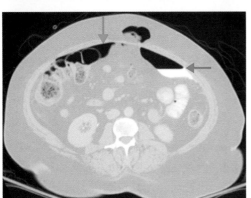

Anastomotic leak

Anastomotic leak is a life-threatening complication after RYGB. In this case, coronal and axial IV and oral contrast-enhanced CT in soft tissue and lung windows demonstrate oral contrast within the gastric pouch (yellow arrow). A defect in the superior wall of the pouch (not directly visible) allowed leakage of contrast into the peritoneal cavity (red arrows). Pneumoperitoneum (blue arrow) and a free gas-contrast level confirm the diagnosis (green arrow). Gas in the anterior abdominal wall may be post-surgical.

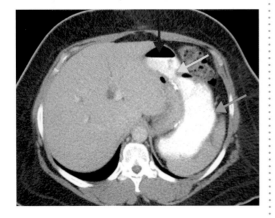

Gastro-gastric fistula

Gastro-gastric fistula (communication between the gastric pouch and the excluded stomach) is one of a few possible explanations for post-operative weight gain. It is usually diagnosed with fluoroscopy or CT, as in this case, in which an IV and oral contrast-enhanced axial image demonstrates a visible communication (yellow arrow) between the gastric pouch (red arrow) and the abnormally opacified excluded stomach (blue arrow). Restoration of near-normal gastric volume allows patients to eat more.

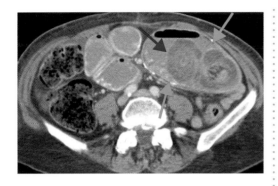

Post-RYGB intussusception

Clinically significant intussusception, usually with the jejunojejunal anastomosis acting as a lead point, may occur after RYGB. In this case, axial and coronal IV contrast-enhanced CT images show the pancreatico-biliary limb (yellow arrow) to be proximally dilated, with the distal loop entering into the common limb (red arrows) at the level of the jejunojejunal anastomosis (blue arrows). Symptomatic post-RYGB intussusception is usually treated surgically.

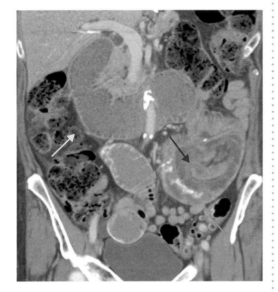

Anastomotic stricture

Gastrojejunal anastomotic stricture is a common post-operative complication of RYGB that may be occult by imaging (as in this case). Often, diagnosis and treatment are endoscopic. The clinical presentation of internal hernia and stricture may be similar, with post-prandial abdominal pain, nausea, and vomiting. This endoscopic image demonstrates a narrowed gastrojejunal anastomosis with perianastomic ulceration (yellow discoloration).

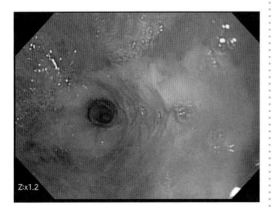

Differential diagnosis of internal hernia

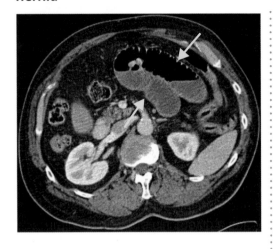

Closed loop SBO

Closed loop SBO has a greater likelihood of both strangulation and torsion than open loop obstruction, and hence, almost always requires surgical management. As demonstrated by axial IV and oral contrast-enhanced CT in this case, imaging features include a U- or C-shaped loop of dilated small bowel (arrows). In most cases, there are two transition points, which indicate obstruction in two locations; however, in some cases, the volvulized loop tapers at both ends into a single transition point.

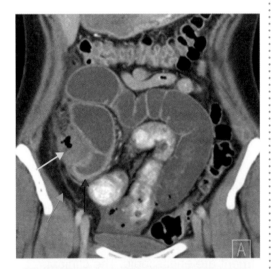

SBO due to Crohn's disease

While the most common causes of obstruction are adhesions and hernia due to prior surgery, obstruction may also be a complication of myriad other conditions including inflammatory bowel disease. Classic findings of open-loop obstruction include dilated loops of small bowel with gas–fluid levels and a single transition point between dilated and decompressed loops. In this case of Crohn's disease, coronal and axial contrast-enhanced CT demonstrate an SBO resulting from transmural inflammation (yellow arrows) at the ileocecal junction, just distal to the tapering terminal ileum (red arrow). There is inflammatory fat stranding in the region of affected bowel, and reactive thickening of the peritoneal lining (blue arrow).

Further reading

Blachar A, *et al*. Internal Hernia: Clinical and Imaging Findings in 17 Patients with Emphasis on CT Criteria. *Radiology* 218: 68–74 (2001).

Bocker J, *et al*. Intussusception: An Uncommon Cause of Postoperative Small Bowel Obstruction after Gastric Bypass. *Obesity Surgery* 14: 116–119 (2004).

Boudiaf M, *et al*. CT Evaluation of Small Bowel Obstruction. *Radiographics* 21: 613–624 (2001).

Carucci L, *et al*. Internal Hernia Following Roux-en-Y Gastric Bypass Surgery for Morbid Obesity: Evaluation of Radiographic Findings at Small-Bowel Examination. *Radiology* 251 (3): 762–770 (2009).

Higa K, *et al*. Internal Hernias after Laparoscopic Roux-en-Y Gastric Bypass: Incidence, Treatment and Prevention. *Obesity Surgery* 13: 350–354 (2003).

Lockhart M, *et al*. Internal Hernia after Gastric Bypass: Sensitivity and Specificity of Seven CT Signs with Surgical Correlation and Controls. *AJR* 188: 745–750 (2007).

Martin L, *et al*. Review of Internal Hernias: Radiographic and Clinical Findings. *AJR* 186: 703–717 (2006).

Scheirey C, *et al*. Radiology of the Laparoscopic Roux-en-Y Gastric Bypass Procedure: Conceptualization and Precise Interpretation of Results. *Radiographics* 36: 1355–1371 (2006).

Takeyama N, *et al*. CT of Internal Hernias. *Radiographics* 25:997–1015 (2005).

Ximenes M, *et al*. Petersen's Hernia as a Complication of Bariatric Surgery: CT Findings. *Abdominal Imaging* 36: 126–129.

Case 18   62-year-old woman with acute onset of upper abdominal pain radiating
to the back with vomiting and obstipation

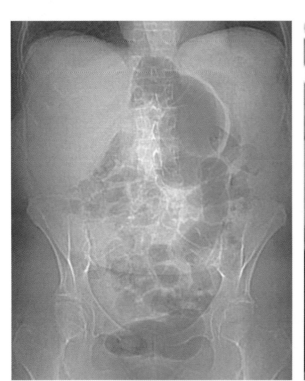

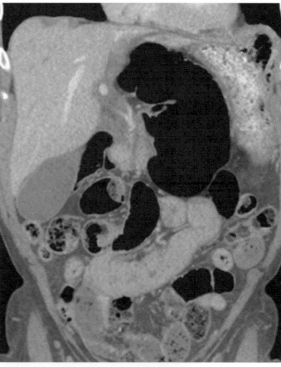

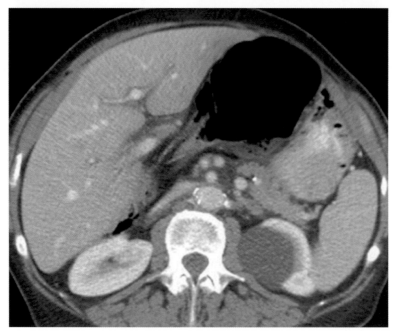

Diagnosis:
Foramen of
Winslow
hernia
containing
incarcerated
cecum

CT topogram (left image) and coronal IV and oral contrast-enhanced CT (middle image) show dilated, gas-filled cecum (yellow arrows) in the left upper abdomen displacing the stomach (red arrows) to the left. Axial contrast-enhanced CT (right image) shows the dilated gas-filled cecum in the lesser sac displacing the stomach posterolaterally. Stretched mesenteric vessels (blue arrow) pass posterior to the portal vein and anterior to the inferior vena cava (IVC) through the foramen of Winslow.

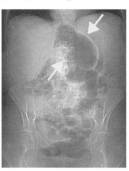 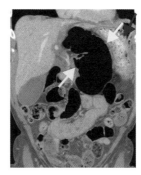 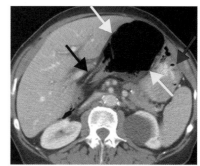

Discussion

- The foramen of Winslow is a normal communication between the greater and lesser sacs. The borders include the IVC posteriorly, the caudate lobe superiorly, and the duodenum inferiorly.
- The foramen of Winslow hernia is a congenital internal hernia that represents 8% of all internal hernias. Most foramen of Winslow hernias involve small intestine (60–70%), while the rest involve cecum and ascending colon. Rarely these hernias contain gallbladder, transverse colon, or omentum. Risk factors for herniation include an enlarged foramen, long small bowel mesentery, hypermobile right colon, and elongated right hepatic lobe.
- Clinically, patients may present with symptoms of proximal bowel obstruction due to mass effect on the stomach. Symptoms are sometimes relieved by bending forward.
- Characteristic CT findings include interposition of mesenteric fat and vessels between the IVC and liver hilum, air-distended bowel in the lesser sac with beaking directed towards the foramen of Winslow, displacement of the right colon from the right hemiabdomen, and anterolateral displacement of the stomach.

Clinical
synopsis

Emergent diagnostic laparoscopy revealed a foramen of Winslow hernia with incarcerated cecum in the lesser sac. As this could not be reduced laparoscopically, the patient underwent open hernia reduction with resection of the ischemic-appearing right hemicolon. Pathologic analysis confirmed mucosal necrosis and ischemic changes of the cecum.

Self-assessment

- *How do you differentiate a foramen of Winslow hernia from a left paraduodenal hernia?*

- An encapsulating membrane is seen with a left paraduodenal hernia and not with a foramen of Winslow hernia.
- The entry point of a left paraduodenal hernia is more inferior and to the left of the spine, with the inferior mesenteric vein (IMV) anteriorly and upwardly displaced in the neck of the hernia sac. The entry point of the foramen of Winslow hernia is superior and to the right of the spine, bordered by the liver hilum anteriorly.
- Mass effect on the transverse colon is more commonly seen in left paraduodenal hernia.

- *What are the characteristic CT findings of foramen of Winslow hernia?*

- Presence of mesenteric fat and vessels between the IVC and liver hilum.
- Air-filled loops in the lesser sac with a beak directed toward the foramen of Winslow.
- Absence of the ascending colon in its normal position in the right abdomen.
- Anterior and lateral displacement of the stomach.

Differential diagnosis of foramen of Winslow hernia

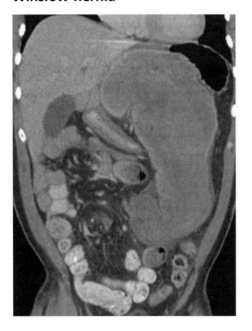

Cecal volvulus

If a foramen of Winslow hernia contains the cecum, it can look similar on plain film to a cecal volvulus; however, in volvulus, the involved cecum will not be in the lesser sac. IV and oral contrast-enhanced CT shows a dilated cecum in the left upper quadrant displacing the gas-filled stomach superiorly.

Further reading

Azar, A. *et al.* Ileocecal Herniation through the Foramen of Winslow: MDCT Diagnosis. *Abdominal Imaging*. 35:574–577 (2010).

Grisham, A. *et al.* Image of the Month: Foramen of Winslow Hernia. *Archives of Surgery*. 146(11):1329–1330 (2011).

Martin, L. *et al.* Review of Internal Hernias: Radiographic and Clinical Findings. *American Journal of Roentgenology*. 186:703–717 (2006).

Takeyama, N. *et al*. CT of Internal Hernias. *Radiographics*. 25:997–1015 (2005).

Wojtasek, D. *et al*. CT Diagnosis of Cecal Herniation through the Foramen of Winslow. *Gastrointestinal Radiology*. 16:77–79 (1991).

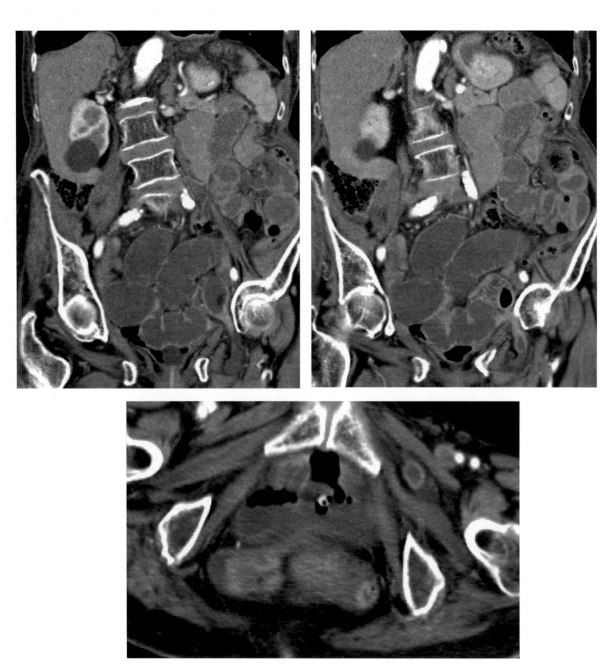

Diagnosis: **Incarcerated left obturator hernia**

Coronal and axial CT images with oral and IV contrast demonstrate multiple dilated loops of small bowel with tapering (yellow arrows; left and middle images) at the level of the obturator foramen. The incarcerated loop (yellow arrow; right image) is visible between the pectineus (red arrow) and obturator externus (blue arrow) muscles. Fluid (green arrow) in the hernia sac raises concern for strangulation.

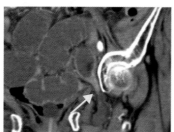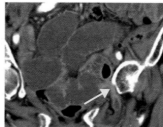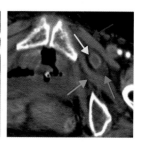

Discussion

Overview of external hernia

- External hernias are characterized by herniation of bowel outside of the normal confines of the peritoneal cavity. They are typically asymptomatic and often electively repaired. External hernia repair is the most commonly performed general surgical procedure in the United States.
- Complications of external hernia include bowel obstruction, incarceration (irreducible sac), and strangulation (ischemia).
- An obturator hernia is a relatively uncommon form of external hernia most commonly occuring in elderly females. Bowel obstruction is common. Recognition of obturator hernia is important as a strangulated obturator hernia has the highest mortality rate of all hernias. Obturator hernias occur in between the pectineus and obturator externus muscles, as demonstrated in the above case.

Imaging of external hernia

- CT is the imaging modality of choice for evaluation of suspected external hernia.
- External hernias that are difficult to palpate due to patient body habitus or anatomic location (as in obturator hernia) may be readily diagnosed by CT. CT can distinguish an abdominal wall hernia from other palpable masses including abdominal wall neoplasms, rectus sheath hematomas, varices, and inguinal lymphadenopathy.
- Complications of external hernia, including small bowel obstruction and ischemia, are well evaluated by CT. CT findings of early bowel compromise include adjacent fat stranding or fluid in the hernia sac. CT findings of ischemia include pneumatosis intestinalis, portal venous gas, or pneumoperitoneum;

however, it is important to note that pneumatosis and portal venous gas may also be "benign" (i.e., non-ischemic in etiology).

| Clinical synopsis | The patient underwent laparoscopic reduction of the incarcerated hernia. The defect was repaired with mesh. There was no evidence of bowel ischemia at the time of surgery. |

Self-assessment

- *Which external hernias are seen more commonly in elderly females?*

- Pelvic hernias (sciatic, obturator, and perineal hernias) are seen more commonly in elderly females due to acquired pelvic floor weakness.

- *What is a Richter's hernia?*

- Herniation of only the antimesenteric wall of the bowel is a Richter's hernia. This most frequently occurs with femoral hernias.

- *What is an interparietal hernia?*

- An interparietal hernia is a rare acquired hernia that is typically found in the inguinal region. The hernia sac fails to exit into the subcutaneous tissue, and instead, travels along the abdominal wall musculature. Interparietal hernias are often complicated by incarceration.

Spectrum of external hernias

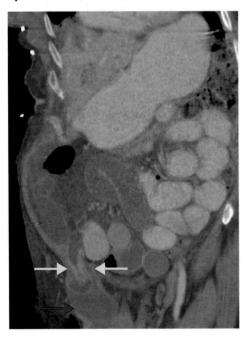

Inguinal hernia causing small bowel obstruction

Inguinal hernias may be direct or indirect, depending on the relationship to the inferior epigastric vessels. Indirect hernias are more common and may be congenital or acquired. Indirect hernias arise lateral to the inferior epigastric vessels. In boys, the processus vaginalis fails to obliterate and abdominal contents pass through the inguinal canal. In adults, acquired indirect inguinal hernias arise from weakness and dilatation of the internal inguinal ring. A hernia that passes into the scrotum is termed "complete." Direct inguinal hernias are always acquired. Herniated contents pass through a defect in the transversalis fascia that is medial to the epigastric vessels. Because direct hernias are posterior to the spermatic cord, they should not reach the scrotum. Coronal oral and IV contrast-enhanced CT shows a loop of small bowel passing through the right inguinal canal (yellow arrows). Multiple loops of dilated small bowel are seen proximally. Fluid in the hernia sac (red arrow) raises concern for strangulation. This was an indirect inguinal hernia, although the lateral relationship of the hernia sac relative to the epigastric vessels is not shown on this image.

Femoral hernia

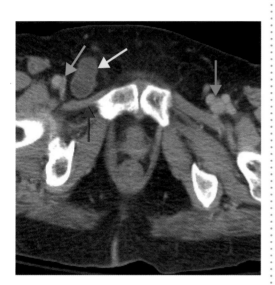

Femoral hernias are less common than inguinal hernias and have a female predominance. They are often right-sided and are located poster-ior to the inguinal ligament and medial to the femoral vein, which may be compressed. It can be difficult to reliably distinguish inguinal from fem-oral hernias; however, compression of the femoral vein is highly suggestive of femoral hernia. Dis-tinction is important as surgical approach is dif-ferent and femoral hernias have a higher risk of strangulation. Axial unenhanced CT shows a loop of bowel (yellow arrow) external to the pectineus muscle (red arrow) and medial to the femoral vessels. The right femoral vein (blue arrow) is compressed relative to the normal left-sided vein (green arrow).

Umbilical hernia

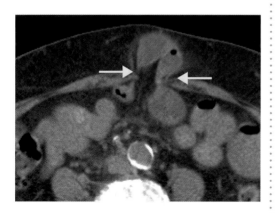

Most umbilical hernias formed in infancy close spontaneously. In adults, they are generally acquired, with risk factors including multiple pregnancies, obesity, ascites, and abdominal masses. They are far more common in women. There is a high frequency of incarcer-ation. Axial unenhanced CT shows a loop of small bowel exiting a defect in the anterior abdominal wall (arrows) in the region of the umbilicus. There is focal proximal dilation concerning for obstruction.

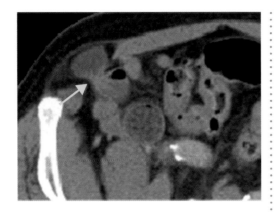

Spigelian hernia

Spigelian hernia is a rare acquired hernia lateral to the rectus muscle and below the umbilicus. Contents herniate through a defect in the linea semilunaris, the fibrous union of the rectus sheath and oblique muscles. There is a high risk of incarceration. Axial enhanced CT shows a loop of small bowel (arrow) protruding lateral to the rectus abdominus. The herniated contents are contained by the external oblique aponeurosis. Spigelian hernias are generally interparietal, extending between layers of the anterior abdominal wall musculature rather than deep to the subcutaneous fat.

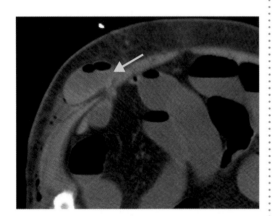

Incisional hernia

While most incisional hernias develop several months after surgery, they can also occur in the early postoperative period. Risk factors include old age and obesity. Axial IV contrast-enhanced CT shows a small bowel obstruction characterized by multiple dilated loops of small bowel with gas–fluid levels. The cause is herniation of a loop of small bowel (arrow) through the right anterior abdominal wall, via an incision from recent laparoscopic surgery. Subcutaneous gas is present, consistent with postsurgical changes.

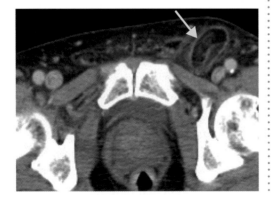

Fat-containing femoral hernia

An external hernia may contain fluid, bowel, bladder, mesentery, or any other intra-abdominal contents. Axial contrast-enhanced CT shows a circumscribed, ovoid, fat-containing structure (yellow arrow) medial to the left common femoral artery and vein. There is a congested central vessel. This was an inflamed epiploic appendage that had herniated into the femoral canal.

Further reading

Aguirre, D.A. *et al.* Abdominal Wall Hernias: Imaging Features, Complications, and Diagnostic Pitfalls at Multi-Detector Row CT. *Radiographics*. 25:1501-1520 (2005).

Lee, G. *et al.* CT Imaging of Abdominal Hernias. *American Journal of Roentgenology*. 161:1209-1213 (1993).

Rutkow, I.M. Demographic and Socioeconomic Aspects of Hernia Repair in the United States in 2003. *Surge Clin North Am*. 83(5):1045-1051 (2003).

Suzuki, S., Furui, S., Okinaga, K. *et al.* Differentiation of Femoral versus Inguinal Hernia: CT Findings. *AJR: American Journal of Roentgenology*. 189(2) (2007), W78–83.

Zarvan, N. *et al.* Abdominal Wall Hernias: CT Findings. *American Journal of Roentgenology*. 164:1391-1395 (1995).

61-year-old woman presenting with diffuse abdominal pain, nausea, and vomiting after 1 day of obstipation

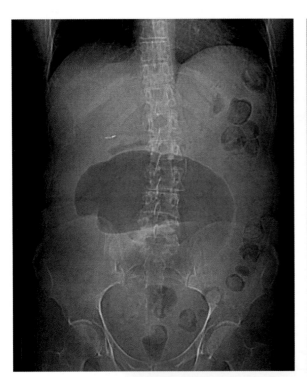
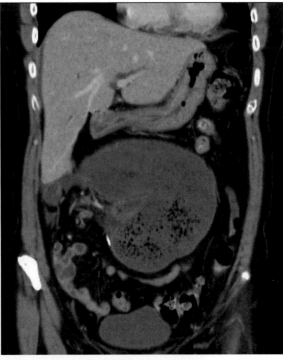

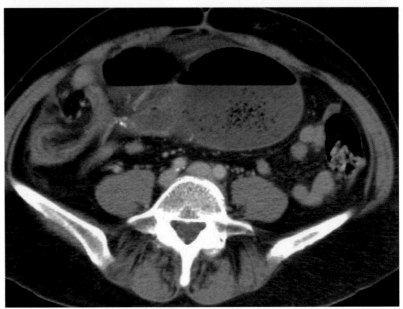

Diagnosis: CT scout image (left image) shows a dilated, gas-filled viscus with haustral
Cecal volvulus folds in the midline (yellow arrows). Coronal (middle image) and axial (right
image) contrast-enhanced CT images show displacement of the dilated, fluid-
filled cecum into the upper abdomen. There is an associated "whirl" sign (an
area of swirling of the bowel and its mesentery, denoted by the red arrows) at
the site of the twist, best seen on the axial image.

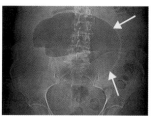 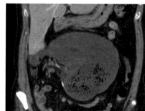 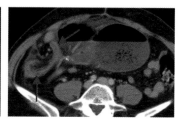

Discussion

Overview of cecal volvulus

- Cecal volvulus accounts for 25–40% of all cases of colonic volvulus and 1% of intestinal obstructions.
- Inadequate fixation of the right colon to the retroperitoneum, allowing increased mobility of the right colon, is the main underlying cause. The other requirement is restriction of the bowel at a fixed point, such as from scarring, adhesions, or an abdominal mass that serves as a fulcrum for rotation.
- As in small bowel obstruction, patients may present with colicky abdominal pain, nausea, vomiting, and obstipation.

Imaging of cecal volvulus

- Cecal volvulus has a characteristic appearance on conventional radiography: a dilated loop of bowel with haustral markings, usually located in the left upper quadrant. The cecum, however, may be displaced anywhere in the abdomen. The loop may look like a coffee bean, similar to the radiographic sign that characterizes sigmoid volvulus.
- Secondary signs of bowel ischemia should always be sought, including free air, portal venous gas, and cecal pneumatosis.
- Small bowel proximal to the cecum is usually dilated.
- After radiography, CT may be useful for diagnosing complications. CT findings include abnormal position of a markedly dilated cecum (typically the left upper

quadrant, less commonly the right upper quadrant). Both bowel and mesentery are twisted, causing the "whirl" sign of swirling mesenteric vessels.

- Contrast enema can confirm the diagnosis, characteristically showing a focal obstruction of the right colon with a beak-like narrowing at the site of twisting. Contrast enema is contraindicated in the setting of perforation, however.

Treatment of cecal volvulus

- Treatment of cecal volvulus is surgical. Delay in diagnosis and treatment of cecal volvulus carries significant risk of morbidity and mortality.

Clinical synopsis

The patient underwent emergency exploratory laparotomy with ileocecectomy. Pathology revealed transmural chronic inflammation.

Self-assessment

- *What is a cecal bascule?*

- Cecal bascule is a variant of cecal volvulus in which the cecum is folded anteriorly without twisting. This is seen as a dilated loop in the mid abdomen.

- *Name the three most common causes of large bowel obstruction.*

- Colon cancer
- Colonic volvulus
- Diverticulitis

Spectrum of cecal volvulus

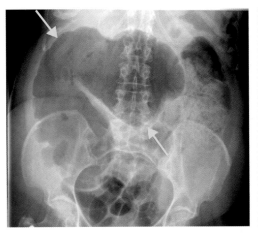

Uncomplicated cecal volvulus

Uncomplicated cecal volvulus is volvulus without ischemia or infarction. Although the dilated loop in cecal volvulus is classically found in the left upper quadrant, the cecum can be located anywhere in the abdomen. Secondary signs of ischemia, including pneumatosis, portal venous gas, and pneumoperitoneum, are absent. Radiograph of the abdomen shows a dilated loop of bowel with haustral markings in the right upper quadrant (arrows).

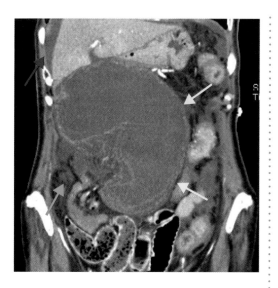

Cecal volvulus with ischemia

Cecal volvulus can be complicated by ischemia of the affected bowel. Coronal enhanced CT shows a large dilated loop of featureless bowel projecting from the right lower to the left upper quadrant. The bowel wall is thickened and hypoenhancing (yellow arrows) and there is perihepatic ascites (red arrow). The mesentery appears congested (blue arrow). These findings are concerning for ischemia.

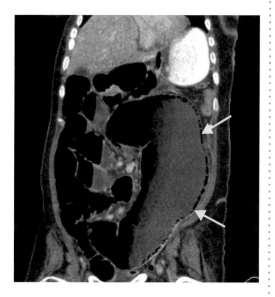

Cecal volvulus with infarction

Coronal enhanced CT shows numerous dilated small bowel loops in the right hemiabdomen, consistent with small bowel obstruction. In the left hemiabdomen, there is a dilated loop of bowel with non-enhancing walls and pneumatosis intestinalis (arrows). Although pneumatosis can be "benign" (i.e., not related to bowel infarction), these findings are concerning for bowel ischemia/ infarction given the mural non-enhancement. This is a surgical emergency with high morbidity and mortality. Lung windows may be helpful for detecting subtle pneumatosis intestinalis, free gas in the abdomen denoting perforation, and gas within the mesenteric and portal veins that has escaped from the infarcted bowel wall.

Differential diagnosis of cecal volvulus

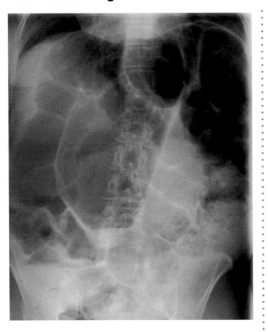

Sigmoid volvulus

Sigmoid volvulus accounts for 60–75% of all cases of colonic volvulus and is most commonly seen in elderly patients and those with neuro-psychiatric disorders. These patients often have chronic constipation from medications and immo-bility. Radiograph demonstrates marked disten-tion of the ahaustral sigmoid colon (in contrast to the cecum, the sigmoid does not have haustra) in a "coffee bean" configuration, with an inverted "U" shape pointing from the left lower to the right upper quadrant. There is large bowel obstruction, characterized by proximal colonic dilatation and absence of rectal gas.

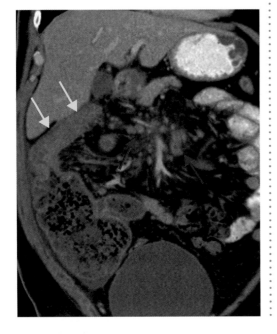

Colon adenocarcinoma

Colon carcinoma is the leading cause of large bowel obstruction. Cancers of the sigmoid are most likely to cause obstruction in comparison to more proximal malignancy, as the diameter of the sigmoid colon is relatively narrow. Coronal enhanced CT shows a relatively long segment of colon with thickened walls at the hepatic flexure (yellow arrows). There are multiple enlarged lymph nodes in the mesentery (red arrows), which favors the diagnosis of colon cancer over other causes of wall thickening. Colon cancer may mimic diver-ticulitis or colitis, especially if tumor extends transmurally into the adjacent fat.

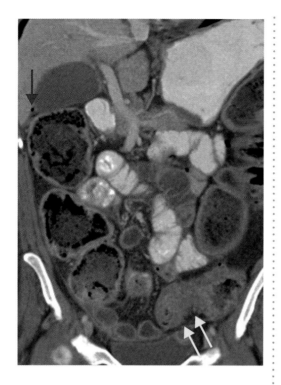

Diverticulitis

Diverticulitis accounts for approximately 10% of cases of large bowel obstruction and may be caused by inflammation, adhesions, pericolic fibrosis, or compression by intramural or extramural abscess. Diverticulitis may appear similar to colon cancer on CT. Although the findings of pericolic stranding, length of abnormal colon that is more than 10 cm long, fluid at the base of the mesentery, and vascular engorgement favor diverticulitis over colon cancer, these two entities may appear identical. Therefore, after treatment for suspected diverticulitis, patients should undergo colonoscopy. Coronal enhanced CT shows thickening and hyperemia of the walls of the sigmoid colon (yellow arrows). Colonic obstruction resulted in marked distention of the cecum with subsequent perforation, denoted by foci of free gas (red arrow).

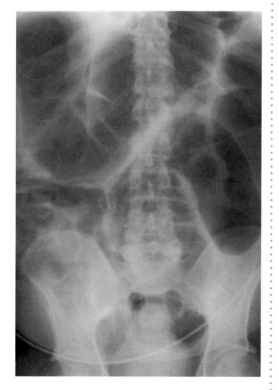

Colonic pseudo-obstruction

Colonic pseudo-obstruction, also called Ogilvie's syndrome, clinically resembles a mechanical obstruction with pain and abdominal distention. Although intramural ganglion damage is seen in chronic pseudo-obstruction, the underlying cause is not clear. Abdominal radiographs are nonspecific, showing distention of the colon. CT imaging demonstrates extensive proximal colonic dilatation without an obstructing lesion at the transition point, typically at or near the splenic flexure. Non-surgical treatment with nasogastric tube, enemas, and neostigmine are usually effective. There is a high risk for perforation if the cecum is markedly dilated, and colonoscopic decompression may be indicated. The acute form, seen in the setting of severe medical illness and major surgery, is typically transient and more likely to perforate. The chronic form usually recurs and is seen in patients with chronic constipation. Abdominal radiograph shows marked dilatation of the colon without a clear transition point to denote mechanical obstruction.

Further reading

Adler, Yolanda *et al*. Pseudo-obstruction in the Geriatric Population. *Radiographics*. 6:995–1005 (1986).

Chintapalli, Kedar *et al*. Diverticulitis versus Colon Cancer: Differentiation with Helical CT Findings. *Radiology*. 210:429–435 (1999).

Choi, JS *et al*. Colonic Pseudo-obstruction: CT findings. *American Journal of Roentgenology*. 190:1521–1526 (2008).

Johnson, CD, Schmit, GD. Mayo Clinic Gastrointestinal Imaging Review. Mayo Clinic Scientific Press (2005)

Levsky, Jeffrey *et al*. CT Findings of Sigmoid Volvulus. *American Journal of Roentgenology*. 194:139–143 (2010).

Moore, Carolyn J. *et al*. CT of Cecal Volvulus: Unraveling the Image. *American Journal of Roentgenology*. 177:95–98 (2001).

Padidar, A. *et al*. Differentiating Sigmoid Diverticulitis from Carcinoma on CT Scans: Mesenteric Inflammation suggests Diverticulitis. *American Journal of Roentgenology*. 163:81–81 (1994).

Peterson, Christine *et al*. Volvulus of the Gastrointestinal Tract: Appearances at Multi-modality Imaging. *Radiographics*. 29:1281–1293 (2009).

Rosenblat, Juliana M. *et al*. Findings of Cecal Volvulus at CT. *Radiology*. 256:169–175 (2010).

Taourel, P. *et al*. Helical CT of Large Bowel Obstruction. *Abdominal Imaging*. 28: 267–275 (2003).

Case 21   60-year-old male with history of non-small-cell lung cancer on bevacizumab (Avastin) presenting with abdominal pain

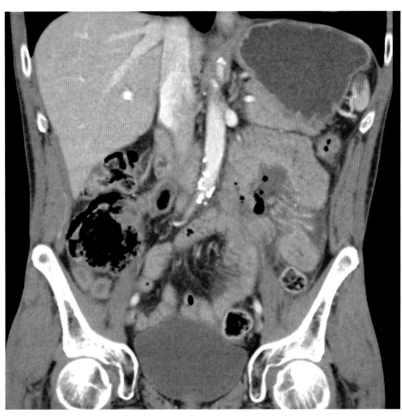

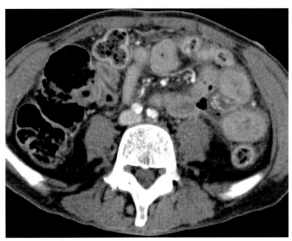
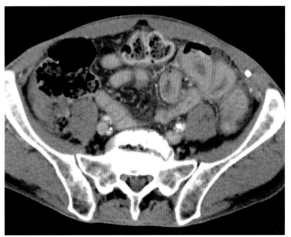

Diagnosis:
Bevacizumab-
associated
bowel
perforation

Coronal (left image) and axial (middle and right image) contrast-enhanced CT images show focal perforation at the duodenojejunal junction with diffuse wall thickening (yellow arrow) and extraluminal gas and fluid (red arrows). Scattered foci of antidependent, extraluminal gas are seen throughout the peritoneal cavity (blue arrows).

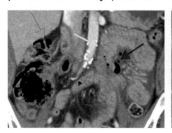 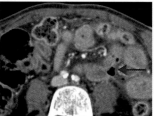 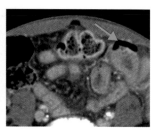

Discussion

Overview of bevacizumab

- Bevacizumab (Avastin; Genentech, South San Francisco, CA) is an anti-angiogenic monoclonal antibody that inhibits the vascular endothelial growth factor (VEGF) receptor on the surface of endothelial cells.
- Tumor growth and the establishment of metastases are dependent on the formation and proliferation of new blood vessels, a process that is termed angiogenesis. Angiogenesis is induced by VEGF, which promotes neovascularization and tumor growth.
- By targeting the endothelial VEGF receptor, bevacizumab and other anti-VEGF agents inhibit neovascularization and abnormal blood vessel remodeling.
- Bevacizumab is currently approved for use in patients with several types of advanced cancer in conjunction with standard chemotherapy, including colon cancer, breast cancer, renal cell carcinoma, non-small-cell lung cancer, and glioblastoma multiforme.

Adverse effects seen in patients on bevacizumab

- VEGF is crucial to endothelial integrity and wound healing; therefore, inhibition of VEGF by bevacizumab predisposes patients to several serious and possibly fatal adverse events, including hemorrhage, neutropenia, bowel perforation, wound or anastomotic dehiscence, hypertensive crisis, and posterior reversible encephalopathy syndrome (PRES). In addition to increased risk of hemorrhage, bevacizumab also predisposes to venous and arterial thrombotic complications.
- Bevacizumab-associated complications vary significantly amongst patients receiving different classes of chemotherapy, which suggests a synergistic and complex interaction between bevacizumab and specific chemotherapeutic agents.

Bevacizumab-associated bowel perforation

- Bevacizumab-associated bowel perforation is a well-documented, albeit relatively uncommon, complication, occurring in approximately 0.3% of patients receiving bevacizumab, with a relative risk of 2.5 compared to similar patients not on the drug.
- The etiology of bevacizumab-associated bowel perforation is not completely understood and may be secondary to treatment-induced necrosis of bowel. Other theories include damage to gastrointestinal microvasculature in association with impaired endothelial healing.
- Treatment of bevacizumab-associated bowel perforation includes permanent discontinuation of bevacizumab. Depending on clinical status, either surgical intervention or conservative treatment with antibiotics and bowel rest may be performed.

Self-assessment

- *Where are common sites of bevacizumab-associated perforation?*

  - Bowel perforation associated with bevacizumab can occur at sites of residual cancer, surgical anastomotic sites, or non-affected bowel secondary to ulceration.

- *What other anti-angiogenic drugs are implicated in bowel perforation?*

  - Other anti-VEGF agents implicated in bowel perforation include sunitinib (Sutent; Pfizer, Cambridge, USA), which is used to treat gastrointestinal stromal tumor and metastatic renal cell carcinoma, and sorafenib (Nexavar; Bayer, Berlin, Germany), which is used to treat advanced metastatic renal cell carcinoma.

Spectrum of bevacizumab-associated complications

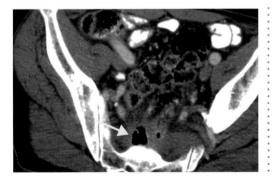

Bevacizumab-associated perforation secondary to anastomotic dehiscence

This example shows a 68-year-old male with rectal cancer, status post lower anterior resection, who presented with lower back pain. Axial (upper image) and sagittal (lower image) enhanced CT demonstrates locules of extraluminal gas in the presacral soft tissues (arrows), representing an abscess due to anastomotic dehiscence.

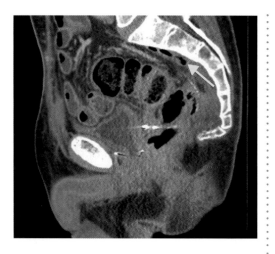

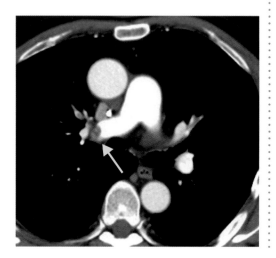

Bevacizumab-associated pulmonary embolism

Anti-angiogenic therapies have been associated with increased incidence of arterial and venous thromboembolic events including pulmonary embolism. Monitoring and surveillance for thromboembolic events, including hemorrhage and infarcts, is warranted in patients taking these therapies. Axial CT pulmonary angiogram in a patient on bevacizumab demonstrates a filling defect in the right main pulmonary artery (arrow).

Differential diagnosis of bevacizumab-associated bowel perforation

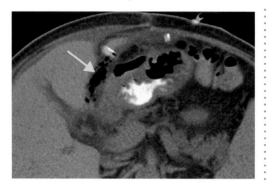

Bowel perforation secondary to peptic ulcer disease

Bowel perforation secondary to peptic ulcer disease often occurs in the duodenal bulb and is associated with *Helicobacter pylori* infection. Axial CT with oral contrast only demonstrates focal extraluminal gas (arrow) in the region of the proximal duodenum, associated with adjacent mural thickening.

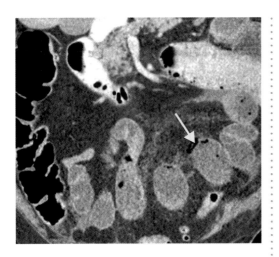

Ischemic bowel

Ischemic bowel, caused by a multitude of primary conditions, is categorized as occlusive (thromboembolic) or non-occlusive (low-flow state). Coronal enhanced CT demonstrates focal pneumatosis (arrow) and adjacent fluid associated with a loop of bowel in the left lower quadrant in this 71-year-old patient who developed ischemic bowel after aortic valve repair and CABG.

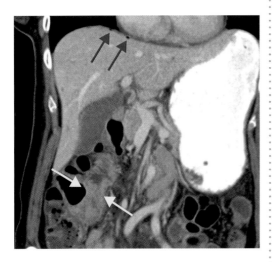

Traumatic small bowel laceration

Coronal enhanced CT in a patient who experienced bicycle trauma demonstrates focal segmental high-attenuation mural thickening of a loop of small bowel (yellow arrows), with adjacent mesenteric stranding. There are punctate foci of subdiaphragmatic pneumoperitoneum (red arrows). The patient was taken to surgery where numerous mesenteric bruises/hematomas were noted, along with a focal laceration of small bowel and associated hematoma.

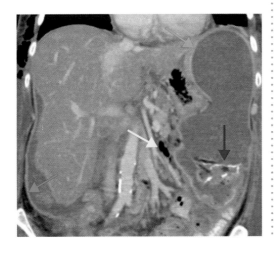

Bowel perforation secondary to anastomotic dehiscence

Coronal enhanced CT demonstrates pneumoperitoneum (yellow arrow) tracking from the left colon anastomosis (red arrow). A very large fluid collection in the left upper quadrant (blue arrow) with adjacent thickened peritoneum displaces the stomach medially. There is diffuse ascites with thickened peritoneum (green arrow), consistent with peritonitis/pyoperitoneum.

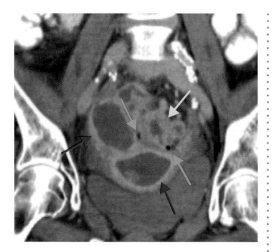

Bowel perforation due to colon cancer

Although perforation of the colon is rarely associated with malignancy, it is still important to consider if extraluminal gas is seen in conjunction with colon wall thickening. Perforation associated with colon cancer may be due to neoplasm extending through the bowel wall, or proximal perforation due to an obstructing mass. Coronal enhanced CT demonstrates nodular thickening of the sigmoid colon (yellow arrow). Adjacent multi-loculated abscesses (red arrows) and foci of extraluminal gas (blue arrows) are due to perforated colon cancer.

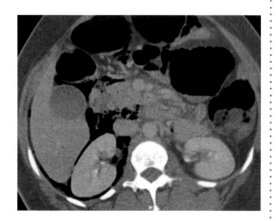

Bowel perforation due to esophagogastroduodenoscopy (EGD)

Perforation secondary to EGD is a rare occurrence, reported in one series with an incidence of 0.033%; however, mortality after perforation was 17%, with a morbidity of 40%. Axial CT demonstrates extensive pneumoperitoneum and retroperitoneal gas surrounding the right kidney in a patient who had recently undergone EGD, consistent with a duodenal perforation.

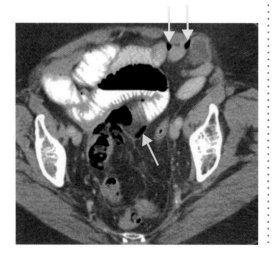

Bowel perforation due to colonoscopy

Similar to perforation after EGD, bowel perforation after colonoscopy is rare but carries a high morbidity and mortality. Axial CT in a patient following colonoscopy demonstrates extraluminal foci of gas in the anterior abdomen and adjacent to the sigmoid (arrows) and mild stranding of the peri-sigmoid fat.

Further reading

Chikarmane, S. A., B. Khurana, K. M. Krajewski, A. B. Shinagare, S. Howard, A. Sodickson, J. Jagannathan, *et al.* 2012. What the emergency radiologist needs to know about treatment-related complications from conventional chemotherapy and newer molecular targeted agents. *Emergency Radiology* 19(6):535–546.

Hapani, S., D. Chu, and S. Wu. 2009. Risk of gastrointestinal perforation in patients with cancer treated with bevacizumab: a meta-analysis. *Lancet Oncol* 10:559–568.

Hurwitz, H. I., L. B. Saltz, E. Van Cutsem, J. Cassidy, J. Wiedemann, F. Sirzen, G. H. Lyman, and U. P. Rohr. 2011. Venous thromboembolic events with chemotherapy plus bevacizumab: a pooled analysis of patients in randomized phase II and III studies. *J Clin Oncol* 29:1757–1764.

Merchea A., D. C. Cullinane, M. D. Sawyer, C. W. Iqbal, T. H. Baron, D. Wigle, M. G. Sarr, M. D. Zielinski. 2010. Esophagogastroduodenoscopy-associated gastrointestinal perforations: a single-center experience. *Surgery* 148(4):876–880.

Saif, M. W., A. Elfiky, and R. R. Salem. 2007. Gastrointestinal perforation due to bevacizumab in colorectal cancer. *Ann Surg Oncol* 14:1860–1869.

Torrisi, J. M., L. H. Schwartz, M. J. Gollub, M. S. Ginsberg, G. J. Bosl, and H. Hricak. 2011. CT findings of chemotherapy-induced toxicity: what radiologists need to know about the clinical and radiologic manifestations of chemotherapy toxicity. *Radiology* 258:41–56.

Case 22   88-year-old woman with bradycardia and 1 day of abdominal pain and hematochezia

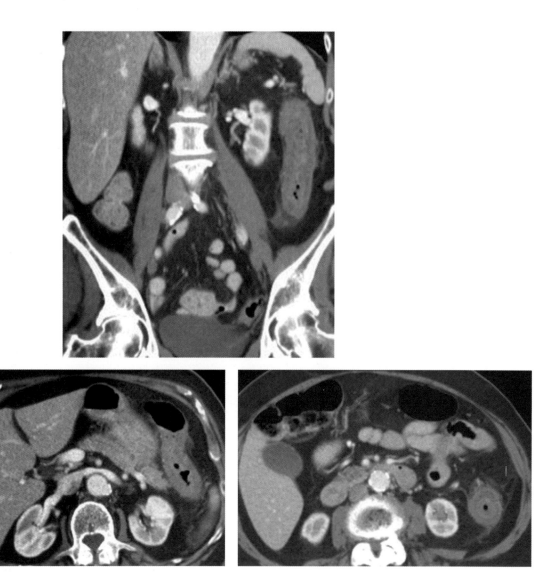

Diagnosis:
Ischemic colitis secondary to low-flow state

Coronal (left image) and axial (middle and right images) IV and oral contrast-enhanced CT demonstrates marked wall thickening (yellow arrows) of the descending colon from the splenic flexure (a watershed area) with adjacent fat stranding. There is atherosclerosis of the abdominal aorta (red arrow) and its branches, without acute vascular cutoff.

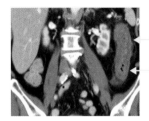 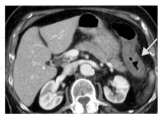 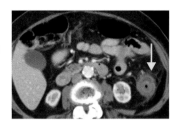

Discussion

Overview of mesenteric ischemia

- Mesenteric ischemia is caused by insufficient blood supply to the intestine and features a wide range of clinical and imaging manifestations, with a reported mortality of 50–90%.
- Mesenteric ischemia may be due to numerous occlusive, nonocclusive, or mechanical etiologies.
  - Occlusive (thromboembolic) mesenteric ischemia is caused by arterial embolism in 85% of cases and venous occlusion in the remainder.
  - Nonocclusive mesenteric ischemia is seen in low-flow states, such as systemic hypotension or cardiogenic etiologies (e.g., myocardial infarction, congestive heart failure, or valvular abnormalities).
  - Mechanical causes of mesenteric ischemia can be seen in the setting of bowel obstruction or trauma.
  - Less common causes of mesenteric ischemia include chemotherapeutic agents, radiation, or toxic ingestion.

Imaging of mesenteric ischemia

- CT is the modality of choice to evaluate for suspected mesenteric ischemia, although the CT findings in bowel ischemia are nonspecific and can be varied, including hypoattenuating or hyperattenuating wall thickening, dilation, abnormal (or absent) mural enhancement, mesenteric stranding and ascites, pneumatosis, and portal venous gas.
- The most common CT finding in acute bowel ischemia is bowel wall thickening, which is also the least specific finding.
- The "double halo" sign represents enhancement of the mucosa and muscularis propria, with edema of the submucosa.

- Thinning of the bowel wall or "paper-thin" wall can be seen with transmural necrosis due to loss of intestinal musculature tone.
- Mesenteric fat stranding, mesenteric fluid, and ascites are other early findings of bowel ischemia, but can also be seen in infectious or inflammatory processes. Bowel dilatation with air-fluid levels may be seen as the bowel wall loses muscle tone.
- Lack of enhancement of the bowel wall is a helpful, relatively specific sign of inadequate blood supply to the intestine. Pneumatosis and portomesenteric venous gas are less common but highly specific for bowel ischemia.
- Mesenteric ischemia may cause hypo- or hyperattenuation of the bowel wall.
- Filling defects in the mesenteric arteries and veins should be routinely sought on studies performed with IV contrast when bowel ischemia or infarction is identified. Absent or diminished flow in a mesenteric vessel is highly specific but not sensitive for mesenteric ischemia.

Clinical synopsis

The patient's symptoms improved with bowel rest and supportive measures including IV fluids. The patient had persistent bradycardia, for which a permanent pacemaker was placed.

Self-assessment

- *What are the two presentations of ischemic colitis?*

  - Transient ischemia, with reversible lesions limited to the mucosa and submucosa. This is managed conservatively and usually has a favorable clinical outcome. Signs suggestive of infarction (as below) are absent.
  - Gangrenous infarction, with transmural necrosis. Bowel must be resected, and there is high morbidity and mortality. Signs such as non-enhancement, "paper-thin" bowel wall, pneumatosis intestinalis, perforation, and mesenteric or portal venous gas are characteristic of infarction in the appropriate clinical setting.

- *What are some findings that favor mesenteric vasculitis over mesenteric thromboembolism?*

  - Vasculitis features diffuse, non-segmental bowel involvement (e.g., involvement of both small and large bowel or both jejunum and ileum).
  - Involvement of the duodenum favors vasculitis.
  - Skipped segments not conforming to a vascular distribution favor vasculitis.

Spectrum of mesenteric ischemia

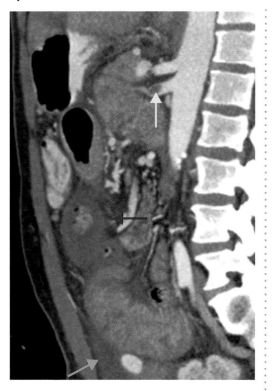

Mesenteric artery thromboembolism

Acute occlusion of the superior mesenteric artery (SMA) from thrombosis or embolization is the most common cause of acute mesenteric ischemia, accounting for approximately 60–70% of cases. The most common predisposing condition is cardiogenic thromboembolism from atrial fibrillation or ventricular aneurysm. Other etiologies include atherosclerosis, aortic thromboembolism, and aortic or mesenteric artery dissection. Sagittal CT with IV and oral contrast shows a filling defect (yellow arrow) within the proximal SMA, representing an acute thrombus. There is bowel wall thickening (red arrow) with a small amount of ascites (blue arrow).

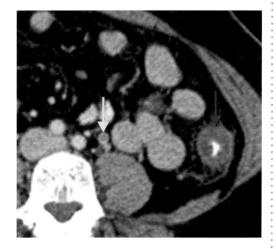

Mesenteric venous thrombosis

Mesenteric venous occlusion may be seen in the setting of recent surgery, neoplasm, infection, inflammation, or in other hypercoagulable states. Because of extensive collateral circulation, proximal venous thrombosis is less likely to cause severe bowel ischemia than distal venous thrombosis. Axial CT image with intravenous and oral contrast shows a hypodense thrombus in the inferior mesenteric vein (IMV; yellow arrow), with wall thickening of the descending colon (red arrow). There is adjacent mesenteric venous congestion and mild fat stranding.

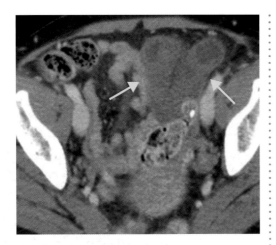

Strangulating, closed-loop bowel obstruction

Intestinal ischemia, or strangulation, occurs in approximately 10% of mechanical small bowel obstructions. Closed-loop obstructions are most often caused by adhesions or hernias, and the closed loop is prone to volvulus. Venous outflow obstruction with mesenteric congestion is followed by arterial ischemia. On CT, closed loop obstruction has a C- or U-shape and radial distribution of dilated fluid-filled bowel around prominent mesenteric vessels that converge toward the point of torsion. Two transition points to normal bowel may be identified. Axial IV contrast-enhanced CT shows a U-shaped loop of poorly enhancing small bowel with wall thickening (arrows) in the left lower quadrant, consistent with closed-loop bowel obstruction. At surgery, the patient was found to have adhesive bands.

Pneumatosis intestinalis and portomesenteric venous gas

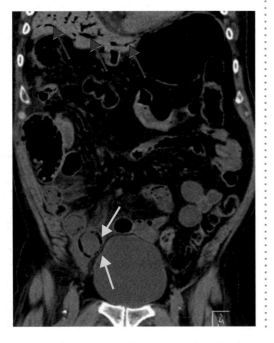

In the setting of bowel ischemia, pneumatosis and portomesenteric gas are strongly associated with transmural infarction or gangrene. It is important to recognize that, in the absence of ischemia, these findings may result from iatrogenic, traumatic, inflammatory, infectious, and neoplastic causes. Lung windows may be helpful in assessing for subtle pneumatosis. Coronal unenhanced CT shows pneumatosis of the ileum (yellow arrow) and extensive portal venous gas (red arrows). There is mesenteric congestion adjacent to the involved loops. Portal venous gas may be distinguished from pneumobilia by its extension to the peripheral aspect of the liver. Gas-containing bile ducts in pneumobilia are more central.

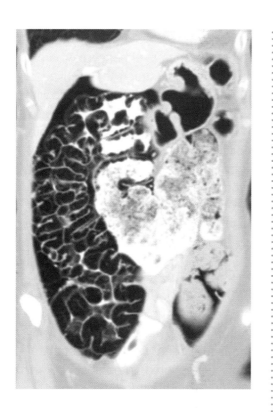

Pneumatosis intestinalis related to chemotherapy and steroids

Corticosteroids are the most common cause of medication-related pneumatosis. Steroids may result in atrophy of lymphoid tissue (Peyer patches), which compromises the integrity of the submucosa. This permits dissection of intraluminal gas into the intestinal wall. Several chemotherapeutic agents, including anti-angiogenic agents such as bevacizumab, cause pneumatosis by a similar mechanism. With these medications, however, the submucosa is likely compromised by microvascular ischemia rather than lymphoid atrophy. Pneumatosis is an indication for suspending bevacizumab. Pneumatosis cystoides coli is an idiopathic, benign condition with bubble-like pneumatosis of the colon. In non-ischemic pneumatosis, patients are typically asymptomatic and other CT signs of ischemia are absent. Coronal enhanced CT in lung windows shows copious gas within the colonic wall with near obliteration of the lumen.

Differential diagnosis of mesenteric ischemia

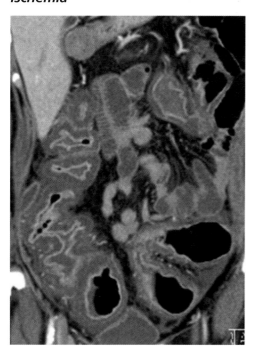

Infectious enterocolitis

Bowel infection tends to involve a long segment and, depending upon the cause, both small and large bowel may be affected. The haustral folds are typically maintained, unlike in ischemia. Clinical, laboratory, or pathologic correlation may be necessary for a definitive diagnosis. In this patient with diarrhea due to *C. difficile* pseudomembranous colitis, IV and oral contrast-enhanced CT shows thickening of the entire colonic wall with mucosal hyperemia.

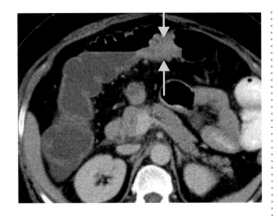

Colon carcinoma

Irregularity and heterogeneous enhancement are typical of colon cancer. In contrast, the involved segment in ischemia is typically homogeneous with smooth thickening. Bowel obstruction is more commonly caused by neoplasms than by ischemia. Enlarged pericolic lymph nodes should raise suspicion for colorectal cancer. Axial IV and oral contrast-enhanced CT shows "apple core" narrowing and heterogeneous enhancement of a focal segment (arrows) of transverse colon, with fluid-filled, slightly dilated obstructed proximal colon.

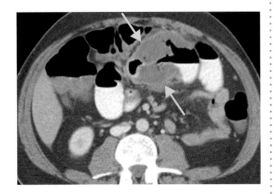

Small bowel lymphoma

Involvement of the small bowel with lymphoma typically features asymmetric, homogeneously enhancing wall thickening, although smooth wall thickening can also be seen. A characteristic feature of small bowel lymphoma is the absence of luminal obstruction despite marked bowel wall thickening (1.5–7 cm), leading to the classic "aneurysmal dilatation" of bowel. Axial IV and oral contrast-enhanced CT demonstrates marked, irregular, homogeneously enhancing mural thickening of a small bowel segment (arrows). There is relative sparing of the luminal diameter given the degree of wall thickening.

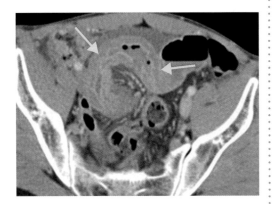

Submucosal hemorrhage

Anticoagulation is the most common cause of non-traumatic small bowel hematoma. Imaging findings of submucosal hemorrhage can mimic bowel ischemia, including homogeneous bowel wall thickening, a "double halo" or "target" sign on contrast-enhanced exams, and ascites (although the ascites due to submucosal hemorrhage may be higher in attenuation due to the presence of blood products). Short segment involvement with marked bowel wall thickening >1 cm favors submucosal hemorrhage. Clinical history (e.g., anticoagulation) may also help in the diagnosis. Axial enhanced CT demonstrates segmental mural thickening (arrows) and adjacent ascites, which are both nonspecific findings.

Further reading

Abbas, M. *et al*. Spontaneous Intramural Small-Bowel Hematoma: Imaging Findings and Outcome. *American Journal of Roentgenology*. 179:1389–1394 (2002).

Balthazar, E. *et al*. Closed-Loop and Strangulating Instestinal Obstruction: CT Signs. Radiology. 185:769–775 (1992).

Furukawa, A. *et al*. CT Diagnosis of Acute Mesenteric Ischemia from Various Causes. *American Journal of Roentgenology*. 192:408–416 (2009).

Ha, H. *et al*. Differentiation of Simple and Strangulated Small-Bowel Obstruction: Usefulness of Known CT Criteria. *Radiology*. 204:507–512 (1997).

Ho, L.M. *et al*. Pneumatosis Intestinalis in the Adult: Benign to Life-Threatening Causes. *American Journal of Roentgenology*. 188:1604–1613 (2007).

Kim, J.K. *et al*. CT Differentiation of Mesenteric Ischemia Due to Vasculitis and Thromboembolic Disease. *Journal of Computer Assisted Tomography*. 25(4):604–611 (2001).

Macari, M. *et al*. CT of Bowel Wall Thickening: Significance and Pitfalls of Interpretation. *American Journal of Roentgenology*. 176:1105–1116 (2001).

Macari, M. *et al*. Intestinal Ischemia Versus Intramural Hemorrhage: CT Evaluation. *American Journal of Roentgenology*. 180:177–184 (2003).

Rha, S.E. *et al*. CT and MR Imaging: Findings of Bowel Ischemia from Various Primary Causes. *Radiographics*. 20:29–42 (2000).

Taourel, P. *et al*. Helical CT of Large Bowel Obstruction. *Abdominal Imaging*. 2:267–275 (2003).

Taourel, P. *et al*. Imaging of Ischemic Colitis. *Radiologic Clinics of North America*. 46: 909–924 (2008).

Wiesner, W. *et al*. CT of Acute Bowel Ischemia. *Radiology*. 226:635–650 (2003).

Wiesner, W. *et al*. Pneumatosis Intestinalis and Portomesenteric Venous Gas in Intestinal Ischemia: Correlation of CT findings with Severity of Ischemia and Clinical Outcome. *American Journal of Roentgenology*. 177:1319–1323 (2001).

Zalcman, M. *et al*. Helical CT signs in the Diagnosis of Intestinal Ischemia in Small-Bowel Obstruction. *American Journal of Roentgenology*. 175:1601–1607(2000).

Case 23 45-year-old female presented with fever, leukocytosis, and pelvic pain

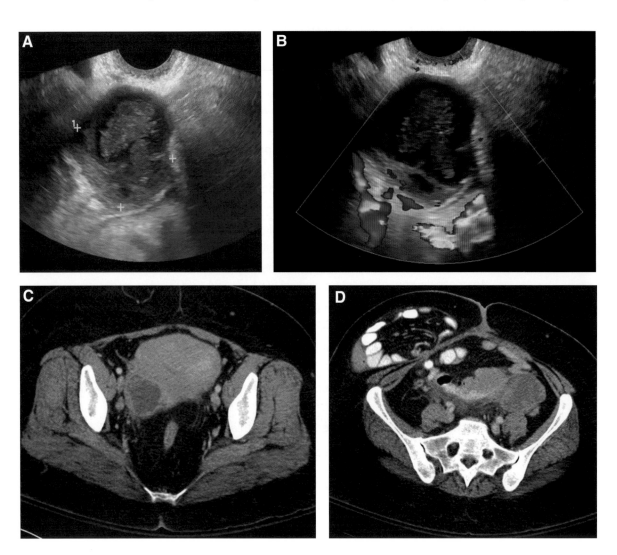

Diagnosis: Sagittal grayscale transvaginal ultrasound image of the right adnexa
Tubo-ovarian (A) demonstrates a complex right adnexal lesion (yellow arrows) that meas-
abscess (TOA) ures up to 5 cm. The lesion was inseparable from the ovarian parenchyma
at real-time imaging. Sagittal grayscale transvaginal ultrasound image with
color Doppler overlay (B) demonstrates peripheral blood flow.

Contrast-enhanced axial CT of the pelvis in the same patient demonstrates
corresponding bilateral adnexal complex fluid collections (red arrows) and
midline inflammatory fat stranding (blue arrow). Incidentally, there is a fibroid
uterus and an uncomplicated bowel-containing right ventral hernia.

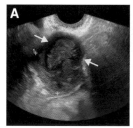 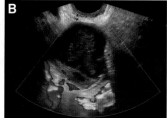 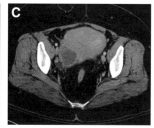 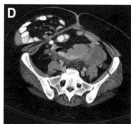

Discussion

Tubo-ovarian abscess (TOA) is pyogenic infection of the ovary and/or the fallopian tube.

- TOA is considered the most severe form of pelvic inflammatory disease (PID).
  Clinical signs and symptoms include abdominal or pelvic pain, fever,
  leukocytosis, and palpable mass.
- Causes of TOA include prior pelvic surgery, older intra-uterine devices such as
  the Dalkon shield, and infertility treatments.
- If left untreated, TOA is associated with abscess rupture, peritonitis, adhesion
  formation, chronic pelvic pain, and impaired fertility.

Ultrasound is the imaging test of choice for suspected TOA.

- The sensitivity of ultrasound is approximately 82% and specificity is up to 90%.
- The typical appearance of TOA is a predominantly hypoechoic, complex cystic,
  thick-walled adnexal mass.
- CT or MRI can be helpful problem-solving modalities. CT is used if ultrasound
  demonstrates nonspecific or atypical findings, or if initial therapy is ineffective.
  In comparison to ultrasound, MRI is capable of demonstrating smaller
  amounts of fluid and may better demonstrate fluid-filled fallopian tubes and
  abscesses in some cases.

Treatment decisions vary based on clinical picture.

- Medical management includes administration of broad-spectrum IV antibiotics
  with anaerobic coverage.

- If there is no clinical improvement within 2–3 days, ultrasound- or CT-guided drainage may be performed.
- Laparotomy may be indicated if ruptured TOA is suspected, if perforated viscus cannot be excluded from the differential diagnosis, or if hysterectomy or salpingo-oopherectomy is necessary.

Clinical synopsis

The patient underwent CT-guided drainage of bilateral TOAs, and approximately 100 mL of purulent fluid was aspirated from the right-sided collection.

Self-assessment

- *Name two imaging findings that may distinguish TOA from abscesses caused by other pelvic processes such as appendicitis or diverticulitis.*

- Anterior displacement of a thickened broad ligament and ill-defined uterine border suggest adnexal origin.

Spectrum of tubo-ovarian abscess

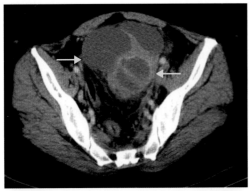

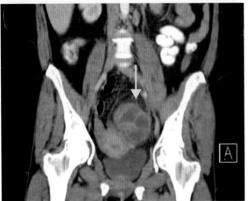

CT imaging of TOA

CT is utilized to determine extent of disease and assess complications. It is also indicated when the patient is not responding to antibiotic therapy or for planning in cases where drainage catheter placement is being considered. Internal foci of gas are specific for abscess; however, they are not often seen in TOA. Secondary CT findings include adjacent fat stranding, indistinct margins of nearby bowel loops, and thickening of the broad ligament. Axial and coronal contrast-enhanced CT images of the pelvis demonstrate a thick-walled, septated, low-density adnexal mass (arrows).

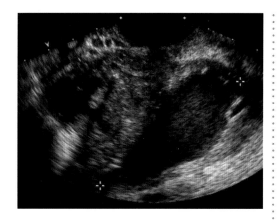

Ultrasound imaging of TOA

Grayscale sagittal transvaginal ultrasound imaging in a 26-year-old woman with a history of chronic pelvic inflammatory disorder shows a dilated, thick-walled, debris-filled structure (calipers), consistent with pyosalpinx. Additional ultrasound imaging findings of pyosalpinx (not shown) include incomplete septa originating from one wall that do not reach the other side and the "beads on a string appearance" due to flattening and degeneration of endosalpingeal fold remnants.

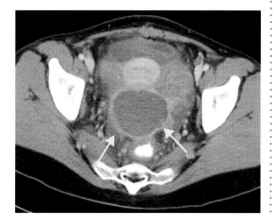

TOA in a patient with Crohn's disease

Two axial contrast-enhanced CT images from a patient with Crohn's disease demonstrate a large central pelvic abscess (arrows) with lateral extension in a tubular configuration suggesting involvement of both fallopian tubes.

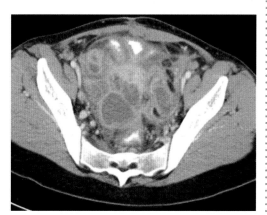

Differential diagnosis of tubo-ovarian abscess

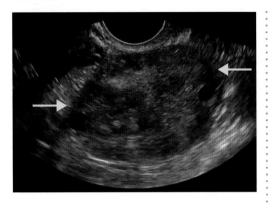

Ovarian torsion

The sonographic distinction between torsion and other adnexal masses can be difficult or even impossible unless there is high clinical suspicion. Patterns of Doppler flow are not specific. A lead point mass may be present, adding further confusion to the imaging appearance. A mass acting as a lead point is more common in adults than in children, who often experience torsion without underlying ovarian disease. Grayscale sagittal transvaginal US image of the right ovary shows an enlarged ovary (arrows) with peripheral follicles in this patient with ovarian torsion.

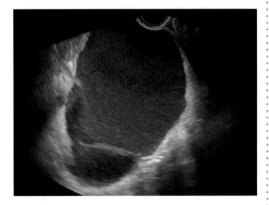

Endometrioma

Endometriomas are composed of ectopic endometrial tissue that is found outside of the uterus. There may be internal septations and wall nodularity. MR imaging (not shown) demonstrates a T1 hyperintense lesion with "shading" on T2-weighted imaging, representing hemorrhagic material that has accumulated due to cyclical bleeding. Grayscale transverse transvaginal ultrasound image of the right adnexa shows a large right ovarian mass with homogeneous low-level internal echoes in a patient with an ovarian endometrioma.

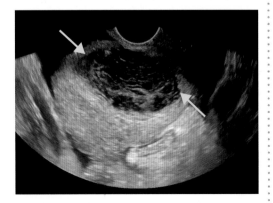

Hemorrhagic cyst

Hemorrhagic cysts occur because of hemorrhage into an ovarian cyst (follicular or corpus luteum) and may be associated with hemoperitoneum if the cyst ruptures. On MRI (not shown), these cysts may demonstrate T1 intermediate to high signal blood products. Treatment is supportive. Grayscale sagittal transvaginal ultrasound image of the left adnexa demonstrates the typical appearance of a hemorrhagic cyst (arrows) with reticular, lacy fibrin strands and internal clot.

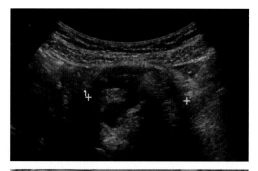

Ovarian neoplasm (germ cell tumor; dermoid)

Ovarian dermoids are benign and account for 10–15% of ovarian neoplasms. They consist of mature tissue from at least two germ cell layers. Grayscale transverse transvaginal ultrasound of the right adnexa (upper image) demonstrates a solid and cystic right adnexal mass (calipers) with posterior acoustic shadowing ("tip of the iceberg" sign). Axial T1 pre-contrast imaging without (middle image) and with (lower image) fat saturation demonstrates the same mass positioned in the anterior central pelvis (arrows). There are areas of T1 shortening within the mass that lose signal with fat suppression, consistent with mature cystic teratoma (ovarian dermoid).

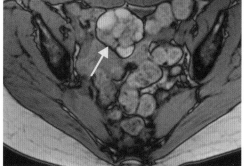

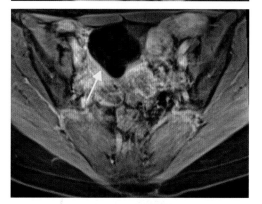

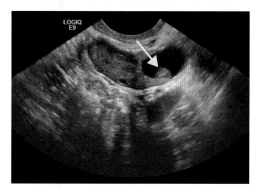

Ovarian epithelial neoplasm (serous cystadenoma)

The majority of ovarian neoplasms (>90%) originate from epithelial cells, with serous cystadenoma/cystadenocarcinoma being the most common. MRI is often obtained for further characterization of an ovarian mass. Ovarian malignancies typically demonstrate solid enhancing components on MR. Grayscale sagittal transvaginal ultrasound image of the left ovary demonstrates an exophytic, hypoechoic mass with a mural nodule (arrow), pathologically proven to be a serous cystadenoma. The solid nodule demonstrated vascularity on color Doppler (not shown).

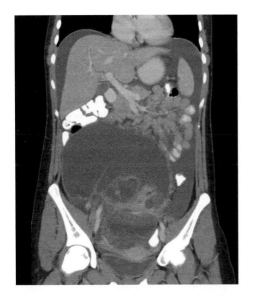

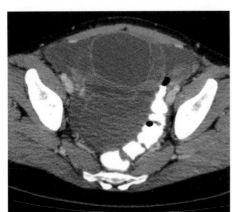

Ovarian epithelial neoplasm (mucinous cystadenoma)

Mucinous ovarian tumors are the second most common epithelial neoplasm. The tumors are variable in size but are often large, with extension into the upper abdomen as seen in this case. On ultrasound, findings include multilocular cystic masses with low-level echoes. MRI of the mass may demonstrate variable signal intensity on both T1- and T2-weighted imaging, with a "stained glass" appearance. Coronal and axial contrast-enhanced CT of the abdomen and pelvis demon-strates a large, multiloculated cystic mass with enhancing septations, and extensive low-density peritoneal fluid.

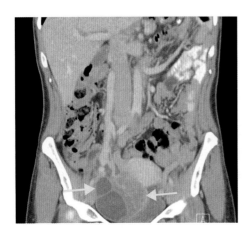

Ovarian neoplasm (metastasis; Krukenberg tumor)

The most common malignancies to metastasize to the ovary are colon and gastric carcinoma. Specifically, Krukenberg tumors have signet cells that secrete mucin. They can be distinguished from primary ovarian malignancies by bilaterality, dense stromal reaction (which is often T1 and T2 hypointense), and mucinous components (which demonstrate T2 hyperintensity). Contrast-enhanced coronal CT demonstrates a complex, cystic and solid mass in the right adnexa (arrows) in a patient with a history of gastric cancer, consistent with Krukenberg tumor.

Further reading

Bennet *et al.*, "Gynecologic Causes of Acute Pelvic Pain: Spectrum of CT Findings," *Radiographics* 2002, 22:785.

Jung *et al.*, "CT and MR Imaging of Ovarian Tumors with Emphasis on Differential Diagnosis," *Radiographics* 2002, 22:1305–1325.

Kaakaji *et al.*, "Sonography of Obstetric and Gynecological Emergencies," *AJR* 2000, 174:651.

Shulman *et al.*, "Percutaneous Catheter Drainage of Tuboovarian Abscess," *Obstet Gynecol* 1992, 80:55.

28-year-old female presented with abnormal vaginal bleeding and a positive pregnancy test

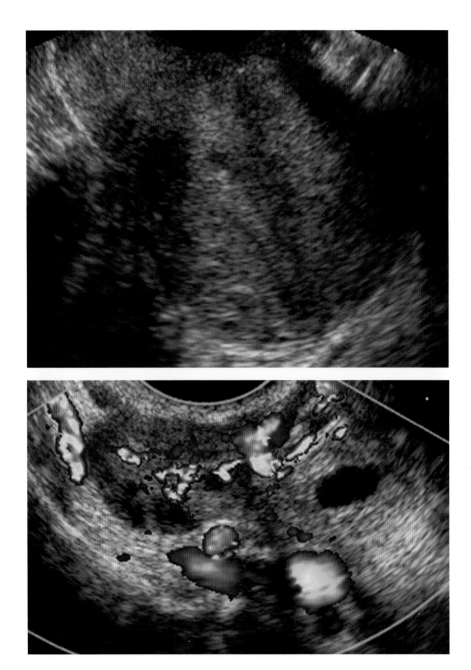

Diagnosis:
Ectopic
pregnancy

Grayscale transvaginal transverse ultrasound view of the uterus demonstrates no intrauterine gestational sac. The echogenic endometrial stripe is thin and linear (yellow arrow). Transvaginal ultrasound of the right adnexa with color Doppler overlay demonstrates an echogenic, ring-shaped ectopic gestational sac in the right adnexa (red arrow) that is separate from and medial to the right ovary (blue arrow). There is Doppler flow within the wall.

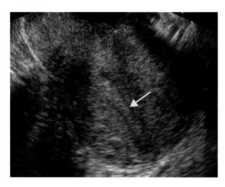 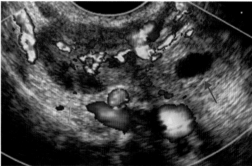

Discussion

Ectopic pregnancy is the most common cause of pregnancy-related mortality in the first trimester.

- Approximately 2% of all pregnancies are ectopic.
- Risk factors include prior ectopic pregnancy, history of gynecologic surgery, infertility, in vitro fertilization, endometriosis, history of placenta previa, intrauterine device, and smoking.
- A history of pelvic pain along with a positive beta human chorionic gonadotropin (β-hCG) level should trigger an evaluation for ectopic pregnancy.

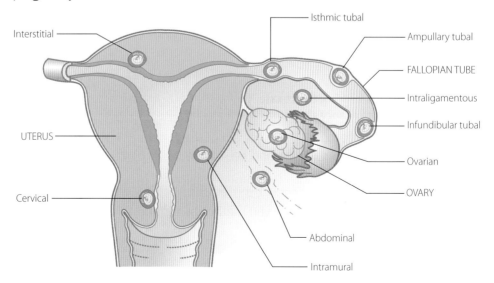

In addition to measurement of the β-hCG level, initial evaluation must include pelvic ultrasonography.

- The fallopian tube is the most common location for an ectopic pregnancy (95%).
- Within the fallopian tube, the ampulla is the most common site (70–80%).
- Unusual sites that are important to consider are the uterine cornua and cervix.

The most common sonographic sign of ectopic pregnancy is the "tubal ring" sign, which is an adnexal mass that does not contain a yolk sac or embryo (seen in 89–100% of ectopic pregnancies). This sign is also highly specific.

- An adnexal mass containing a yolk sac or embryo with a heartbeat is less common, but pathognomonic for ectopic pregnancy.
- Doppler flow at the periphery of a tubal ring (the "ring of fire" sign) is not specific for ectopic pregnancy and may be seen with physiologic corpus lutea. Corpus lutea are common in normal intrauterine pregnancies. Demonstrating that a non-ovarian adnexal lesion is separable from the ovary on real-time exam with pressure from the ultrasound transducer raises specificity by differentiating it from a primary ovarian mass such as a corpus luteum.

It is important to remember that a positive β-hCG without a detectable intrauterine gestational sac or with a nonspecific-appearing endometrial fluid collection (sometimes referred to as a "pseudo-gestational sac") does not equate to ectopic pregnancy.

- If the patient is clinically stable, a follow-up study should be scheduled in 3–7 days (depending on the clinical setting), as these findings may be seen in early intrauterine pregnancies.
- If the radiologist is not mindful of this consideration, some patients may be treated with methotrexate with resultant loss of desired pregnancy at this stage.

Following treatment with methotrexate, falling ß-hCG is a more accurate indicator of treatment success in ectopic pregnancy than ultrasound appearance.

- An ectopic pregnancy successfully treated with methotrexate may initially increase in size and even vascularity before involuting.

Clinical synopsis   The patient received methotrexate and the serum β-hCG level fell to zero.

Self-assessment

- *What is the most common location for an ectopic pregnancy?*

- *Name three signs of ectopic pregnancy in order of specificity.*

- *True or false: following methotrexate administration, an ectopic pregnancy may enlarge and Doppler flow may increase.*

- The ampullary portion of the fallopian tube.

- Adnexal ring containing a yolk sac or live embryo, empty tubal adnexal ring, complex adnexal mass.

- True. Falling β-hCG is a more reliable indicator of therapeutic success than changing sonographic appearance.

Spectrum of ectopic pregnancy

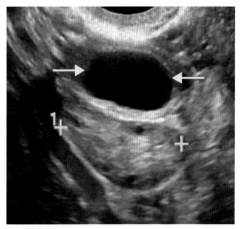

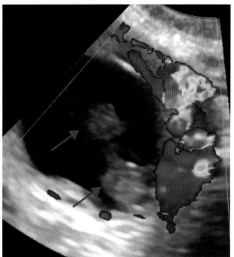

Twin ectopic pregnancy

This patient presented with pelvic pain and a positive pregnancy test. Transvaginal ultrasound demonstrates a cystic lesion (yellow arrows) superficial to the right ovary (between calipers), which was shown to contain two embryo-like structures (red arrows). There is Doppler flow within the wall. No cardiac activity was identified. In a patient with a serum β-hCG level <4000 mIU/mL, if an ectopic pregnancy is less than 3.5 to 4 cm in diameter and lacks embryonic cardiac activity, the patient may receive methotrexate therapy rather than surgical intervention. In select cases, watchful waiting is the initial strategy chosen by the obstetrician-gynecologist.

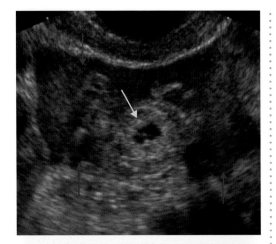

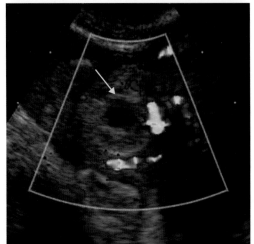

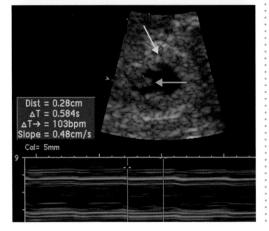

Ruptured ectopic pregnancy

This patient presented with pelvic pain, vaginal bleeding, and a positive pregnancy test. Grayscale and color Doppler ultrasound demonstrates a cystic structure in the right adnexa (yellow arrows), with extensive surrounding complex hemorrhagic fluid (red arrows). The cystic structure contained an embryo with heart rate of 103 beats per minute (blue arrow). Ruptured ectopic pregnancy is considered a surgical emergency.

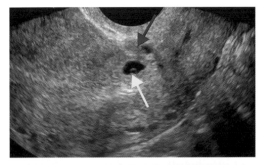

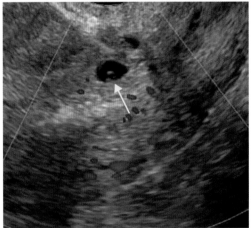

Cesarean section scar ectopic pregnancy

This patient with a prior history of cesarean section presented with pelvic pain and a positive pregnancy test. Grayscale and color Doppler ultrasound demonstrate a normally shaped intra-uterine gestational sac with a yolk sac (yellow arrow) located in the lower uterine segment, with bulging, thin covering anterior myometrium (red arrow), at the cesarean section myometrial scar. No embryo or heartbeat was present. Feared complications of cesarean section scar ectopic include uterine rupture and massive hemorrhage. Treatments include injection of methotrexate or potassium chloride into the gestational sac (along with systemic methotrexate therapy), and surgical resection or hysterectomy.

Differential diagnosis of ectopic pregnancy

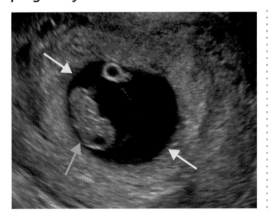

Intrauterine pregnancy

The presence of an intrauterine pregnancy and normal adnexa (not shown) reliably excludes an ectopic pregnancy. Grayscale ultrasound of a normal intrauterine pregnancy shows an intrauter-ine gestational sac (yellow arrows), which contains a yolk sac (red arrow) and an embryo (blue arrow).

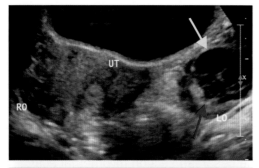

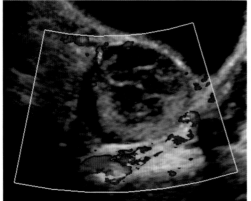

Hemorrhagic corpus luteum (hemorrhagic cyst)

It is important to consider physiologic corpus lutea, which are frequently present in normal intrauterine pregnancies, in the differential diagnosis of ectopic pregnancy. Hemorrhagic corpus lutea share imaging features with other hemorrhagic ovarian cysts, such as web-like internal echoes. This 25-year-old female with a negative pregnancy test presented with pelvic pain. Grayscale ultrasound with color Doppler demonstrates a complex cystic structure (yellow arrow) arising from the left ovary (red arrow), with surrounding flow seen on color Doppler. This was inseparable from the ovary at real-time exam.

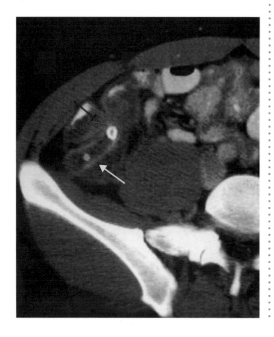

Acute appendicitis

In a young female patient presenting with abdominal or pelvic pain, acute appendicitis should always be considered; however, a pregnancy test should generally be obtained prior to imaging. Ultrasound may be the initial investigation of choice in many young patients with suspected appendicitis – it can be very effective in experienced hands to identify an abnormal appendix, especially in thin patients. CT is highly sensitive and specific and is often employed if the normal appendix is not evident by ultrasound. In a patient with pelvic pain, axial contrast-enhanced CT demonstrated a blind-ending tubular structure with mucosal hyperenhancement (yellow arrow), surrounding stranding, and an obstructing appendicolith (red arrow).

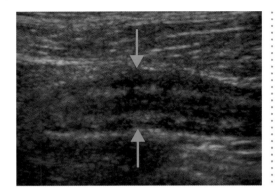

Right lower quadrant transabdominal ultrasound in a different patient demonstrates a hypoechoic, blind-ending, tubular structure with thickened walls (blue arrows). This was noncompressible, with mural hyperemia (not shown).

Further reading

Atri M, Leduc C, Gillett P, *et al.* Role of endovaginal sonography in the diagnosis and management of ectopic pregnancy. *Radiographics* 1996; 16: 755–774.

Bhatt S, Ghazale H, Dogra VS. Sonographic evaluation of ectopic pregnancy. *Radiol Clin North Am* 2007; 45: 549–560.

Blaivas M, Lyon M. Reliability of adnexal mass mobility in distinguishing possible ectopic pregnancy from corpus luteum cysts. *J Ultrasound Med* 2005; 24: 599–603.

Dogra V, Paspulati RM, Bhatt S. First trimester bleeding evaluation. *Ultrasound* 2005; 21: 69–85.

Eyvazzadeh AD, Levine D. Imaging of pelvic pain in the first trimester of pregnancy. *Radiol Clin North Am* 2006; 44: 863–877.

Levine D. Ectopic pregnancy. *Radiology* 2007; 245: 385–397.

Lin EP, Bhatt S, Dogra V. Diagnostic clues to ectopic pregnancy. *Radiographics* 2008; 28: 1661–1671.

Lipscomb GH, Stovall TG, Ling FW. Nonsurgical treatment of ectopic pregnancy. *N Engl J Med* 2000; 343: 1325–1329.

Paspulati RM, Bhatt S, Nour S. Sonographic evaluation of first-trimester bleeding. *Radiol Clin North Am* 2004; 42: 297–314.

Webb EM, Green GE, Scoutt LM. Adnexal mass with pelvic pain. *Radiol Clin North Am* 2004; 42: 329–348.

Case 25   38-year-old female with abdominal pain

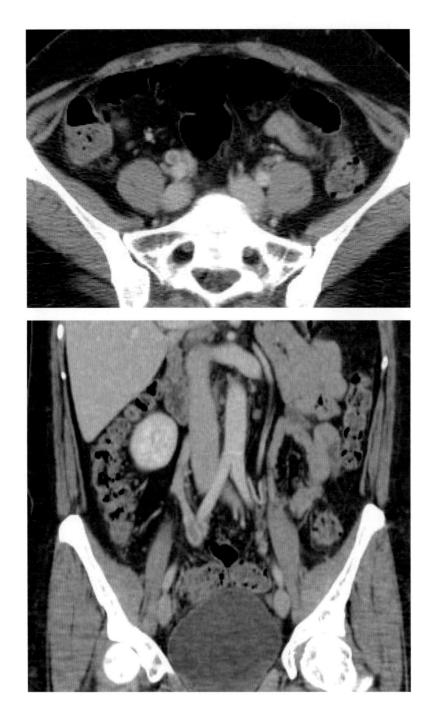

Diagnosis: **Gonadal (ovarian) vein thrombosis**

Contrast-enhanced axial (left image) and coronal (right image) CT demonstrate a non-occlusive, linear filling defect in the right gonadal vein (arrows).

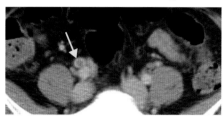 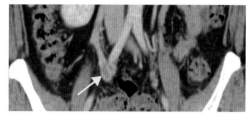

Discussion

Overview of ovarian vein thrombosis

- Ovarian vein thrombosis is a rare but serious condition that may occur in the postpartum period or in patients with PID, malignancy, or recent pelvic surgery.
- Patients with ovarian vein thrombosis may be asymptomatic or present with vague abdominal pain and fever; if the condition is untreated, pulmonary embolism, sepsis, or even death may result.
- Mainstays of treatment include intravenous antibiotics and therapeutic anticoagulation. In some cases, surgery may be indicated to treat the underlying condition.
- Ovarian veins arise from the broad ligament and extend superiorly in the retroperitoneum, anterior to the psoas muscle. The right gonadal vein enters the IVC directly, whereas the left gonadal vein drains into the left renal vein.

Ovarian vein thrombosis can be detected using ultrasound or cross-sectional imaging modalities such as CT or MRI.

- Ultrasound is often used as the first-line imaging test, given its wide availability – however, it has lower sensitivity and specificity than MRI or CT. The typical ultrasound appearance is an enlarged vein with an intraluminal, echogenic filling defect.
- On contrast-enhanced CT, a gonadal vein thrombus may appear as a central filling defect within the opacified vein. When occluded, the thrombosed vein may appear as a non-enhancing tubular structure in the retroperitoneum. In some cases, the vein may be enlarged with surrounding inflammatory fat stranding. Multiplanar imaging helps distinguish the ovarian vein from other tubular structures such as the appendix, ureter, and bowel.
- MRI findings include a variable-signal-intensity filling defect on T1-weighted contrast-enhanced images and an intermediate to high signal thrombus with a dark peripheral rim (hemosiderin) on T2-weighted images.

Self-assessment

- *Why does gonadal vein thrombosis most often affect the right-sided vein?*

- The right-sided vein is affected in up to 90% of cases. This is likely multifactorial, due to longer length, less competent valves, and decreased retrograde flow relative to the left-sided veins.

- *What is the limitation of CT in assessing the extent of ovarian vein thrombosis?*

- Mixing of contrast within the IVC at the level of the renal veins can cause false positive filling defects within the vessel on CT. MRI can be used to assess the superior extent of ovarian vein thrombosis at the level of the IVC.

Spectrum of gonadal vein thrombosis

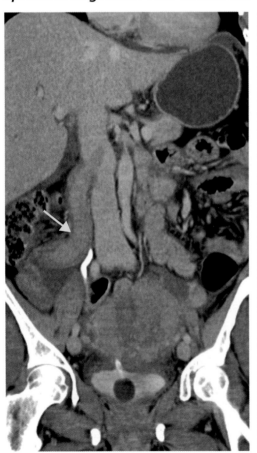

Severe gonadal vein thrombosis

A 25-year-old female patient presented with pain after C-section. Contrast-enhanced coronal (upper), axial (middle), and sagittal (lower) CT images demonstrate a markedly dilated right ovarian vein (arrows) with thrombus extending to the confluence of the right ovarian vein with the IVC. Note that the right ovarian vein drains directly into the IVC, while the left gonadal vein drains into the left renal vein. The index case is a more subtle example.

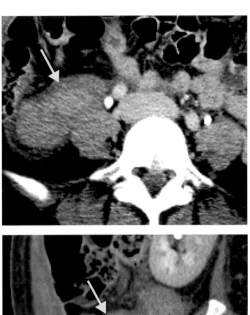

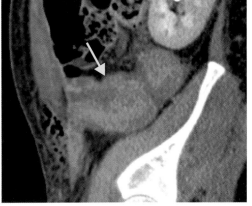

Differential diagnosis of gonadal vein thrombosis

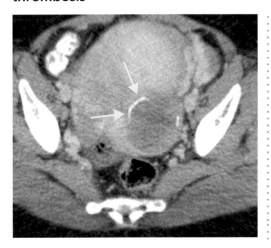

Degenerating fibroid

This 44-year-old female presented with pelvic pain and vaginal bleeding due to a degenerating uterine fibroid. Contrast-enhanced axial pelvic CT demonstrates non-uniform enhancement of a left-sided fibroid due to hypodense central necrosis. The rim is partially calcified (arrows).

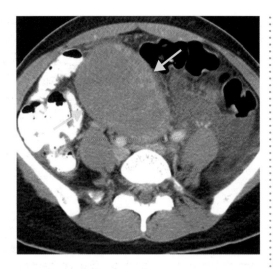

Gynecological malignancy

This 54-year-old female presented with abdominal pain. Axial contrast-enhanced CT demonstrates a large, heterogeneous mass (arrows) in the right hemipelvis with nodular enhancement along its left lateral margin. This mass was found to arise from the right ovary (not pictured). Systematic identification of pelvic blood vessels may help distinguish organ-based masses from thrombosed veins.

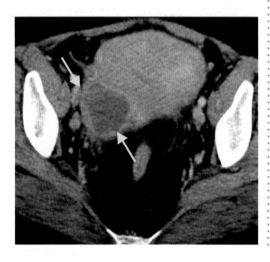

Tubo-ovarian abscess

This 45-year-old female presented with fever, leukocytosis, and pelvic pain from a tubo-ovarian abscess. Axial contrast-enhanced pelvic CT demonstrates a right-sided complex adnexal fluid collection with thick, enhancing walls (arrows). The right ovary could not be separately identified. Both tubo-ovarian abscess and gonadal vein thrombosis may be non-enhancing, hypo-attenuating, serpiginous, and masslike.

Further reading

Bennet *et al.*, "Gynecologic Causes of Acute Pelvic Pain: Spectrum of CT Findings," *Radiographics* 2002, 22: 785.

Karaosmanoglu *et al.*, "MDCT of the Ovarian Vein: Normal Anatomy and Pathology" *AJR* 2009, 192: 295–299.

Sharma, P., Abdi, S., "Ovarian Vein Thrombosis" *Clinical Radiology* 2012, 67: 893–898.

Case 26   25-year-old female presented with nausea, vomiting, and
left abdominal pain

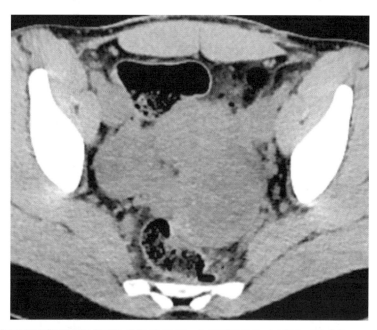

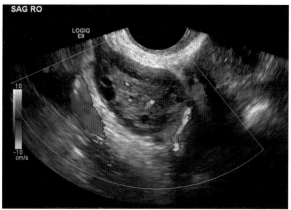

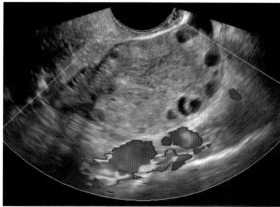

Diagnosis: **Left ovarian torsion in a patient with polycystic ovarian syndrome (PCOS)**	Axial noncontrast abdominal CT demonstrates enlargement of both ovaries (arrows) in this patient with a history of polycystic ovarian syndrome (PCOS). The left ovary is slightly larger than the right. Grayscale and color Doppler ultrasound images of each ovary (right ovary: middle image; left ovary: right image) in the same patient demonstrate enlarged ovaries with multiple small peripheral follicles ("string of pearls" sign). The left ovary appears enlarged and heterogeneously echogenic compared to the right, with absent blood flow.

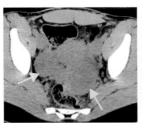 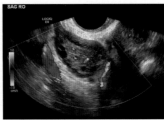 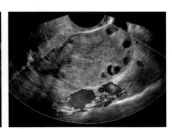

Discussion

Ovarian torsion is most common in women of reproductive age, and 20% of cases occur during pregnancy.

- Ovarian masses (acting as "lead points") and other conditions that result in ovarian enlargement predispose to torsion. In cases without a lead point, ligamentous laxity or vascular tortuosity may be risk factors. The risk of ovarian torsion during the first trimester of pregnancy is increased due to the corpus luteum, which acts as a lead point.
- Women undergoing fertility treatments are also at increased risk due to enlargement of numerous follicles, especially with concomitant ovarian hyperstimulation syndrome (OHSS).
- Torsion of the normal ovary can occur in prepubescent females because of adnexal hypermobility, usually on the right side.

Ovarian torsion may have a nonspecific clinical presentation of pelvic pain, nausea, and vomiting. Symptoms may be intermittent.

- There is symptomatic overlap with many mimickers, including appendicitis, gastroenteritis, pelvic inflammatory disease, ectopic pregnancy, and ruptured ovarian cyst.

Ultrasound is the most sensitive imaging modality for ovarian torsion, and, hence, the modality of choice in most scenarios where torsion is suspected.

- As a general rule, ovarian torsion is extremely rare when the ovary is normal in size, echogenicity, and position. The most common imaging finding is

asymmetric enlargement of one ovary due to venous congestion, with peripheralization of follicles.
- A cystic or mass-like structure interposed between the uterus and bladder is highly suggestive of torsion.
- Free pelvic fluid is present in up to two-thirds of cases.
- Common CT and MR imaging features include fallopian tube thickening, smooth wall thickening of a cystic adnexal mass that appears twisted, ascites, uterine deviation to the side of the abnormal adnexa, and an adnexal mass rotated out of the pelvis to the contralateral side of midline.

Color and spectral Doppler analysis is neither sensitive nor specific, but is routinely performed.
- Normal ovaries may have no detectable Doppler signal due to technical factors, while blood flow or even hyperemia may be seen in an ovary that is undergoing intermittent torsion with transient vascular obstruction.
- The sonographic "twisted vascular pedicle" or "whirlpool" sign is highly suggestive of torsion. A twisted pedicle may only be visible with Doppler overlay. Absence of flow in the twisted pedicle, or flow in only the artery and not the vein may be seen in cases of torsion.

The most common treatment for ovarian torsion is laparoscopic surgery with manual detorsion and removal of any underlying mass that has acted as a lead point.
- In patients who have experienced torsion, there is a 10% increased incidence of torsion in the contralateral adnexa at another point in time.

Clinical synopsis Laparoscopy confirmed left ovarian torsion, and the left ovary was detorsed.

Self-assessment

- *List three risk factors for ovarian torsion.*

- *True or false:* demonstrating absence or presence of blood flow by color and spectral Doppler ultrasound has proven reliable for definitive diagnosis or exclusion of ovarian torsion.

- Ovarian mass, OHSS from hormonal therapy for in vitro fertilization, pregnancy (with a corpus luteum acting as a lead point), adnexal hyper-mobility, vascular tortuosity.

- False. Detectable flow may be present in a torsed ovary and absent in a non-torsed ovary.

- *What is the most reliable sonographic sign of ovarian torsion?*

- The "whirlpool" sign of a twisted vascular pedicle. Another classic ultrasound sign is a large, echogenic ovary with peripheralized follicles.

Spectrum of ovarian torsion

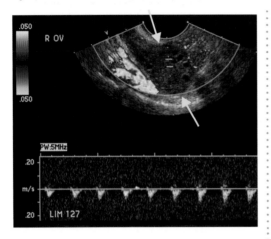

Right ovarian torsion with preserved arterial flow

Color and spectral Doppler ultrasound in a patient with right-sided pelvic pain demonstrates asymmetric enlargement and hyperechogenicity of the right ovary (arrows). There is diminished arterial perfusion with absence of diastolic flow of the right ovary. In torsion, venous congestion leads to ovarian edema, which is generally followed by progressive arterial compromise.

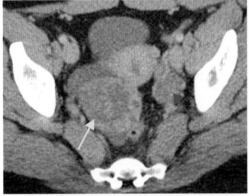

Right ovarian torsion with complete absence of flow

This 25-year-old female presented with acute right lower quadrant pain. Contrast-enhanced axial CT demonstrates a markedly enlarged, heterogeneous right ovary (yellow arrow) with surrounding fluid. The left ovary (red arrow) is normal in size. Color Doppler ultrasound demonstrates an enlarged, avascular, heterogeneously echogenic right ovary with small peripheral follicles. The diagnosis of ovarian torsion was confirmed intraoperatively.

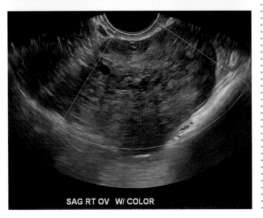

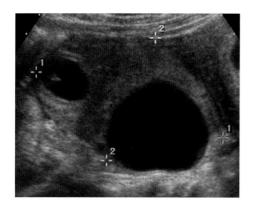

Torsion in a patient with ovarian hyperstimulation syndrome (OHSS)

This patient with a history of pharmacologic ovarian stimulation for treatment of infertility presented with pelvic pain. Grayscale transvaginal ultrasound image demonstrates an enlarged (9 cm) right ovary containing multiple hypoechoic cysts and intervening edematous stroma. OHSS is a serious complication of pharmacologic ovulation induction. Early in the course, there is mild ovarian enlargement with abdominal discomfort. Later, there is marked enlargement of the ovaries, with pelvic pain, abdominal distention, nausea, and vomiting. The typical sonographic finding is bilaterally enlarged ovaries with multiple large cysts that produce a "spoke wheel" appearance. Pregnant patients with OHSS have a greater risk of torsion (16%) than those who are not pregnant. Separation of the cystic elements by the markedly edematous stroma may indicate torsion of the hyperstimulated ovary.

Right ovarian torsion in a pregnant patient

This 15-week-pregnant 26-year-old female with right ovarian torsion presented with acute pelvic pain. Axial (upper image) and coronal T2-weighted MRI demonstrate an enlarged, edematous, torsed right ovary (yellow arrows) in the right posterior pelvis. A corpus luteum is seen as an intermediate-signal-intensity ring within the ovary (red arrow). Gestational sac (blue arrows) is partially visualized.

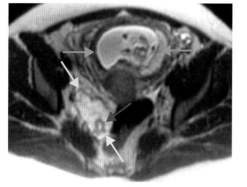

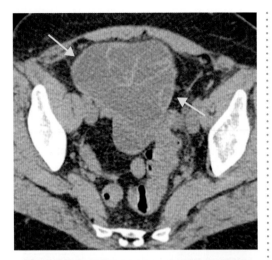

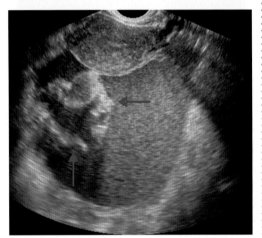

Left ovarian torsion mimicking neoplasm

In a 46-year-old female with acute-onset left abdominal pain, axial unenhanced CT demonstrates a midline multicystic lesion (arrows) with internal septations. Grayscale ultrasound demonstrates a predominantly cystic mass with diffuse low-level echoes and solid elements (red arrows) arising from the left ovary. Intraoperative and histologic findings demonstrated infarcted and hemorrhagic ovarian tissue.

Differential diagnosis of ovarian torsion

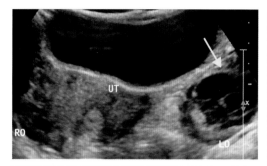

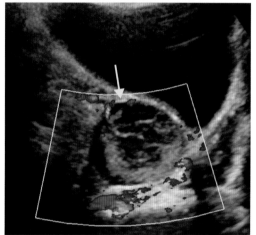

Hemorrhagic cyst

Hemorrhagic ovarian cysts are sometimes referred to as a "great imitator" owing to their various imaging appearance. They typically result from bleeding into a corpus luteum or follicular cyst and mainly occur in premenopausal women. The appearance depends on stage of bleeding, which follows a predictable pattern: active hemorrhage, clot formation, retraction, and resolution. The most typical sonographic appearance of hemorrhagic cyst is an avascular cyst with a fine reticular pattern or "fishnet" appearance, which is produced by crossing fibrin strands. A retracting blood clot may be seen as an echogenic focus within an otherwise anechoic cyst. A fluid-fluid or fluid-debris level may be visualized when blood products separate. Follow-up ultrasound is usually performed in 6 to 8 weeks to ensure resolution. In a patient with pelvic pain, grayscale and color Doppler ultrasound demonstrate a complex cystic structure (yellow arrows) arising from the left ovary (LO), with a characteristic fine reticular internal echo pattern.

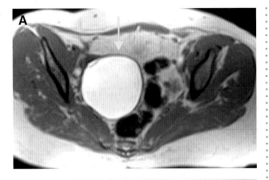

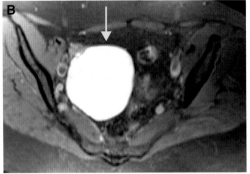

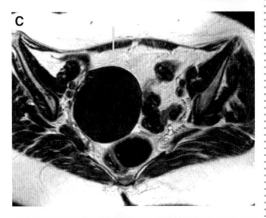

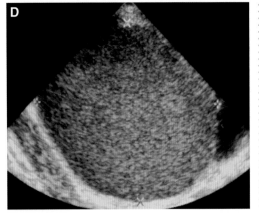

Endometrioma

An endometrioma is a cyst that contains blood products produced by extra-uterine endometrial tissue. Endometriomas usually arise from the ovary and are often bilateral. The finding of an endometrioma should prompt a thorough search of the pelvis for other ectopic endometrial deposits. Axial T1-weighted MR images without (A), and with, fat suppression (B), demonstrate a round, homogeneously hyperintense pelvic mass (arrows). High signal persisting on fat suppression indicates that the hyperintense contents are blood products rather than fat. The mass is low signal on the T2-weighted image (C). Grayscale transvaginal ultrasound image (D) demonstrates the typical sonographic appearance of a rounded mass with diffuse, low-level echoes.

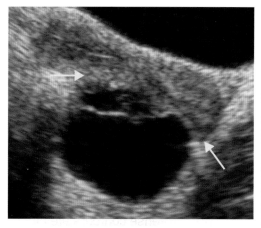

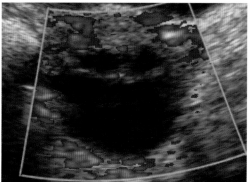

Serous cystadenoma

Ovarian cystadenomas are benign epithelial neoplasms that occur in women of reproductive age. They are bilateral in up to 20% of cases. Typically, imaging shows large, unilocular, thin-walled cystic lesions with thin septations or papillary projections. Cystadenocarcinomas are the malignant counterparts of serous cystadenoma. Resection is the treatment of choice for both benign and malignant epithelial lesions. Grayscale and spectral Doppler transvaginal ultrasound demonstrate a complex cyst with an internal septation arising from the left ovary (arrows). Blood flow is demonstrated in the ovarian parenchyma and within the septation.

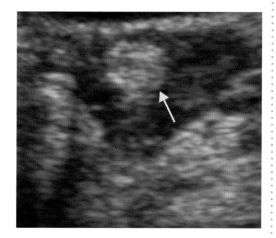

Dermoid cyst

"Dermoid cyst" is a synonym for "mature cystic ovarian teratoma." Dermoids are the most common benign ovarian tumor in females younger than 45 years of age. Detection of fat within the ovary in a young female by any imaging modality is highly suggestive of dermoid. Grayscale transvaginal ultrasound demonstrates a well-circumscribed echogenic focus in the left ovary (arrow), with minimal posterior acoustic shadowing. This finding is known as a "dermoid plug" or "Rokitansky nodule." This echogenic area within the dermoid is thought to represent sebaceous material within the cystic cavity.

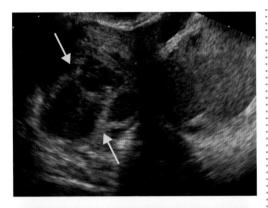

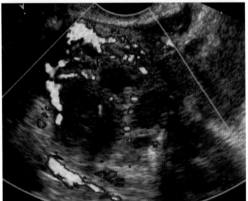

Pelvic inflammatory disease (tubo-ovarian abscess)

Pelvic inflammatory disease is infection of the adnexa and uterus typically caused by sexually transmitted disease. Acute complications include tubo-ovarian abscess, pyosalpinx, and peritonitis. Pelvic sonograms are frequently normal in early infection and in uncomplicated cases. In severe or advanced cases, sonographic findings include endometrial thickening with or without endometrial fluid and gas, ovarian enlargement with indistinctness of the ovarian borders, uterine enlargement with indistinctness of the uterine contour, and free intraperitoneal fluid. Grayscale and color Doppler transvaginal ultrasound in a patient with right lower quadrant pain and fever demonstrate a complex cystic structure (arrows) with internal echoes and thick septations, with mural and septal vascularity.

Further reading

Chang HC, Bhatt S, Dogra VS. Pearls and pitfalls in diagnosis of ovarian torsion. *Radiographics.* 2008;28(5):1355–1368.

Bennett GL, Slywotzky CM, Giovanniello G. Gynecologic causes of acute pelvic pain: spectrum of CT findings. *Radiographics.* 2002; 22(4): 785–801.

Rha SE, Byun JY, Jung SE, *et al.* CT and MR imaging features of adnexal torsion. *Radiographics.* 2002; 22(2): 283–294.

Chiou SY, Lev-Toaff AS, Masuda E, Feld RI, Bergin D. Adnexal torsion: new clinical and imaging observations by sonography, computed tomography, and magnetic resonance imaging. *J Ultrasound Med.* 2007;26(10): 1289–1301.

Singh A, Danrad R, Hahn PF, Blake MA, Mueller PR, Novelline RA. MR imaging of the acute abdomen and pelvis: acute appendicitis and beyond. *Radiographics.* 2007;27 (5):1419–1431.

Hiller N, Appelbaum L, Simanovsky N, Lev-Sagi A, Aharoni D, Sella T. CT features of adnexal torsion. *AJR Am J Roentgenol.* 2007;189(1):124–129.

Durfee SM, Frates MC. Sonographic spectrum of the corpus luteum in early pregnancy: gray-scale, color, and pulsed Doppler appearance. *J Clin Ultrasound* 1999; 27(2): 55–59.

Albayram F, Hamper UM. Ovarian and adnexal torsion: spectrum of sonographic findings with pathologic correlation. *J Ultrasound Med.* 2001; 20(10): 1083–1089.

Madrazo BL, Cordes JF, Cacciarelli AA. Ultrasound case of the day: right adnexal torsion. *Radiographics.* 1992; 12(1): 201–202.

Pena JE, Ufberg D, Cooney N, Denis AL. Usefulness of Doppler sonography in the diagnosis of ovarian torsion. *Fertil Steril.* 2000; 73(5): 1047–1050.

Vijayaraghavan SB. Sonographic whirlpool sign in ovarian torsion. *J Ultrasound Med.* 2004; 23(12): 1643–1649.

Case 27   62-year-old male presented with scrotal pain

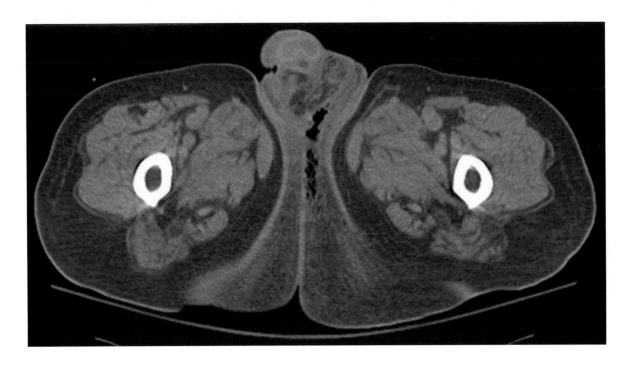

Diagnosis:
Fournier
gangrene

Contrast-enhanced axial CT demonstrates fat stranding and gas (arrow) extending to the perineum and left medial gluteal region via Colles' fascia.

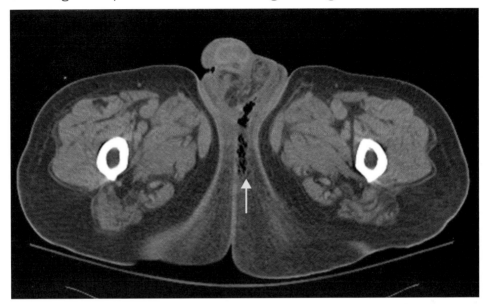

Discussion

Fournier gangrene has a high mortality rate and is considered a surgical emergency.

- Patients may present with scrotal swelling, abdominal pain, pruritus, crepitus, and fever.
- The most important predisposing factors include diabetes mellitus and alcohol abuse. Other risk factors include localized trauma, indwelling catheters, HIV infection, and radiation or chemotherapy.
- Common causal organisms are aerobic bacteria such as *E. coli* and Streptococcal species, and anaerobes such as *B. fragilis*.
- Treatment includes intravenous antibiotics and immediate surgical debridement.

Understanding perineal anatomy including the fascial planes is important in recognizing spread of infection.

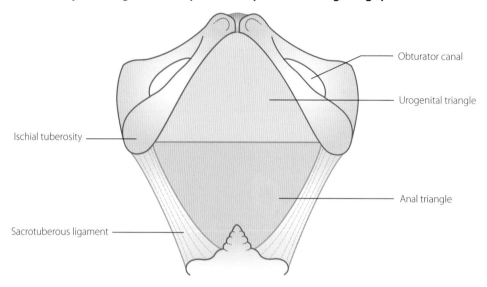

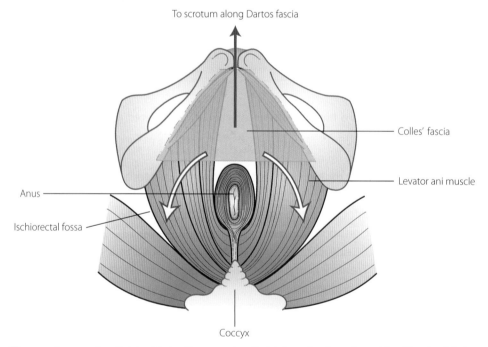

- The perineum is divided into the urogenital triangle (bordered by the ischial rami laterally and pubis anteriorly) and anal triangle (bordered by the coccyx posteriorly and sacrotuberous ligaments laterally).
- Disease arising from the anal triangle may spread along Colles' fascia into the ischiorectal fossa and then into the buttocks and thighs.
- Disease may also spread anteriorly via the Dartos fascia to involve the scrotum and penis.

Although Fournier gangrene is often diagnosed clinically, imaging can play a key role in diagnosis and assessment of extent.

- Radiographs may demonstrate subcutaneous gas before crepitus is evident on physical exam (though the absence of radiographically apparent gas does not exclude the diagnosis).
- Ultrasound may show scrotal wall thickening with edema, dirty shadowing from subcutaneous gas, and reactive hydroceles.
- CT findings include thickening of the fascial planes, fluid collections, abscesses, and subcutaneous gas; CT may help differentiate Fournier gangrene from cellulitis and soft-tissue edema.

Clinical synopsis
The patient was treated with IV antibiotics and underwent emergent surgical debridement.

Self-assessment

- *Name three infectious or inflammatory processes that can lead to Fournier gangrene.*

- *Why are the testes often normal in cases of Fournier gangrene that involve the scrotum?*

- Perianal abscess, anal fissures, intra-abdominal or retroperitoneal infection (e.g., diverticulitis), and fistulous tracts from bowel.

- The blood supply to the testes (testicular branches from the aorta) is separate from the supply to the scrotum (pudendal branches from the internal iliac artery). If the testes are involved, direct spread of infection from an intra-abdominal or retroperitoneal source should be considered.

Spectrum of Fournier gangrene

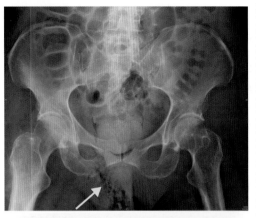

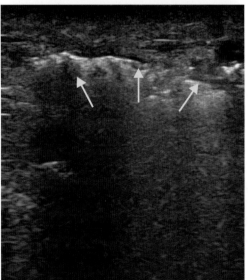

Radiographic and ultrasound findings of Fournier gangrene

In this 64-year-old with swollen labia and pelvic pain, a frontal radiograph of the pelvis demonstrates multiple foci of gas and soft tissue thickening in the right groin (arrow), extending inferiorly to the right labia. Corresponding ultrasound of the right labia demonstrates skin edema and multiple echogenic gas bubbles with dirty posterior acoustic shadowing (arrows). These findings were compatible with Fournier gangrene, and the patient underwent immediate surgical debridement.

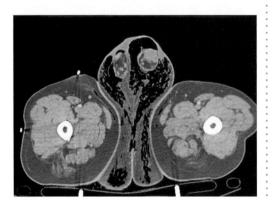

Severe Fournier gangrene

Axial contrast-enhanced CT shows a markedly enlarged scrotal sac containing a large amount of gas that extends into the perineum and bilateral medial gluteal regions via Colles' fascia.

Differential diagnosis of Fournier gangrene

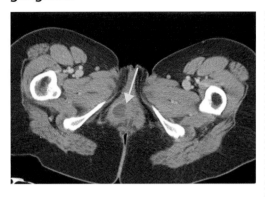

Bartholin gland cyst

Bartholin glands are derived from the urogenital sinus and are located at the posterolateral introitus. Bartholin gland cysts (retention cysts) may develop from chronic inflammation and retention of secretions, and may also become infected. They are distinguished from Fournier gangrene by their limited extent and characteristic location. In this 45-year-old female with pelvic pain, contrast-enhanced CT of the pelvis demonstrates a 2 cm right-sided Bartholin gland cyst (arrow) with marginal enhancement suggestive of inflammation.

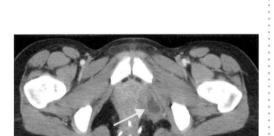

Perianal abscess

Perianal and perirectal disease occurs in up to 80% of patients with Crohn's disease, and is often a late complication. Other typical findings of Crohn's disease include abscesses, ulcers, fissures, and luminal stenoses. In this 23-year-old female with Crohn's disease and perianal abscess, contrast-enhanced axial CT of the pelvis demonstrates a 3 cm complex fluid collection in the left ischiorectal fossa (arrow) that extends to the level of the levator ani but remains external to the pelvis.

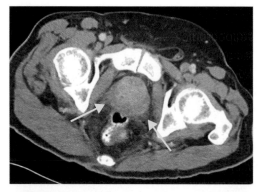

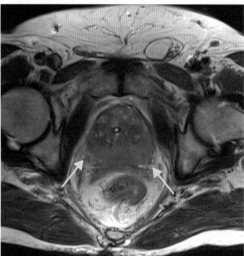

Prostatitis

Prostatitis may result from ascending urinary tract infection or occur after biopsy. Risk factors are similar to those for Fournier gangrene and include diabetes, chronic catheterization, and bladder obstruction from prostatic enlargement. In this 73-year-old male with fever and urosepsis from acute prostatitis, axial contrast-enhanced CT of the pelvis (upper image) demonstrates an enlarged, heterogeneous prostate gland with surrounding fat stranding (arrows). Axial T2-weighted MRI (lower image) confirms the findings of an enlarged prostate with adjacent fat stranding and regions of increased T2 signal.

Further reading

Levenson RB, Singh AK, Novelline RA. Fournier Gangrene: Role of Imaging. *Radiographics* 2008; 28:519–528.

Gore RM, *et al.* CT Features of Ulcerative Colitis. *AJR Am J Roentgenol* 1996; 167:3–15.

Prasad SR, Menias CO, Narra VR, *et al.* Cross-sectional Imaging of the Female Urethra: Technique and Results. *Radiographics* 2005; 25:749–761.

Case 28   30-year-old male presented with a palpable left testicular mass

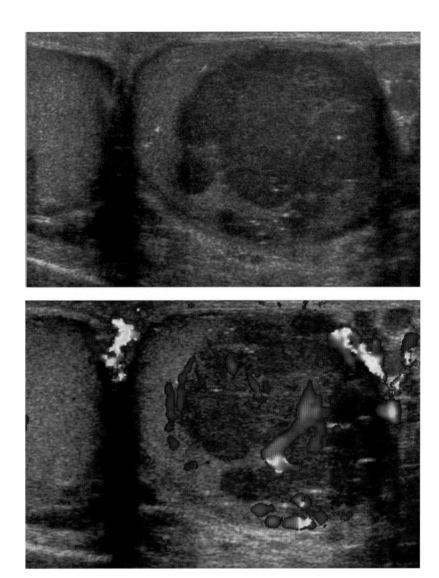

Diagnosis: **Seminoma and testicular microlithiasis** — Grayscale and color Doppler ultrasound demonstrate a large, solid, lobulated, hypoechoic, left testicular mass, which demonstrates internal vascularity. Small specular reflectors within the mass and within the normal parenchyma represent microlithiasis (arrows).

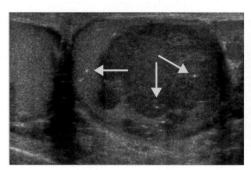 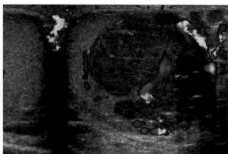

Discussion

Primary testicular tumors are the most common malignancy in young adult males.

- Testicular neoplasms commonly present as painless testicular enlargement or palpable scrotal masses.
- Germ cell tumors account for 95% of testicular masses, and are usually malignant.
- The most common germ cell tumor in adults is seminoma, which usually presents between 30 and 45 years of age.
- Nonseminomatous germ cell tumor (NSGCT) subtypes include choriocarcinoma, teratoma, yolk sac tumor, embryonal cell carcinoma, and mixed germ cell tumor. Serum markers such as alpha-fetoprotein (AFP), lactate dehydrogenase (LDH), and the beta subunit of human chorionic gonadotropin (β-hCG) are elevated in patients with different tumor subtypes.
- Seminomas are less aggressive than NSGCT, and are usually confined within the tunica albuginea at the time of diagnosis. They are highly radiosensitive and chemosensitive, hence their better prognosis.

Lymphoma and leukemia commonly involve the testis, and should be strongly considered in older patients with testicular masses, especially if bilateral.

- Metastasis should be considered in patients with a known primary malignancy.
- Uncommonly, intra-testicular masses may be benign: benign adrenal rests occur in patients with congenital adrenal hyperplasia, and sarcoidosis may affect the testes as well.

Ultrasound is the test of choice for the diagnosis of testicular neoplasm, with sensitivity near 100%. CT is used to evaluate for metastasis, usually to retroperitoneal lymph nodes.

- Most testicular neoplasms are hypoechoic and hypervascular relative to the normal testicular parenchyma.
- Ultrasound cannot definitively differentiate among types of testicular germ cell tumor; however, seminomas are generally homogeneous, while NSGCT are heterogeneous, with cystic areas and calcification.
- Non-neoplastic testicular lesions that can potentially be confused with tumors, such as hematomas, abscesses, and infarcts, are differentiated from neoplasms by lack of internal vascularity.

Microlithiasis is an uncommon condition caused by calcification of collagenous material within the seminiferous tubules.

- The testicular ultrasound criterion for diagnosis is five or more echogenic foci within the testicular parenchyma on a single field of view.
- The strength of the association between testicular microlithiasis and malignancy is controversial, as the prevalence of microlithiasis in asymptomatic patients is unknown.
- In a recent meta-analysis, Tan *et al.* demonstrated that asymptomatic patients in whom microlithiasis was incidentally detected had a low absolute risk of malignancy, while the summary risk ratio was 8.5-fold higher in patients with risk factors such as cryptorchidism (which raises risk of testicular neoplasm by about 30-fold), subfertility, or personal history of germ cell tumor.

Clinical synopsis   CT of the chest, abdomen, and pelvis demonstrated no metastatic disease. The patient underwent left radical orchiectomy, and histopathology was consistent with seminoma. Radiotherapy was followed by routine surveillance, which, to date, has shown no disease recurrence.

Self-assessment

- *Name three benign lesions that can appear as a focal hypoechoic testicular mass.*

  - Hematoma, abscess, infarct, ectopic adrenal rest, sarcoidosis.

- *Are testicular neoplasms usually benign or malignant?*

  - Testicular neoplasms are usually malignant.

- *What is the most common germ cell tumor occurring in adult males?*

  - Seminoma.

Differential diagnosis of testicular seminoma

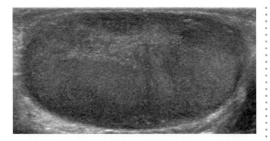

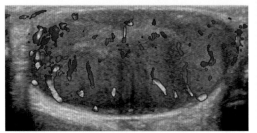

Testicular acute myelogenous leukemia (AML)

This patient with a past medical history of AML presented with a painless scrotal mass. Grayscale and color Doppler ultrasound images of the left testicle demonstrate heterogeneous echotexture with increased Doppler flow. Biopsy demonstrated AML.

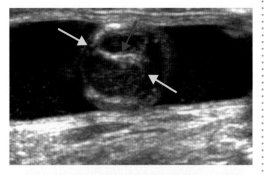

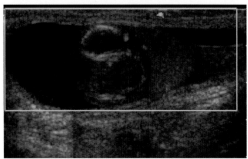

Testicular teratoma

Pure testicular teratomas represent up to 9% of all testicular tumors, and most commonly present as painless scrotal masses. Testicular teratomas are NSGCTs that are classified by patient age and degree of differentiation (mature or immature). While mature teratomas are usually indolent, immature teratomas may be present in malignant mixed germ cell tumors. This 22-year-old male presented with a right scrotal mass. Grayscale and color Doppler ultrasound of the right testicle demonstrate a complex, predominantly hypoechoic testicular mass (yellow arrows) with linear hyperechoic septa (red arrow) and minimal internal flow. A large hydrocele is present.

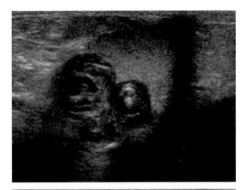

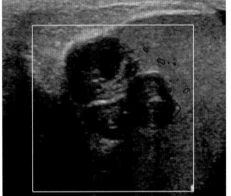

Epidermoid cyst

Epidermoid cysts are benign tumors that contain ectodermal derivatives. They appear as hypo-echoic masses with hyperechoic, calcified rims or multiple concentric internal laminations ("onion skinning"). It is important to recognize a sus-pected epidermoid cyst prior to surgery, as treat-ment is typically testis-sparing enucleation rather than orchiectomy. Grayscale and color Doppler ultrasound demonstrate a hypoechoic testicular mass with a concentric lamellar pattern.

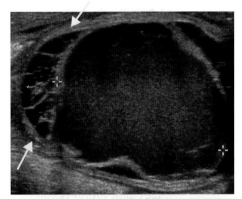

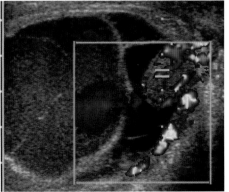

Hematoma

Despite the vulnerable anatomic position of the testes, testicular trauma is relatively uncommon. Testicular injuries can be divided into three broad categories based on trauma mechanism: (1) blunt trauma, (2) penetrating trauma, and (3) degloving trauma. Traumatic injuries are typically seen in males aged 15–40 years. Grayscale and color Doppler ultrasound of the left scrotum in a patient with pain and swelling after trauma shows a hematoma with a dense echogenic rim, lace-like internal septations peripherally (yellow arrows), and low-level internal echoes centrally (calipers). This complex collection is separate from the left testicle (not pictured). The epididymis demon-strates increased Doppler flow, consistent with reactive hyperemia.

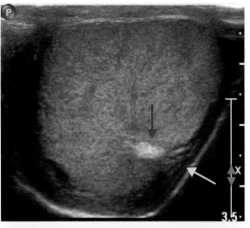

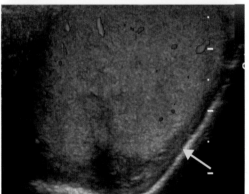

Testicular scar

This patient with a past medical history of left testicular torsion and orchiopexy presented with gradually increasing left scrotal discomfort and swelling. Grayscale and color Doppler ultrasound images of the left testicle demonstrate a hypo-echoic, hypovascular rim of post-surgical scar tissue (yellow arrows) surrounding the normal left testicle. The small hyperechoic focus on the image at left is the normal mediastinum testis (red arrow). Blood flow within the testicle is normal.

Further reading

Adham WK, Raval BK, Uzquiano MC, Lemos LB. Best cases from the AFIP: bilateral testicular tumors: seminoma and mixed germ cell tumor. *Radiographics*. 2005 May–June;25(3):835–839.

Benson CB, Doubilet PM, Richie JP. Sonography of the male genital tract. *AJR Am J Roentgenol*. 1989 Oct.;153(4):705–713.

Dogra VS, Gottlieb RH, Oka M, Rubens DJ. Sonography of the scrotum. *Radiology*. 2003 Apr.;227(1):18–36. *Epub* 2003 Feb, 28, 2003.

Fernández-Pérez GC, Tardáguila FM, Velasco M, Rivas C, Dos Santos J, Cambronero J, Trinidad C, San Miguel P. Radiologic findings of segmental testicular infarction. *AJR Am J Roentgenol*. 2005 May;184(5):1587–1593.

Kim W, Rosen MA, Langer JE, Banner MP, Siegelman ES, Ramchandani P. US MR imaging correlation in pathologic conditions of the scrotum. *Radiographics*. 2007 Sept.-Oct.;27(5):1239–1253.

Tan IB, Ang KK, Ching BC, Mohan C, Toh CK, Tan MH. Testicular microlithiasis predicts concurrent testicular germ cell tumors and intratubular germ cell neoplasia of unclassified type in adults: a meta-analysis and systematic review. *Cancer*. 2010 Oct. 1;116(19):4520–4532.

Woodward PJ, Sohaey R, O'Donoghue MJ, Green DE. From the archives of the AFIP: tumors and tumorlike lesions of the testis: radiologic—pathologic correlation. *Radiographics*. 2002 Jan.–Feb.;22(1):189–216.

19-year-old male presented with acute onset right scrotal pain

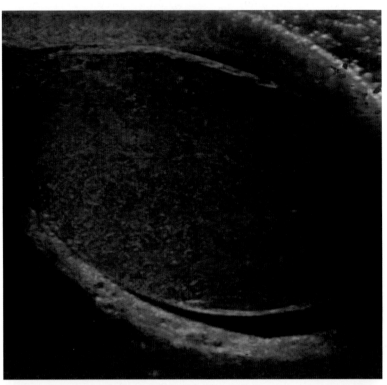

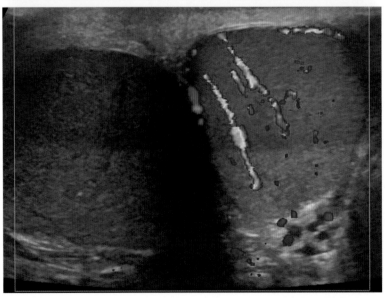

Diagnosis:
Testicular torsion

Sagittal grayscale ultrasound image of the right testis (left image) and transverse image of both testes with Doppler overlay (right image) demonstrate diffuse hypoechogenicity of the right testis and no demonstrable blood flow. There is a small, simple, reactive right hydrocele (arrow). The left testis is normal in echotexture, with normal Doppler flow.

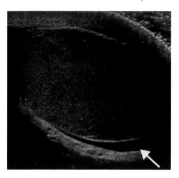 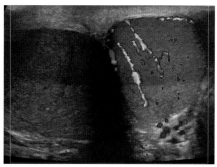

Discussion

Testicular torsion most often affects pubescent boys and young adult males.

- Typical symptoms include pain that may radiate into the groin and lower abdomen, nausea and vomiting, and swelling of the scrotum.
- On physical examination, there is often marked tenderness, and the testis may be oriented in a transverse lie.

The normal testis is anchored to the wall of the scrotum by a broad posterior attachment that prevents excessive rotation. Testes with "bell clapper" deformity are predisposed to torsion.

- The "bell clapper" deformity is a congenital anomaly in which the normal testicular–scrotal attachment is absent, so that the testis is suspended in the scrotal sac by its vascular pedicle.

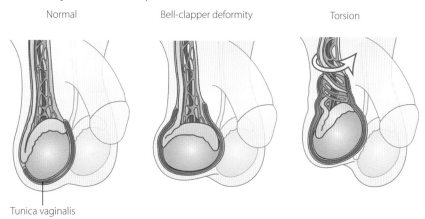

- Forceful contraction of the cremasteric muscles can be the precipitating event in testicular torsion, resulting in elevation and rotation of the testis.

Diagnosis is difficult to make on the basis of grayscale ultrasound alone. In the early stages of torsion, the grayscale appearance of the affected testis is frequently normal. Color Doppler ultrasound with spectral analysis is the most accurate and important imaging modality in the evaluation of testicular torsion.

- The normal testis is homogeneously hyperechoic. If the testis appears heterogeneous or hypoechoic on gray scale imaging, it is almost certainly nonviable.
- Torsion may also be associated with a small reactive hydrocele and thickening of the scrotal skin.
- The most important finding is absence of testicular vascularity. Demonstration of testicular flow does not completely exclude torsion, because some flow can be seen in patients who have incomplete or intermittent torsion (usually in an atypical pattern).

If surgery occurs within six hours of symptom onset, the majority of testes will maintain viability.

- With prompt diagnosis and surgical detorsion, there is a good chance that the testis can be salvaged.
- If surgery is delayed beyond 24 hours, infarction resulting in irreversible necrosis may occur.
- Between 6 and 24 hours after symptom onset, the chance of testicular salvage progressively diminishes.

Clinical synopsis   The patient underwent scrotal exploration with right testicular detorsion. Bilateral orchiopexies were performed.

Self-assessment

- *What congenital anomaly predisposes to testicular torsion?*

  - Bell clapper deformity, where the normal broad posterior attachment of the testis to the scrotum is congenitally absent.

- *What is the surgical salvage rate for a testis that has been torsed for 24 hours?*

  - Essentially zero percent. If detorsion occurs within 6 hours, the majority of testes remain viable. Between 6 and 24 hours, the salvage rate decreases progressively.

- *True or false: the diagnosis of early torsion is easily made with grayscale ultrasound without color Doppler overlay.*

  - False. Doppler overlay is necessary in the early stages to demonstrate diminished or absent testicular blood flow.

Spectrum of testicular torsion

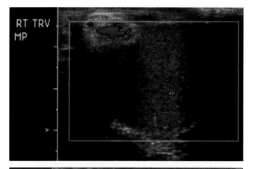

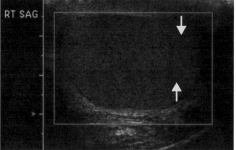

Incomplete torsion

Grayscale and color Doppler ultrasound of the right testicle in a patient with right scrotal pain shows decreased testicular vascularity, with some preserved flow (upper image). Sagittal ultrasound (lower image) demonstrates subtly decreased echogenicity of the lower pole parenchyma, which indicates ischemia (arrows).

Differential diagnosis of testicular torsion

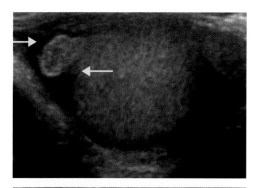

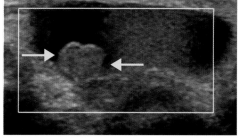

Torsion of the appendix testis

The appendix testis is an embryonic remnant of the mesonephric and paramesonephric ducts. Torsion of the appendix testis occurs predominantly in pre-pubescent boys (aged 7–14 years), and is more frequently left-sided. The classic physical exam finding is the "blue dot" sign of a firm nodule with bluish discoloration on the superior aspect of the testis. On ultrasound, the normal appendix testis is about 5 mm in size, and is situated between the epididymis and the testis. In contrast to testicular torsion, torsion of the appendix testis is usually treated nonoperatively. Pain resolves within 2 to 3 days. Grayscale ultrasound without and with color Doppler overlay in a patient with acute right-sided scrotal pain demonstrates an enlarged, heterogeneous testis appendix (arrows), adjacent to the normal testis. Color Doppler overlay demonstrates no Doppler flow. There is a small reactive hydrocele.

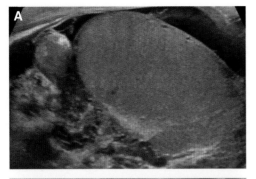

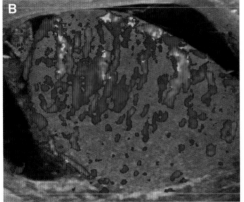

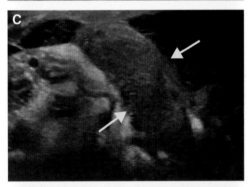

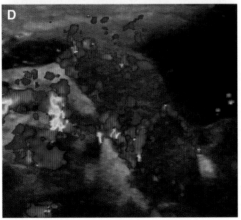

Epididymo-orchitis

Epididymo-orchitis is infection of the testicle and epididymis. In epididymo-orchitis, infection usually spreads from the bladder or prostate gland via the vas deferens and the lymphatics of the spermatic cord to the epididymis, and then to the testis. Orchitis without epididymitis is rare. Grayscale (A) and color Doppler (B) ultrasound of the left testicle in a patient with subacute left scrotal pain demonstrate mildly hyperechoic testicular parenchyma and increased vascular flow. Grayscale (C) and color Doppler (D) ultrasound of the left epididymis demonstrate a diffusely enlarged, hypervascular epididymis (arrows).

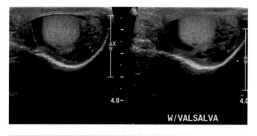

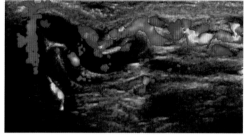

Varicocele

A varicocele is an abnormally enlarged pampiniform venous plexus. Varicoceles are more frequently left-sided because the left gonadal vein drains into the left renal vein at about a 90-degree angle. The right gonadal vein drains into the larger IVC at an acute angle and usually experiences less backflow pressure. If a patient experiences sudden onset of varicocele, or has an isolated right-sided varicocele or a varicocele that is irreducible in the supine position, he should be evaluated for retroperitoneal pathology that is compressing the gonadal vein (e.g., retroperitoneal mass, fibrosis). Grayscale ultrasound of the left testicle (upper image) in a patient with painless left scrotal swelling demonstrates abnormal dilatation of the veins in the pampiniform plexus of the spermatic cord (calipers) that is exaggerated with the Valsalva maneuver. Ultrasound with Doppler overlay (lower image) demonstrates vascular flow within the serpiginous veins.

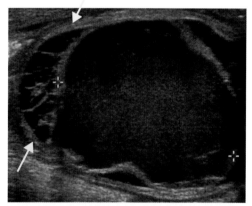

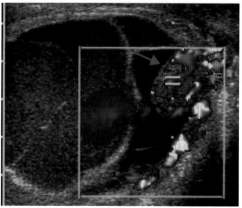

Traumatic scrotal hematoma

The amount of swelling and ecchymosis associated with scrotal hematoma may vary, and the size of the hematoma does not necessarily correlate with the severity of testicular injury. In cases of scrotal trauma, the tunica albuginea should be examined carefully for disruption, which is indicative of testicular rupture. Conversely, contusion without fracture of the tunica albuginea may be accompanied by significant bleeding that requires surgical intervention. Grayscale and color Doppler ultrasound of the left scrotum in a patient with pain and swelling after trauma shows a hematoma with a dense echogenic rim, lace-like internal septations peripherally (yellow arrows), and low-level internal echoes centrally (calipers). This complex collection is separate from the left testicle (not pictured). The epididymis (red arrow) demonstrates increased Doppler flow, consistent with reactive hyperemia.

Further reading

Arce JD, *et al.* Sonographic diagnosis of acute spermatic cord torsion. *Pediatric Radiology*. 2002;32: 485–491.

Baud C, *et al.* Spiral twist of the spermatic cord: a reliable sign of testicular torsion. *Pediatric Radiology*. 1998;28: 950–954.

Dogra VS, Gottlieb RH, Oka M *et al.* Sonography of the scrotum. *Radiology*. 2003; 227 (1): 18–36.

Karamazyn B, *et al.* Clinical and sonographic criteria of acute scrotum in children: A retrospective study of 172 boys. *Pediatric Radiology*. 2005;35: 302–310.

Paushter D. Testicular Torsion. *Emedicine*. July 20, 2004.

Vijayaraghavan SB. Sonographic differential diagnosis of acute scrotum: Real-time whirlpool sign, a key sign of torsion. *J Ultrasound Med*. 2006;25: 563–574.

Case 30   48-year-old male with oliguria 2 days after renal transplant

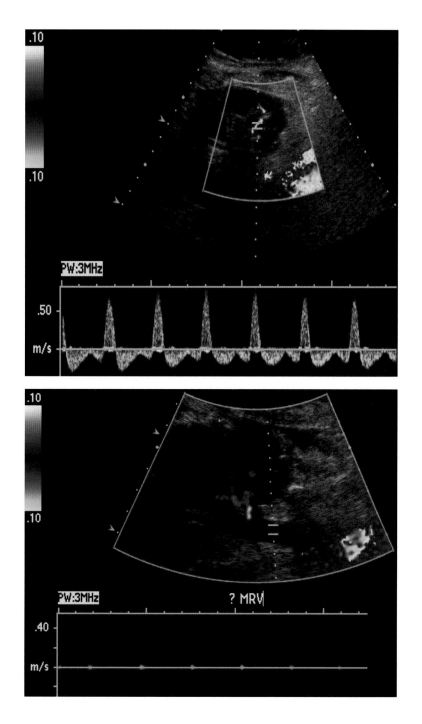

Diagnosis:
Renal vein thrombosis in a transplanted kidney

Ultrasound with color Doppler shows a right lower quadrant transplanted kidney, which is edematous and hypoechoic. Spectral Doppler of the lower pole interlobar artery (yellow arrow) reveals elevated intrarenal resistive indices and reversal of flow during diastole (red arrow). No Doppler flow is detected within the main renal vein (blue arrow).

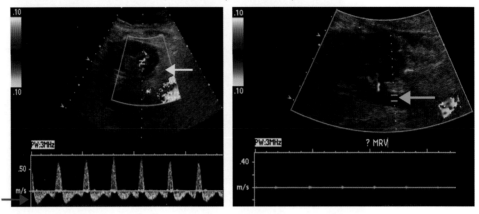

Discussion

Transplanted kidneys are typically placed in an extraperitoneal location in the right iliac fossa with end-to-side or end-to-end anastomosis with the external iliac vasculature.

- Donor organs may be cadaveric (cadaveric renal transplant, CRT), from a living related donor (LRT), or from a living nonrelated donor (LNRT). As a donated organ, the left kidney is preferred for its longer renal vein that is easier to anastomose. The type of graft that is available for harvest dictates the type of arterial anastomosis.
- From cadaveric donors, a Carrel patch (a small piece of aorta around the origin of the renal artery) may be harvested along with the graft, and anastomosed to the recipient external iliac artery in an end-to-side fashion. The preferred method for restoring ureteral drainage is ureteroneocystostomy, in which the ureter is anastomosed directly to the urinary bladder. If the cadaveric donor is under 5 years of age, both donor kidneys may be transplanted into a single recipient using the donor aorta and vena cava for vascular anastomosis ("en bloc" pediatric transplant).

Early recognition of complications is essential for graft and patient survival.

- In evaluating patients who have had a renal transplant, a systematic approach should be utilized. Complications may be categorized by affected anatomic site: the transplant perinephric space, the renal parenchyma, the urinary collecting system, and the renal vasculature.
- When sonographic findings are nonspecific, the clinical and laboratory data are often very helpful in narrowing the differential diagnosis; however, biopsy may ultimately be necessary for a more definitive diagnosis.

- Perinephric space: postoperative fluid collections containing pus, blood, lymphatic fluid, or urine are common in the transplant perinephric space. Ultimately, these collections may require sampling for diagnosis, as the sonographic appearances overlap. Clinical significance depends on size, composition, location, and degree of mass effect.
- Renal parenchyma: parenchymal abnormalities have a nonspecific sonographic appearance. Infarct, rejection, and focal pyelonephritis can appear as focal areas of increased or decreased echogenicity.
- Urinary collecting system: complications include urine leak, urinoma, urinary obstruction, and urinary calculi.
- Renal vasculature: renal artery occlusion and renal vein thrombosis are devastating complications of the early postoperative period that can rapidly lead to graft loss. Delayed complications include renal artery stenosis and post-biopsy arteriovenous fistulas and pseudoaneurysms. Renal vein thrombosis is more common than renal artery occlusion and typically occurs in the first few days after transplant. Etiologies include suboptimal technique, compression of the renal vein by a fluid collection, and hypovolemia. The affected kidney may appear enlarged and hypoechoic, with lack of Doppler signal in the renal vein. The intraparenchymal renal artery branches are compressed, and spectral Doppler shows increased resistance, often with reversal of flow away from the kidney during diastole (ordinarily, flow is toward the kidney in all portions of the cardiac cycle). Reversal of diastolic flow can also be seen in severe rejection or acute tubular necrosis, but the finding of absent venous flow is diagnostic for renal vein thrombosis.

Ultrasound is the test of choice for the evaluation of renal transplants both in the perioperative period and in long-term follow-up. A working knowledge of the renal transplant procedure is helpful for interpretation of both normal and abnormal findings. In particular, knowledge of the vascular anatomy is important for evaluating complications involving vessels and anastomoses.

- Spectral Doppler evaluation of the upper, mid, and lower pole interlobar arteries, along with the main renal artery and vein and external iliac artery and vein should be performed. Interlobar arteries should demonstrate brisk upstroke with low diastolic resistance.
- Elevated resistive index (RI) above 0.8 is a nonspecific parameter of renal dysfunction. Increased RI is seen in acute tubular necrosis, renal vein thrombosis, graft infection, compression by fluid collections, and obstructive hydronephrosis. The normal RI (defined as the difference between peak systolic velocity and end diastolic velocity divided by peak systolic velocity) is between 0.6 and 0.8.
- Normal velocity in the main renal artery is <200 cm/sec, and venous structures normally demonstrate monophasic, continuous flow (sometimes with transmitted pulsatility from the arterial system).

Clinical synopsis	The patient was taken to surgery, where the transplant kidney was found to be grossly ischemic and unsalvageable.

Self-assessment

- *True or false: elevated RI indicates a specific cause of renal transplant dysfunction.*

- • False. Elevated RI is seen in many conditions.

- *Name three factors that predispose to renal vein thrombosis in the early postoperative period.*

- • Suboptimal surgical technique, renal vein compression by fluid collections, and hypovolemia.

- *True or false: normal velocity in the main renal artery is <200 cm/sec.*

- • True.

Spectrum of post-renal transplant complications

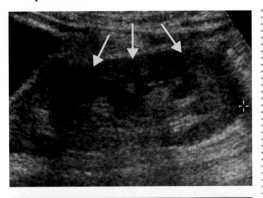

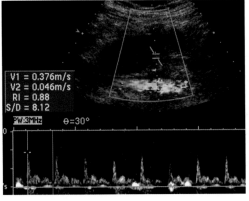

Transplant renal artery stenosis (RAS)

Transplant RAS typically manifests 3–24 months after surgery. Predisposing factors include atherosclerosis within the donor artery and transplantation of pediatric donor arteries into adult patients. The majority of stenoses occur at or near the anastomosis with the iliac artery. This 40-year-old female presented with rising glomerular filtration rate (GFR) 6 years after renal transplant. Grayscale ultrasound with color and spectral Doppler demonstrates mildly hypoechoic renal echotexture (arrows) and elevated resistive index (RI = 0.88) within the interlobar renal artery. Additionally, there was elevated velocity within the main renal artery (300 cm/s, not shown).

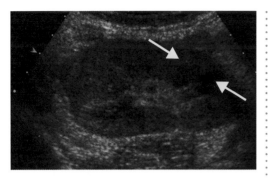

Post-biopsy arteriovenous fistula

Grayscale sagittal ultrasound image of a transplanted kidney demonstrates an ill-defined hypoechoic area within the lower pole (arrows), which was the site of a biopsy 4 years prior. Color Doppler examination demonstrates a corresponding very high flow vascular lesion with both arterial and venous waveforms.

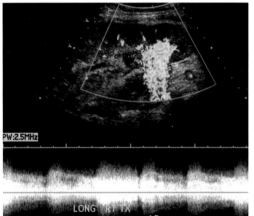

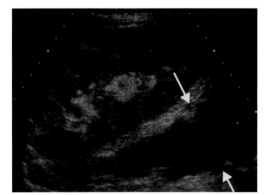

Lymphocele

Lymphoceles are the most common post-transplant collections, occurring in up to 18% of patients with transplanted kidneys. They usually occur 2 to 3 weeks after transplant and are usually anechoic – the presence of internal echoes suggests abscess or hematoma. Laparoscopic marsupialization is considered to be a safe and effective treatment. This 11-year-old female presented 4 months after renal transplant with a new, hypoechoic collection (arrows) posteromedial to the right transplant kidney.

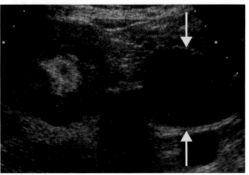

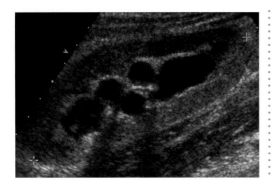

Hydronephrosis

Hydronephrosis of the transplanted kidney in the postoperative period usually results from anastomotic edema at the ureteroneocystostomy site and resolves spontaneously. Grayscale ultrasound in a 13-year-old female 2 days after renal transplantation demonstrates moderate hydronephrosis of the transplanted kidney, which completely resolved within 2 weeks without intervention.

Further reading

Friedewald S, Molmenti E, Friedewald J, *et al.* Vascular and nonvascular complications of renal transplants: sonographic evaluation and correlation with other imaging modalities, surgery, and pathology. *J Clin Ultrasound*. 2005;33:127–139.

Jimenez C, Lopez M, Gonzalez E, Selgas R. Ultrasonography in kidney transplantation: values and new developments. *Transplant Rev (Orlando)*. 2009;23:209–213.

Singh AK, Sahani DV. Imaging of the renal donor and transplant recipient. *Radiol Clin North Am*. 2008;46:79–93.

SECTION 2 THORAX

Section 2.1 Chest Pain

Case 31 39-year-old man presenting to the ER with increasing shortness of breath

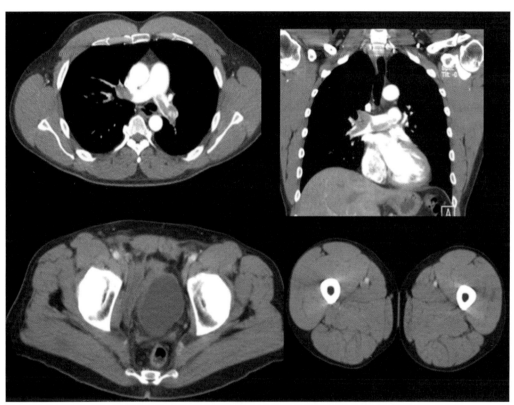

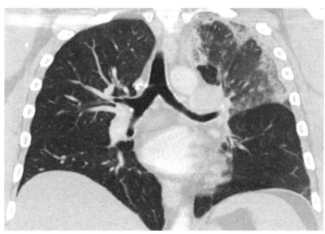

***Diagnosis:*
**Pulmonary
embolism**

Axial and coronal images from a CT pulmonary angiogram including the thighs and pelvis demonstrate central filling defects in the right and left main pulmonary arteries (yellow arrows). There is hypodense thrombus expanding the right external iliac and femoral veins (red arrows). Coronal CT in lung window shows a wedge-shaped, peripheral infarct (blue arrow).

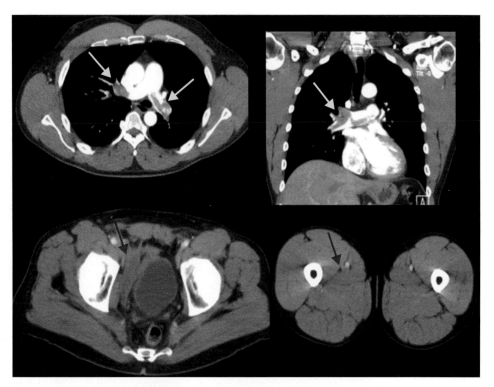

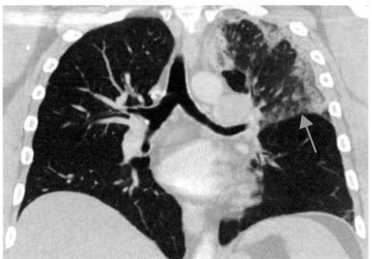

Discussion

Pulmonary embolism (PE) is the third most common cause of death from cardiovascular disease after myocardial infarction and stroke, and is a leading cause of preventable morbidity and mortality in hospitalized patients.

- Estimates of incidence of venous thromboembolism (VTE, defined as PE and deep venous thrombosis, or DVT) range from 300,000 to 600,000 per year.
- Two-thirds of patients with VTE present with DVT, while one-third present with PE.
- While some patients are asymptomatic, up to 25% of patients with PE may have a first presentation of sudden cardiac death.

Establishing a diagnosis of VTE may be challenging given variation in clinical presentation and variable sensitivity and specificity of diagnostic modalities. VTE may be asymptomatic or have subtle clinical manifestations in some cases. History, physical exam, laboratory studies, and imaging play vital and complementary roles.

- Risk factors include inherited thrombophilias, pregnancy, malignancy, obesity, chronic disease, advanced age, iatrogenic factors (hormonal therapies, hospitalization, trauma, and surgery), and immobilization.
- Typical clinical findings in DVT include lower extremity edema, warmth, and erythema. PE tends to present with dyspnea, pleuritic chest pain, tachypnea, syncope, and cough.
- Several clinical probability-scoring systems have been developed – the Wells criteria, with separate systems for determining the probability of DVT and PE, is perhaps the most well known (the Geneva score is also well validated). Based on the presence of risk factors, signs, and symptoms, patients are stratified into low-, intermediate-, and high-probability categories.
- Testing for elevated D-dimer, a fibrin degradation product, is sensitive but not specific for VTE – the negative predictive value is approximately 94%; however, D-dimer may be elevated in other conditions, including renal impairment, pregnancy, and hemorrhage. Thus, the D-dimer assay is used in conjunction with prediction rules such as the Wells criteria to determine the need for further work up including imaging.

Imaging modalities used in the work-up of PE include lower extremity ultrasound to assess for DVT (up to 35% of patients with DVT above the knee have silent PE), nuclear medicine ventilation-perfusion (V/Q) scanning, conventional angiography, and CT pulmonary angiography (CTPA), which is the most commonly used imaging modality in the United States.

- Choice of imaging modality is dependent on multiple clinical factors. American College of Radiology (ACR) appropriateness criteria and other guidelines are available to guide modality selection in cases of suspected PE.

- CTPA should be used in patients with low pretest probability for PE and an abnormal D-dimer result, or in those who have a high pretest probability irrespective of D-dimer result. Clinical validity for CTPA in diagnosing PE is similar to that of conventional pulmonary angiography and V/Q scanning. Strengths of CTPA over other modalities include non-invasiveness, wide availability, convenience, and ability to identify alternative diagnoses. Drawbacks of CTPA include risk of contrast nephropathy and exposure to ionizing radiation.
- Currently, conventional angiography is reserved for cases in which clinical suspicion remains high in the setting of negative CTPA or when intervention is being considered, as in hemodynamically significant PE.
- V/Q scanning is useful in select situations, but is non-diagnostic in many cases and, therefore, usually second-line in the emergency setting.
- In pregnant patients, some guidelines indicate that a chest x-ray to evaluate for alternative diagnoses is the preferred initial approach. If normal, the next indicated study is a perfusion (Q) scan. This is only followed by a ventilation (V) scan to assess for V/Q mismatch indicative of PE if the perfusion scan is abnormal (it should be noted, however, that evidence is limited and these approaches are not incontrovertible).

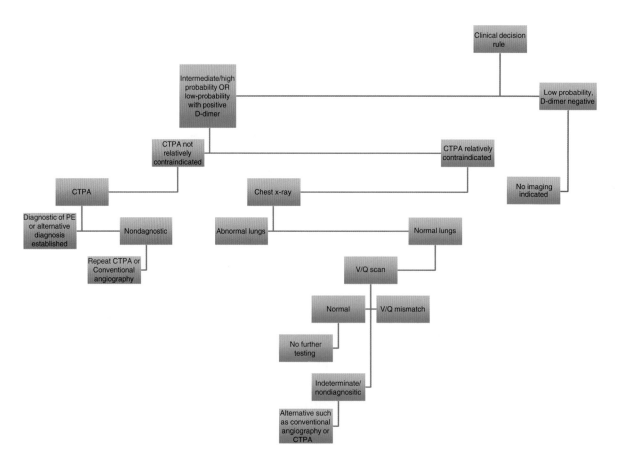

- Signs of acute PE differ from those of chronic PE, and management decisions may depend on whether PE is acute or chronic.
- Signs of acute PE on CTPA include intraluminal filling defects, visibility of thrombus on three or more images, enlarged artery, mosaic perfusion (abnormal lucent areas due to low local perfusion), and associated hemorrhage, infarction, or cavitation. Technical quality of the CTPA study is important to consider; this includes assessment of adequacy of the contrast bolus and whether there is limiting respiratory motion.
- Chronic pulmonary emboli, which can cause secondary pulmonary hypertension and cor pulmonale, tend to be eccentric within the vessel, with webs, calcification, or post-stenotic dilatation. Signs of secondary pulmonary hypertension caused by chronic PE include prominent right ventricle (RV), diameter of right main pulmonary artery >18 mm, diameter of the pulmonary trunk >29 mm, mosaic attenuation, and vascular pruning.
- Enlargement of the RV relative to the left ventricle (RV/LV ratio >0.8–1.0), bowing of the interatrial and interventricular septa, reflux of contrast into the inferior vena cava (IVC) and hepatic veins, or engorgement of the superior vena cava and azygos veins should raise concern for right heart strain; patients with this finding should be referred for echocardiography.

Self-assessment

- *How do CTPA appearances of acute and chronic PE differ?*

- Acute pulmonary emboli are central filling defects that enlarge the vessel. In chronic emboli, eccentric thrombus layers along the vessel wall and may be calcified, with webs, post-stenotic dilatation, and signs of secondary pulmonary hypertension. There may be abrupt cutoff of pulmonary arteries, bronchial artery collaterals, and intimal irregularity in chronic PE.

- *Name three signs that raise concern for right heart strain with acute PE that should prompt referral for echocardiography.*

- RV/LV ratio >0.8–1, bowing of the interatrial or interventricular septa, reflux of contrast into the inferior vena cava and hepatic veins, and engorgement of the superior vena cava and azygos veins.

Differential diagnosis of pulmonary embolism

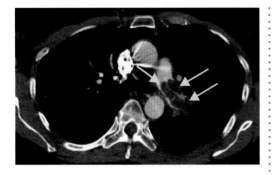

Primary pulmonary artery sarcoma

Pulmonary artery sarcoma is a rare mesenchymal tumor arising from the intima of the pulmonary artery. As show by this axial CTPA, it appears as a filling defect (arrows) that produces nodular enlargement of the pulmonary arteries. There may be enhancement, neovascularity (as in this case), metastasis, or direct extension into the lung parenchyma.

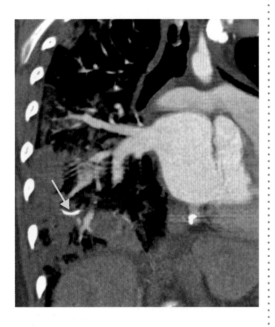

Iatrogenic emboli

PE from iatrogenic causes includes kyphoplasty cement that has leaked into the lumbar veins, angiographic guide wires, broken IVC filters, and pacemaker leads. Mechanical devices are generally retrieved under angiographic guidance, but may be left alone if in a distant vessel. In this case, coronal oblique CT image shows an embolized needle (arrow) in a subsegmental branch of the right lower lobe pulmonary artery. The needle was misplaced during surgery for repair of an atrial septal defect and had to be removed by wedge resection.

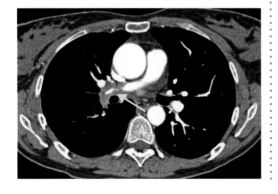

Giant cell arteritis

Giant cell arteritis (GCA) is a vasculitis involving the medium- and large-sized blood vessels. It is a multisystem disease and very rarely involves the pulmonary artery. GCA can clinically present with nonspecific chest pain and dyspnea. Imaging findings include narrowing or aneurysmal dilatation of the pulmonary artery with or without parenchymal abnormality. Treatment is with steroids. Axial

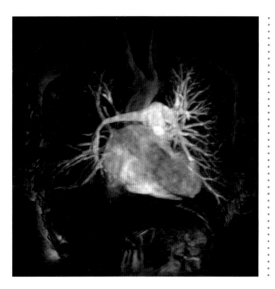

enhanced CT demonstrates mural thickening and diffuse narrowing of the right main pulmonary artery (arrow). Coronal MR MIP demonstrates pruning of the pulmonary arterial tree on the right. Biopsy of the soft tissue surrounding the right main pulmonary artery revealed blood and inflammation. The patient responded to high-dose steroids.

Further reading

Akpinar MG, Goodman LR. Imaging of pulmonary thromboembolism. *Clinics in Chest Medicine* 2008; 29(1): 107–116.

Beckman MG, Hooper WC, Critchley SE, Ortel TL. Venous thromboembolism: a public health concern. *Am J Prev Med*. Apr. 2010; 38(4 Suppl): S495–501.

Bettman MA, Baginski SG, White RD, *et al. ACR Appropriateness Criteria®. Acute Chest Pain – Suspected Pulmonary Embolism*. Available at www.acr.org/~/media/186992e39e754270bb3abbf44a5a5801.pdf. Accessed January 25, 2014.

Castañer E, Gallardo X, Ballesteros E, Andreu M, Pallardó Y, Mata JM, Riera L. CT diagnosis of chronic pulmonary thromboembolism. *Radiographics*. 2009 Jan.–Feb. 2009; 29(1): 31–50.

Chong S, Kim TS, Kim B-T, Cho EY, Kim J. Pulmonary artery sarcoma mimicking pulmonary thromboembolism: integrated FDG PET/CT. *AJR* June 2007; 188: 1691–1693.

Goldhaber SZ, Visani L, De Rosa M. Acute pulmonary embolism: clinical outcomes in the International Cooperative Pulmonary Embolism Registry (ICOPER). *Lancet* 1999; 353: 1386–1389.

Huisman MV, Klok FA. How I diagnose acute pulmonary embolism. *Blood*. 2013 May 30; 121(22): 4443–4448.

Wilbur J, Shian B. Diagnosis of deep venous thrombosis and pulmonary embolism. *Am Fam Physician*. Nov. 15, 2012; 86(10): 913–919.

Case 32   32-year-old male complaining of chest pain after upper endoscopy

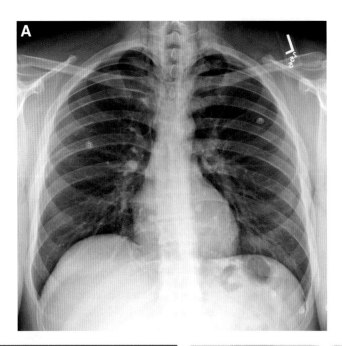

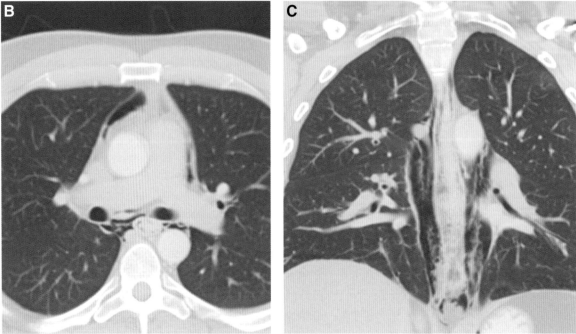

Diagnosis: **Esophageal rupture post upper endoscopy**

Chest radiograph (A) demonstrates streaky lucencies outlining the mediastinum, most prominently seen extending to the lower neck (arrows), consistent with pneumomediastinum. Axial (B) and coronal (C) enhanced CT images confirm the presence of extensive pneumomediastinum (arrows), with a large amount of air surrounding the esophagus. No direct esophageal injury is identified.

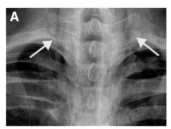 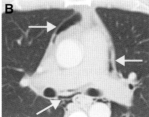 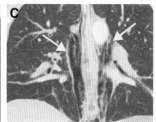

Discussion

Overview and etiology of esophageal rupture

- The esophagus is more prone to rupture in comparison to other hollow viscera due to its lack of supporting adventitia and relatively poor blood supply.
- Iatrogenic perforation is the most common cause of esophageal rupture, which may occur as a complication of upper endoscopy or more invasive surgical procedures. An impacted food bolus may also cause esophageal rupture due to pressure necrosis. Other etiologies of esophageal rupture include malignancy, trauma, esophagitis (infectious, reflux, post radiation), and increased intraluminal pressure (Mallory–Weiss tear).
- The symptoms of esophageal injury (and rupture) are nonspecific, including severe chest pain, dysphagia, and odynophagia.

Imaging of esophageal injury

- Although a water-soluble contrast esophagram is considered the imaging modality of choice for suspected esophageal injury, CT is most often performed due to immediate availability and ability to identify alternative diagnoses for a nonspecific clinical presentation. If esophageal injury is clinically suspected, water-soluble oral contrast can be helpful.
- On CT imaging, pneumomediastinum is almost always seen in the setting of esophageal rupture, even in the absence of direct visualization of an esophageal defect, as in the case above. However, it is important to note that although pneumomediastinum can be the result of esophageal rupture,

alveolar rupture due to barotrauma is overall the most common cause of pneumomediastinum. Pneumomediastinum as an isolated finding is nonspecific and may also occur in patients with asthma, during straining against a closed glottis (parturition, weight lifting, vomiting), after blunt chest trauma, or due to traumatic airway laceration.

- Other CT findings of esophageal injury include direct visualization of a mural defect, extravasation of oral contrast, and periesophageal gas and/or fluid collections. Ancillary signs of esophageal injury include mediastinal fat stranding and pleural effusion.

Treatment and complications of esophageal rupture

- Treatment of esophageal rupture is often surgical. If an impacted food bolus is identified (typically appearing as a mixed-attenuation lesion containing foci of gas), endoscopic removal is the treatment of choice.
- Complications of esophageal perforation include mediastinitis, pneumonia, empyema, and lung abscess, all of which may be apparent on CT.

Clinical synopsis   The patient was admitted to thoracic surgery given CT evidence of extensive pneumomediastinum and was kept NPO for 3 days with improvement of pneumomediastinum on subsequent chest radiographs. An esophagram was also performed and did not reveal contrast leakage. Diet was advanced and patient was discharged home feeling well.

Self-assessment

- *What is the most common cause of pneumomediastinum?*

- Alveolar rupture.

- *What are the different causes of esophageal rupture?*

- Esophagitis, malignancy, iatrogenesis (endoscopy, surgery), foreign body impaction (commonly food), Mallory–Weiss tear, chest trauma.

- *What anatomic features increase the susceptibility of the esophagus to perforation?*

- The lack of adventitia and poor blood supply.

Spectrum of esophageal rupture

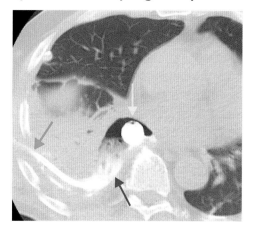

Esophageal perforation after attempted esophagectomy

Axial CT with oral contrast in a patient status post attempted esophagectomy demonstrates a densely opacified esophageal stent (yellow arrow), surrounded by pneumomediastinum. There is leak of oral contrast into the right pleural space (red arrow), consistent with perforation. Note the right-sided surgical pleural drain (blue arrow).

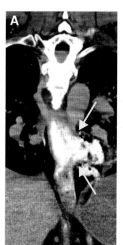
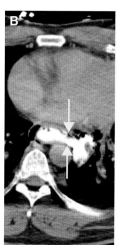

Mallory–Weiss tear / Boerhaave syndrome

A Mallory–Weiss tear is a longitudinal mucosal laceration in the distal esophagus or across the gastroesophageal junction. Boerhaave syndrome is defined by oesophageal rupture. These pathologies most commonly occur in the setting of intense vomiting due to alcohol intoxication. CT may show evidence of esophageal wall hemorrhage or foci of extraluminal gas. Coronal (A) and axial (B) CT images with oral contrast demonstrate a defect of the left lateral wall of the distal thoracic esophagus (arrows) with extravasation of oral contrast material.

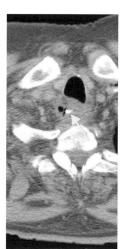
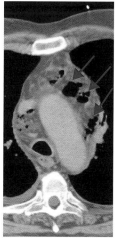

Foreign body impaction complicated by esophageal perforation and mediastinitis and abscess formation

An impacted esophageal foreign body may result in esophageal perforation if it causes direct perfor-ation (most commonly with an ingested bone or other sharp object) or pressure necrosis develops. Mediastinitis and abscess formation may result. Axial enhanced CT images demonstrate an impacted ingested bone perforating the upper esophagus (yellow arrow). Diffuse mediastinal fat stranding is indicative of mediastinitis, and multiple gas collections in the anterior and middle medias-tinum (red arrows) are concerning for abscesses.

Differential diagnosis of esophageal rupture

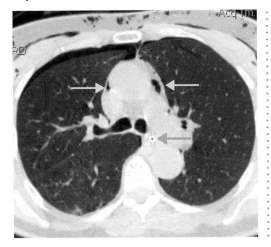

Pneumomediastinum due to alveolar rupture

Blunt trauma to the chest, usually from a motor vehicle accident, may cause pneumomediastinum secondary to alveolar rupture or fracture of the trachea or bronchi. Axial CT demonstrates pneumomediastinum (yellow arrows), subcutaneous emphysema, and bilateral pneumothoraces (red arrows). A nasogastric tube is present in the esophagus (blue arrow). Note the absence of pneumomediastinum directly surrounding the esophagus, suggesting against an esophageal rupture.

Further reading

Young CA, Menias CO, Bhalla S, *et al*. CT Features of Esophageal Emergencies. *Radiographics* 2008; 28:1541–1553.

Zylak CM, Standen JR, Barnes GR, *et al*. Pneumomediastinum Revisited. *Radiographics* 2000; 20:1043–1057.

Case 33   88-year-old female with chest pain and shortness of breath

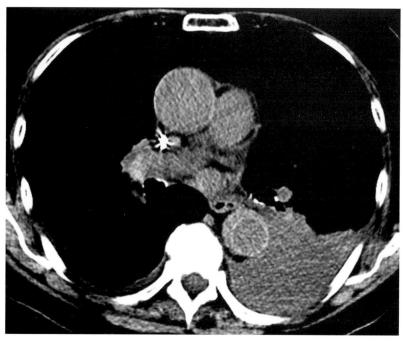

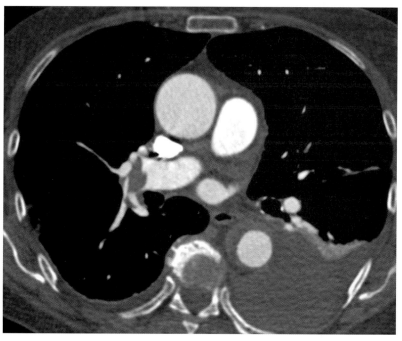

Diagnosis:
**Main right
pulmonary
artery
embolus and
thrombosed
type B aortic
dissection**

Unenhanced (left) and contrast-enhanced (right) axial CT of the chest
shows crescentic high attenuation in the descending thoracic aorta on
unenhanced CT that does not enhance following intravenous contrast
material (yellow arrows). Pulmonary embolus is present in the right main
pulmonary artery (red arrows).

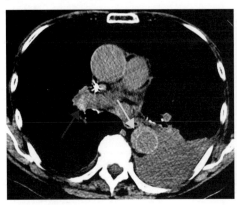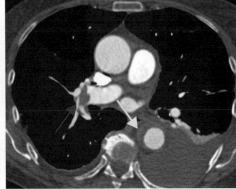

Discussion

Overview of aortic dissection (pulmonary embolism is case 31)

- CT is the modality of choice for evaluating aortic dissection. Most institutions
  perform a low-dose unenhanced CT followed by a contrast-enhanced CT of
  the chest.
- Although aortic dissection occurs most commonly in older hypertensive
  patients, risk factors in younger patients include hypertension, connective
  tissue diseases (e.g., Marfans, Ehlers–Danlos), bicuspid aortic valve, aortic
  coarctation, pregnancy, and cocaine use.
- Approximately 60% of aortic dissections involve the ascending aorta (type A)
  and 40% involve the descending aorta (type B).
- Type A dissection is usually accompanied by substernal chest pain at onset,
  while type B dissection is usually accompanied by interscapular back pain at
  onset. Pain symptoms can migrate as aortic dissection progresses, and can
  abate as the dissection stops.
- Type A dissection is generally managed surgically, and type B dissection is
  generally managed medically. In-hospital mortality is 26% and 11% for type
  A and type B dissection, respectively.

***Clinical
synopsis***

The patient was admitted to the hospital where echocardiography showed
no evidence of right heart strain despite the large burden of pulmonary
embolus. A decision was made not to anticoagulate the patient because of
the aortic dissection. An IVC filter was placed because of the continued

presence of DVT in both lower extremities. The aortic dissection was managed medically with a beta-blocker for blood pressure control. The patient became asymptomatic and was discharged to rehabilitation 5 days later.

Self-assessment

- *What CT findings may be observed on unenhanced CT when aortic dissection is present?*

- The positive intimal flap sign, intramural hematoma, and displaced intimal calcification are findings that may be present on unenhanced CT.

- *Can aortic dissection be excluded on the basis of an unenhanced CT?*

- No. Contrast-enhanced CT must be performed to exclude aortic dissection.

- *How is aortic dissection classified using either the Stanford or DeBakey classification system?*

- Stanford type A dissection is any dissection involving the ascending aorta proximal to the innominate artery regardless of whether it is confined to the ascending aorta or extends beyond it. The DeBakey classification subdivides this group to those with involvement beyond the ascending aorta (type I) and those confined to the ascending aorta (type II). Stanford type B and DeBakey type III describe aortic dissection confined to the aortic arch and/or descending aorta with no involvement proximal to the innominate artery.

- *How is the false aortic lumen differentiated from the true aortic lumen?*

- The most reliable method is to show continuity of the true lumen with the uninvolved aorta. In the involved portion, the false lumen is usually larger and often shows the beak sign (acute angle formed between the intimal flap and the aortic wall). If the dissection is circumferential, the true lumen is always the inner lumen.

- *What complications can occur with aortic dissection?*

- Aortic dissection may rupture into the pericardial sac, mediastinum, pleural cavity, or retroperitoneum. The dissection can occlude arterial branches leading to end-organ ischemia or infarct (e.g., stroke, myocardial infarction, renal infarction, etc.). Complete thrombosis of the false or true lumen can occur.

Spectrum of aortic dissection

The spectrum of aortic dissection ranges from conspicuous intimal flap to subtle thickening of the aortic wall. Dissection may involve both the ascending and descending aorta, or be confined to either. Extent of dissection may be limited to several centimeters within a single segment, or involve the entire aorta and propagate distally into the common iliac arteries. Associated complications of aortic dissection may be absent, or may include aortic rupture, thrombosis, and/or end-organ ischemia/infarction.

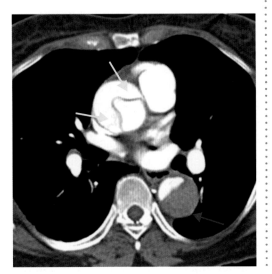

Stanford type A / DeBakey type I aortic dissection

Approximately 60% of aortic dissections involve the ascending aorta. Because ascending aortic involvement is associated with higher mortality when treated medically, dissection involving this segment is generally managed surgically. Axial CT angiogram demonstrates an obvious dissection flap involving the ascending aorta with beak sign in the false lumen (arrow) where the flap meets the aortic wall. The true lumen is the inner lumen. In the descending aorta the false lumen is unperfused and larger than the true lumen (red arrow).

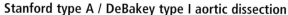

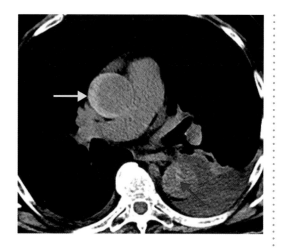

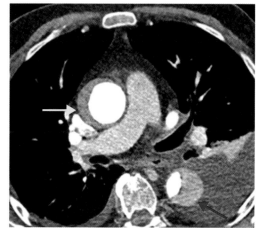

Stanford type A / DeBakey type I aortic dissection

The false lumen of an aortic dissection can thrombose, which may diminish conspicuity of the pathognomonic feature of dissection, the intimal flap. When this occurs, unenhanced CT will reveal smooth, crescentic high attenuation. Following administration of intravenous contrast material, the false lumen will not perfuse. Unenhanced CT (top image) shows crescentic high attenuation intramural hematoma in the ascending aorta (yellow arrow) and the intimal flap sign in the descending aorta (red arrow). Following intravenous contrast material, no significant enhancement is seen in the thrombosed ascending false lumen (yellow arrow). There is some enhancement of the false lumen in the descending aorta indicating slow flow as compared to the true lumen (red arrow).

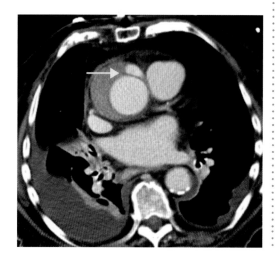

Stanford type A / DeBakey type II aortic dissection

Any aortic dissection involving the ascending aorta is classified as a Stanford type A dissection. The DeBakey classification system separates those confined to the ascending aorta (type II) from those that extend beyond the ascending aorta to involve the arch or descending thoracic aorta (type I). Contrast enhanced CT shows contrast partially opacifying the false lumen of the ascending aorta (yellow arrow). The descending thoracic aorta is uninvolved.

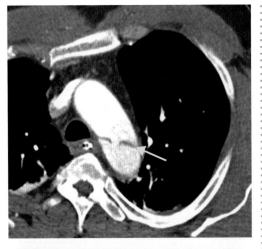

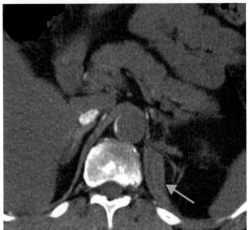

Stanford type B / DeBakey type III aortic dissection

Approximately 40% of aortic dissections do not involve the ascending aorta, and are confined to the aortic arch and/or descending aorta. These dissections are generally managed medically since the mortality associated with surgical management is significantly higher. However, patients with intractable pain, end-organ ischemia, aortic occlusion or rupture generally require surgical or endovascular intervention. Contrast-enhanced CT shows a dissection flap originating in the posterior aortic arch (yellow arrow). Near the aortic hiatus, the false lumen is thrombosed and completely occludes the true lumen (red arrow). Soft tissue attenuation in the left retroperitoneum (blue arrow) indicates this dissection is complicated by aortic rupture.

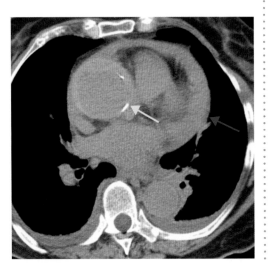

Stanford type A / DeBakey type II aortic dissection

Unenhanced CT is able to diagnose most cases of aortic dissection based on the presence of either intramural hematoma, displaced intimal calcification, and/or visualization of an intimal flap. Unenhanced CT shows displacement of intimal calcification toward the aortic lumen and crescentic high attenuation consistent with intramural hematoma (yellow arrow). This dissection is complicated by rupture into the pericardial sac causing hemopericardium (red arrow). The descending aorta is uninvolved.

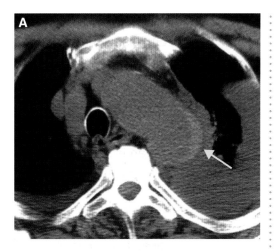

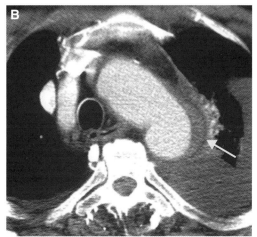

Stanford type B / DeBakey type III aortic dissection

Unenhanced CT (A) shows crescentic high attenuation in the posterior aortic arch (arrow). Following intravenous contrast administration (B), there is no enhancement within the false lumen (arrow) consistent with thrombosis of the false lumen. The ascending aorta is uninvolved. The left pleural effusion is simple fluid attenuation.

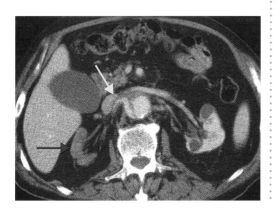

Stanford type B / DeBakey type III aortic dissection

Axial enhanced CT in a patient with dissection involving the post-subclavian aorta shows extension to the abdominal aorta and involvement of the right renal artery (yellow arrow). The right kidney is unperfused and ischemic (red arrow). The left kidney is perfused normally. The patient underwent endovascular fenestration in an attempt to restore right renal perfusion.

Differential diagnosis of aortic dissection

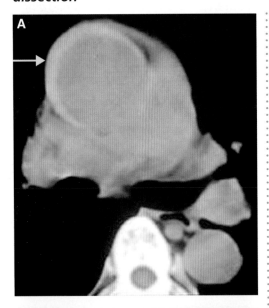

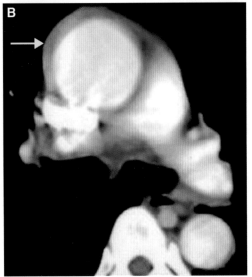

Isolated intramural hematoma

Spontaneous isolated intramural hematoma is distinguished from aortic dissection by the absence of an intimal breach, the distinguishing imaging feature of aortic dissection. Therefore, when there is complete thrombosis of the false lumen of an aortic dissection it is impossible to differentiate dissection from spontaneous intra- mural hematoma. Thankfully, aortic dissection and intramural hematoma are managed similarly. If there is involvement of the ascending aorta, then surgery is generally pursued. If there is absence of ascending involvement, then medical manage- ment is generally pursued. Unenhanced CT (A) shows smooth, crescentic high attenuation within the ascending aorta (arrow) that appears as mild aortic wall thickening after intravenous contrast administration (B; arrow). The patient underwent thoracotomy and ascending aortic graft. Patholo- gic evaluation of the ascending aorta found no intimal breach.

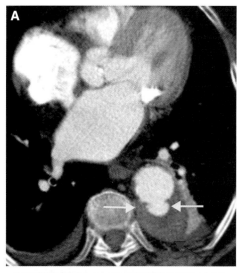

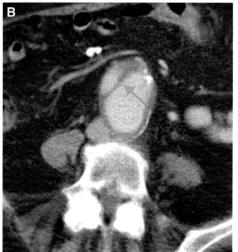

Penetrating atherosclerotic ulcer

This entity is most common in the 8th decade and usually encountered in the setting of marked atherosclerotic disease. The clinical presentation is generally indistinguishable from aortic dissection, and the most common associated finding is localized intramural hematoma. Contrast-enhanced CT (A) shows a focal outpouching from the descending thoracic aorta with overhanging edges consistent with an ulcer (yellow arrows). There is associated localized intramural hematoma indicating acuity (red arrow). Contrast-enhanced CT in a different patient (B) shows the appearance of a chronic penetrating ulcer in the infrarenal abdominal aorta. Overhanging edges of the ulcer can simulate a dissection flap (blue arrow), but the location, localized morphology, and associated findings should readily distinguish this entity from aortic dissection.

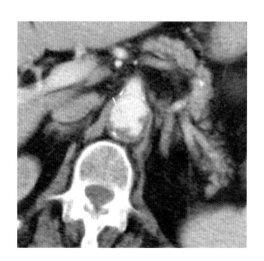

Mural thrombus and atherosclerotic plaque

Mural thrombus and atherosclerotic plaque are commonly encountered in older hypertensive patients, and therefore frequently present among patients undergoing evaluation for aortic dissection. Low attenuation and irregular morphology of this entity help distinguish it from intramural hematoma and aortic dissection. Contrast-enhanced CT shows irregular low attenuation intraluminal thrombus that resides above the intimal calcification (arrow).

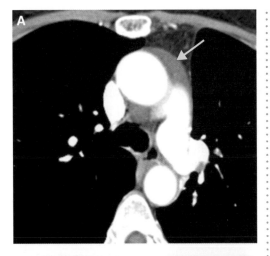

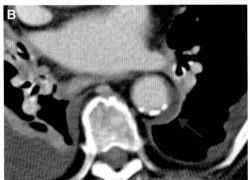

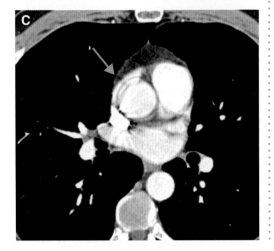

Periaortic processes mimicking aortic dissection

Because aortic dissection involves the peripheral wall of the aorta, periaortic processes can sometimes mimic aortic dissection. Most of these entities are readily excluded by familiarity with anatomic structures and morphologic appearances. Contrast-enhanced CT (A) shows pericardial effusion in the superior pericardial recess adjacent to the ascending thoracic aorta (arrow), which can simulate aortic wall thickening of intramural hematoma. Contrast-enhanced CT in a different patient (B) shows loculated pleural effusion wrapping around the descending thoracic aorta (red arrow), but clearly beyond the calcified aortic wall. Contrast-enhanced CT in a third patient (C) shows the right atrial appendage extending around the proximal ascending aorta (blue arrow).

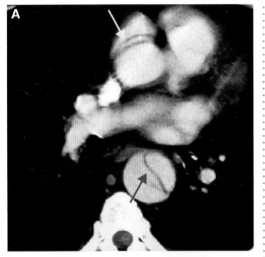

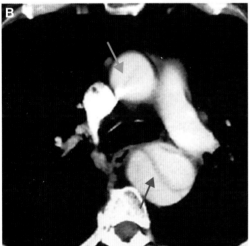

Artifacts

There are classic artifacts at CT imaging that can simulate aortic dissection. Pulsation artifact is caused by the systolic anterior motion of the heart, typically seen on ungated studies. Contrast-enhanced CT (A) shows the typical double wall sign (yellow arrow) that can simulate dissection involving the ascending aorta in a patient who clearly has dissection involving the descending aorta (red arrow). A different axial image from the same study (B) shows streak artifact (blue arrow) across the ascending aorta due to the high iodine concentration in the superior vena cava from the contrast bolus. It's critically important that these artifacts in the ascending aorta be recognized as such given the presence of dissection involving the descending aorta so that the dissection can be properly classified as type A or type B. The ability to differentiate these findings would determine whether this patient undergoes thoracotomy or is medically managed. If there is any uncertainty in the diagnosis, then the patient could return for a gated aortic study with reduced concentration of contrast injection.

Further reading

Castaner E, Andreu M, Gallardo X, Mata JM, Cabezuelo MA, Pallardo Y. CT in non-traumatic acute thoracic aortic disease: typical and atypical features and complications. *Radiographics*. Oct. 2003;23 Spec. No.:S93–110.

Hiratzka LF, Bakris GL, Beckman JA, *et al.* ACCF/AHA/AATS/ACR/ASA/SCA/SCAI/SIR/STS/SVM Guidelines for the diagnosis and management of patients with thoracic aortic disease. *J Am Coll Cardiol.* Apr. 6, 2010;6;55(14):e27–e129.

Macura KJ, Corl FM, Fishman EK, Bluemke DA. Pathogenesis in acute aortic syndromes: aortic dissection, intramural hematoma, and penetrating atherosclerotic aortic ulcer. *AJR Am J Roentgenol.* Aug. 2003;181(2):309-316.

Sakamoto S, Taniguchi N, Nakajima S, Takahashi A. Diagnostic value of nonenhanced multidetector computed tomography for ruling out acute aortic dissection in patients presenting with chest or back pain. *Int J Cardiol.* Sept. 2013;168(2):734-738.

Souza D, Ledbetter S. Diagnostic errors in the evaluation of nontraumatic aortic emergencies. *Semin Ultrasound CT MR.* Aug. 2012;33(4):318-336.

Case 34   29-year-old woman with fever, cough, and pleuritic chest pain

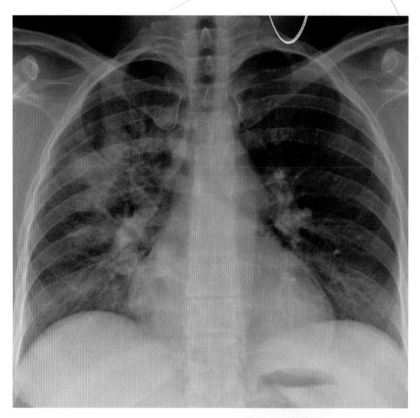

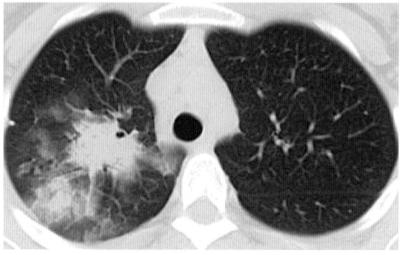

Diagnosis:
**Community-
acquired
pneumonia**

PA chest radiograph (left image) demonstrates a patchy right upper lobe
parenchymal opacity (arrow). Unenhanced axial CT confirms two adjacent
patchy consolidative opacities in the right upper lobe (arrows), consistent with
bronchopneumonia.

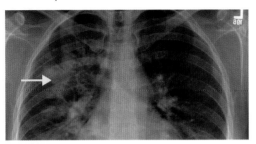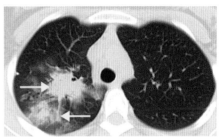

Discussion

Overview and classification of pneumonia

- Pneumonia is infection of the lung parenchyma. Although pneumonia can be
caused by several different viral, bacterial, and fungal pathogens, it is clinically
divided into community-acquired pneumonia (CAP) and other types of
pneumonia associated with current or recent hospitalization. These include:
  - Hospital acquired pneumonia (HAP), which is thought to be due to microaspiration
  of secretions in a hospitalized patient, with high prevalence of antibiotic-resistant
  gram-positive cocci such as methicillin-resistant *Staphylococcus aureus* (MRSA)
  and gram-negative bacilli such as *Pseudomonas aeruginosa*.
  - Healthcare-associated pneumonia (HCAP), which is defined as pneumonia
  in a nursing home resident or a patient with a hospitalization within the past
  90 days. The causative pathogens are similar to those that cause HAP.
  - Ventilator-associated pneumonia (VAP), which occurs within 48 hours of
  mechanical ventilation.
- There are 5.6 million cases of CAP reported each year, with up to 1.1 million
hospitalizations and associated health care costs of up to $8 billion.
- CAP usually starts as an upper respiratory infection, spreading into the distal
airways. There are dozens of microorganisms that can cause CAP; however the
most common are *Streptococcus pneumoniae,* viruses, and atypical bacteria
such as *Mycoplasma pneumoniae.*

Imaging patterns of pneumonia

- Pneumonia can present with several different patterns of imaging, which may
correlate with the causative organism.
- Lobar pneumonia (complete opacification of a single lobe) is typically seen
with *Streptococcus pneumoniae* (pneumococcus) or *Klebsiella pneumoniae.*

- Bronchopneumonia (patchy opacification along the bronchovascular bundle, as in this case) can be seen with atypical organisms, *Staphylococcus aureus*, viral pneumonia, or *Legionella pneumophila*.
- Interstitial pneumonia (diffuse opacification, often partial, of multiple lobes) can be seen with viral pneumonia, *Legionella pneumophila*, and *Pneumocystis jirovecii* pneumonia (previously called *Pneumocystis carinii pneumonia*, or PCP).
- Cavitary pneumonia (pneumonia causing cavitation) can be caused by anaerobic bacteria, *Klebsiella pneumoniae*, *Mycobacterium tuberculosis*, *Staphylococcus aureus*, or fungal pneumonia.

Pneumonia imaging

- Chest radiography is the primary modality to evaluate for clinically suspected pneumonia. A chest radiograph can identify the presence, location, and extent of disease, and can also detect some complications, such as cavitation, abscess, pneumothorax, and effusion.
- CT is an adjunct to the chest radiograph. CT is used for failed medical treatment or lack of radiographic resolution despite clinical improvement. Also, CT can suggest additional or alternative diagnoses.

Pneumonia treatment and follow-up algorithm (in an immunocompetent individual)

- If the patient does respond clinically to medical treatment, a follow-up radiograph is recommended to ensure resolution.
  - For a patient < 50 years old, CAP should clear in 3–4 weeks.
  - For a patient > 50 years old, CAP should clear in 8–12 weeks.
- In cases where the clinical or radiographic findings do not respond to medical treatment, a CT should be performed to evaluate for an alternative explanation.

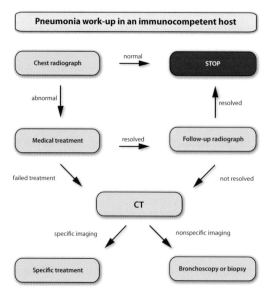

Pneumonia in an immunosuppressed individual

- The immunosuppressed host may have altered immunity due to HIV infection, hematological malignancy, transplant, chemotherapy, chronic corticosteroid use, or diabetes.
- In addition to the infectious organisms discussed on the previous page, opportunistic fungal and viral infections are common in the immunosuppressed, including *Pneumocystis jirovecii* and *Aspergillus fumigatus*. Additionally, reactivation of latent infections such as tuberculosis occurs much more commonly in the immunosuppressed.
- If there is high clinical suspicion for pneumonia in an immunosuppressed patient and the chest radiograph is negative, further imaging with CT is often performed.

Clinical synopsis

This 29-year-old female with community-acquired pneumonia was treated with oral levofloxacin. A follow-up radiograph at 6 weeks showed complete resolution.

Self-assessment

- *What are the common complications of pneumonia?*

  - Empyema and abscess formation are the two most common complications.

- *What is the differential diagnosis of a chronic pulmonary opacity?*

  - The key to diagnosing pneumonia is the chronicity. An acute change is overwhelmingly likely to represent infection. However, chronic pulmonary opacities (which are often first diagnosed as non-resolution of an abnormality originally thought to represent pneumonia) include mucinous adenocarcinoma, cryptogenic organizing pneumonia, hypersensitivity pneumonitis, lymphoma, eosinophilic pneumonia, and vasculitis.

- *What is the difference in pneumonia in the immunocompetent and immunosuppressed host?*

  - Pneumonia is aggressive, difficult to treat, and takes longer to resolve in the immunosuppressed. Opportunistic fungal and viral infections are more common in the immunosuppressed. Additionally, reactivation of latent infections such as tuberculosis occurs much more commonly in the immunosuppressed.

Patterns of pneumonia

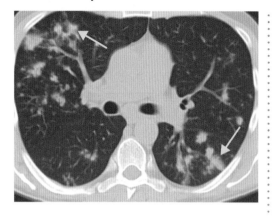

Bronchopneumonia

Bronchopneumonia is acute inflammation of the walls of the bronchioles, characterized by multiple centrilobular nodules in a bronchocentric distribution. Bronchopneumonia is the most common pattern seen with *Staphylococcus aureus*, viral pneumonia, and *Legionella pneumophila*. Axial CT demonstrates patchy centrilobular nodules bilaterally (arrows).

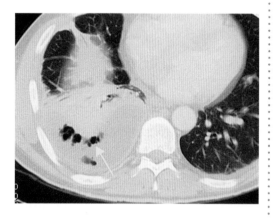

Lobar pneumonia

Lobar pneumonia is the most common pattern of pneumonia in an immunocompetent host, and produces confluent opacification that respects the segmental or fissural anatomy. Lobar pneumonia is the most common pattern seen in *Streptococcus pneumoniae*. Pathophysiologically, there is peripheral, subpleural spread of infection leading to hemorrhagic edema. Axial CT demonstrates a dense right lower lobe opacity with a few central air bronchograms (arrow).

Differential diagnosis of pneumonia

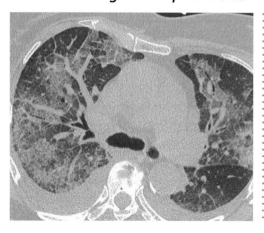

Pulmonary edema

Pulmonary edema is abnormal fluid accumulation in the lung parenchyma and air spaces. It is characterized by smooth interlobular septal thickening and pleural effusions. Short interval repeat radiographs showing improvement can help differentiate from pneumonia. Pulmonary edema changes with volume status, while pneumonia will improve with antibiotic therapy. Axial CT demonstrates peribronchovascular ground glass opacification with bilateral pleural effusions.

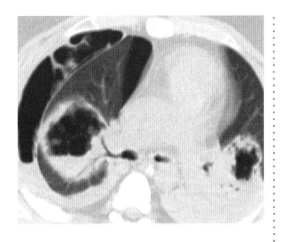

Vasculitis

Granulomatosis with polyangiitis (GPA, formerly known as Wegener's granulomatosis) and Churg Strauss vasculitis can mimic necrotizing pneumonia. Both of these entities can present with nodules that undergo cavitation. Spontaneous pneumothorax can occur if the cavity ruptures to the pleura. In general, leukocytosis and fever are absent even in the presence of extensive disease. Vasculitis is a diagnosis of exclusion, typically made after a patient has failed antibiotic treatment. C-ANCA is very specific for GPA when positive. Axial CT demonstrates bilateral cavitary masses and a right hydropneumothorax.

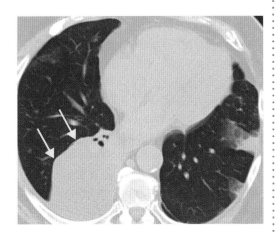

Atelectasis

Collapse of a segment or lobe can mimic consolidation. If intravenous contrast is administered, then atelectasis typically enhances, unlike pneumonia. If an unenhanced CT is performed, then an important clue to the presence of atelectasis is volume *loss* of the affected lung. Axial unenhanced CT demonstrates a right basilar medial opacity. There is displacement of the right oblique fissure posteriorly (arrows), abutting the collapsed right lower lobe, and hyperexpansion of the right middle lobe. Nonspecific patchy opacities in the left lung may represent subsegmental atelectasis.

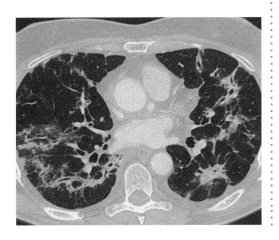

Organizing pneumonia

Organizing pneumonia is characterized histologically by granulation tissue polyps filling the distal airways, and can be seen in response to infection, drug reaction, toxic inhalation, or in the setting of organ transplantation or connective tissue disorders. Cryptogenic organizing pneumonia (COP) is the clinical syndrome of organizing pneumonia without known cause. Treatment is with steroids. Axial CT shows peripheral opacities in a peribronchovascular distribution.

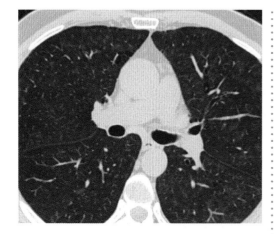

Hypersensitivity pneumonitis

Hypersensitivity pneumonitis (HSP) is an inhalational lung disease caused by a hypersensitivity reaction to an inhaled organic antigen, such as bird protein. Acute HSP is characterized by non-specific ground glass or consolidation. Subacute HSP features characteristic ground glass centrilobular nodules. Mosaic attenuation (geographic areas of relative lucency) may also be seen, due to a combination of altered perfusion and air trapping. Chronic HSP may cause upper-lobe predominant fibrosis. Axial CT demonstrates diffuse centrilobular ground glass nodules in a patient with subacute HSP.

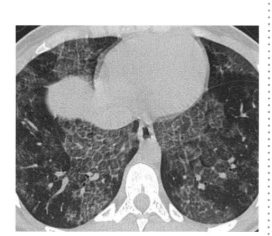

Alveolar proteinosis

Alveolar proteinosis is an idiopathic disorder characterized by filling of alveoli by a proteinaceous, lipid-rich material. The classic CT finding is the "crazy paving" sign, which is characterized by smooth interlobular septal thickening with geographic regions of ground glass attenuation. Note that the "crazy paving" sign is nonspecific and can also be seen in organizing pneumonia and mucinous adenocarcinoma, among other entities. Axial CT demonstrates bilateral geographic regions of ground glass attenuation and superimposed septal thickening representing the "crazy paving" sign.

Further reading

Mandell LA, Wunderink RG, Anzueto A, *et al. Infectious Diseases Society of America/ American Thoracic Society consensus guidelines on the management of community-acquired pneumonia. Infect Dis.* 2007; 44 (Suppl. 2):S27–S72.

Niederman M. In the clinic: community-acquired pneumonia. *Ann Intern Med.* 2009; 151(7):ITC4-1.

Sharma S, Maycher B, Eschun G. Radiological imaging in pneumonia: recent innovations. *Current Opinion in Pulmonary Medicine.* 2007; 13 (3):159-169.

Torres A, *et al.* Pyogenic bacterial pneumonia and lung abscess. In: Mason RJ, Broaddus VC, Martin TR, *et al.*, eds. *Murray & Nadel's Textbook of Respiratory Medicine.* 5th edn. Philadelphia, PA: Saunders Elsevier; 2010: ch. 32.

Van der Poll T, Opal SM. Pathogenesis, treatment, and prevention of pneumococcal pneumonia. *Lancet.* 2009; 374:1543–1556.

Case 35 37-year-old woman with a history of rheumatoid arthritis presenting with non-resolving bilateral effusions and chest pain

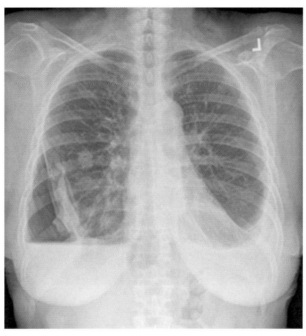

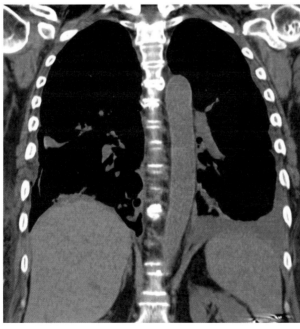

Diagnosis:
Empyema

Frontal chest radiograph demonstrates a left pleural effusion (yellow arrow) and a right hydropneumothorax (red arrow). A right-sided lung nodule is present (blue arrow). Coronal noncontrast CT image better demonstrates the complex left pleural effusion with associated pleural thickening (yellow arrow). Diagnostic thoracentesis confirmed that the effusions were infected.

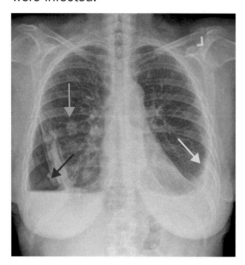 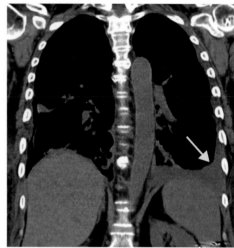

Discussion

Empyema is defined as an infected pleural effusion or collection. There are three stages in the evolution of empyema.

- The first or "exudative" stage is characterized by rapid egress of fluid from the pulmonary interstitial space into the pleural space, which may be augmented by capillary leakage. Evaluation of pleural fluid indicates that the effusion is exudative rather than transudative by Light's criteria, but bacterial cultures are negative.
- Without appropriate treatment, there is progression to the second or "fibropurulent stage", in which the pleural fluid becomes infected and loculated.
- If the collection is not drained, progression to the third stage, the development of a thick "pleural peel," may occur due to transit of fibroblasts from the parietal and visceral pleura into the empyema. This pleural peel may restrict lung movement and must be surgically removed (decorticated) by open thoracotomy or video-assisted thorascopic surgery (VATS).

Empyema is defined as an infected pleural effusion or collection. There are three stages in the evolution of empyema.

- Empyema appears as a loculated effusion with a lenticular appearance.
- CT can be used for confirmation and assessment for underlying pneumonia.

- CT is also the best modality for identification and characterization of complications such as bronchopleural fistula (BPF) and empyema necessitans, defined as extension of the pleural collection out of the pleural space into the chest wall.
- When clinical features and imaging suggest the diagnosis, diagnostic thoracentesis is performed.

Empyemas are treated with aggressive antibiotics.

- Surgical decortication may be helpful in patients who do not respond to antibiotics or in cases of moderate or large empyema, and may include a Clagett window procedure. In the Clagett window procedure, a small thoracotomy is left open for ongoing irrigation with antibiotic solution and drainage. When infection has resolved and granulation tissue has formed, antibiotic solution is instilled into the pleural space and the window may be closed using muscular flaps from the latissimus dorsi.

Clinical synopsis

- The bilateral empyemas did not resolve even after repeated courses of aggressive intravenous antibiotics. The right pneumothorax was caused by previous thoracentesis attempt, and the right-sided lung nodule was thought to be a rheumatoid necrobiotic nodule. The patient underwent bilateral surgical decortication and creation of Clagett windows. Upon resolution of infection, closure was achieved with bilateral latissimus dorsi flaps.
- Noncontrast CT image of the chest in the coronal plane (left image) shows bilateral Clagett windows, which provide communication between the pleural space and the outside. Mixed density packing material is visible (arrows). After resolution of infection, repeat noncontrast coronal CT shows that the Clagett windows have been closed with latissimus dorsi flaps.

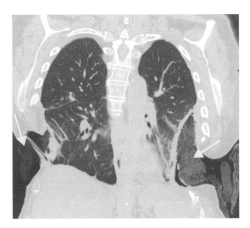 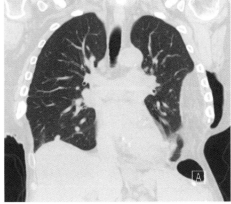

Self-assessment

- *What radiographic view can help determine whether an effusion is loculated?*

- *What is "empyema necessitans?"*

- *Name two signs of BPF that may be seen after pneumonectomy.*

- Decubitus view. Loculated effusion will not layer dependently.

- The term "empyema necessitans" refers to extension of a pleural infection into the chest wall.

- Increased gas and loss of fluid in a previously fluid-filled pneumonectomy space and progressive mediastinal emphysema are signs of BPF.

Spectrum of empyema

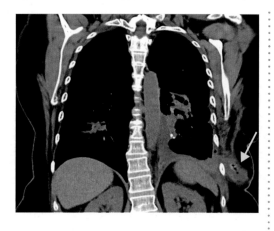

Empyema necessitans

Very rarely, an empyema can directly communicate with the chest wall, either through a previous chest tube tract or a spontaneously developed sinus tract. While the most common pathogens are *M. tuberculosis* and *Actinomyces*, empyema necessitans can also be seen with other bacterial infections. Coronal CT image shows that the left-sided empyema communicates with the left chest wall (arrow).

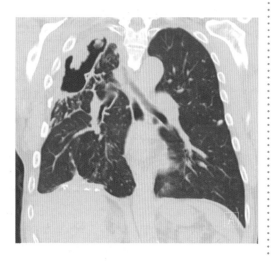

Bronchopleural fistula

A bronchopleural fistula (BPF) is defined as an abnormal communication between a bronchus and the pleural space. A central BPF involves a central, large bronchus, while a peripheral BPF involves a small peripheral bronchus. The most common causes of central BPF are dehiscence of a bronchial stump after lung transplantation, full or partial pneumonectomy, and trauma. Peripheral BPF are caused by necrotizing pneumonia, empyema, trauma, ruptured bullae, and iatrogenic causes such as radiation therapy and thoracentesis. On imaging, increased volume of pleural air (without

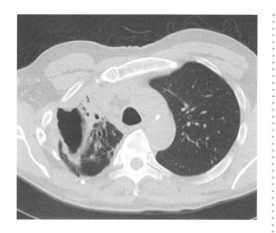

a history of instrumentation) and loss of fluid in a previously filled or filling post-pneumonectomy space are indirect signs of BPF. New gas within an empyema may also suggest fistulization. Direct findings include the fistulous connection itself or extra-luminal air bubbles adjacent to the bronchial stump. Bronchopleural fistulas are very difficult to treat and may require a Clagett window or marsu-pialization of the chest cavity followed by a muscle flap for closure of the chest after the infection resolves. Coronal (upper image) and axial (lower image) unenhanced CT images demonstrate development of a bronchopleural fistula in a patient with chronic *Aspergillus* infection.

Differential diagnosis of empyema

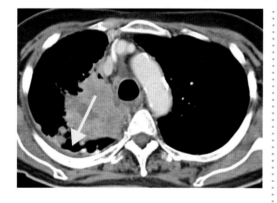

Malignant pleural effusion

Malignant pleural effusions can be seen in lung, breast, ovarian, and gastrointestinal malignancies (among others). These manifest as rapidly increasing pleural effusions and are serosangui-neous in appearance upon thoracentesis. The presence of an exudative pleural effusion without fever or leukocytosis should raise concern for a malignant effusion. In early stages, differentiation between benign and malignant effusion can be made only by pleural fluid analysis. After thora-centesis, the effusion usually rapidly re-accumu-lates. Sometimes, pneumothorax may be present following thoracentesis due to "trapping" of the lung by adhesions. In later stages, distinction by imaging is clearer – malignant effusions tend to be associated with nodularity, mass formation, or enhancement. Axial enhanced CT demonstrates a large right upper lobe mass, with a dependent pleural effusion (arrow) containing nodular enhancement.

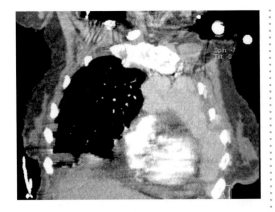

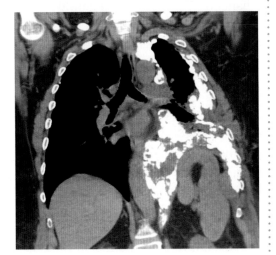

Pleural metastasis

Pleural metastasis is due to secondary dissemination of tumor to the pleura. Enhanced coronal chest CT (upper image) in a patient with metastatic thymoma shows a lobulated, pleural-based soft tissue mass filling the left hemithorax. Non-contrast coronal CT in a different patient with osteosarcoma (lower image) shows a large, lobulated, densely calcified soft tissue mass in the left hemithorax, which represented osteosarcoma metastatic to the pleural space.

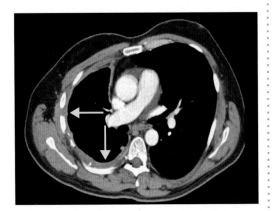

Malignant pleural mesothelioma

Malignant pleural mesothelioma is a rare, primary pleural malignancy. Risk is increased with asbestos exposure. Though calcified pleural plaques do not transform into mesothelioma, their presence may elevate suspicion by indicating prior asbestos exposure. The disease presents as a pleural effusion that later progresses to pleural thickening and nodularity. Nodal involvement and distant metastases are seen in later stages. Direct spread to the chest wall, mediastinal structures, and peritoneal cavity may occur. Treatment includes pleurectomy or extra-pleural pneumonectomy. Unlike empyema, mesothelioma does not present with signs of infection, and volume loss in the affected hemithorax is typical. Enhanced axial chest CT shows marked volume loss in the right hemithorax with circumferential pleural thickening (arrows). Tissue biopsy showed malignant mesothelioma.

Further reading

Ferrer J, Roldán J, Teixidor J, Pallisa E, Gich I, Morell F. Predictors of pleural malignancy in patients with pleural effusion undergoing thoracoscopy. *Chest.* Mar. 2005; 127 (3): 1017–1022.

Gaur P, Dunne R, Colson YL, Gill RR. Bronchopleural fistula and the role of contemporary imaging. *J Thorac Cardiovasc Surg.* 2014; 148 (1): 341-3473 Dec 16. 5.

Gill RR. Imaging of mesothelioma. *Recent Results Cancer Res.* 2011; 189: 27–43.

Light RW. Parapneumonic effusions and empyema. *Proceedings of the American Thoracic Society.* 2006; 3 (1): 75–80.

Pothula V, Krellenstein DJ. Early aggressive surgical management of parapneumonic empyemas. *Chest.* Mar. 1994; 105 (3): 832–836.

Qureshi NR, Rahman NM, Gleeson FV. Thoracic ultrasound in the diagnosis of malignant pleural effusion. *Thorax.* Feb. 2009; 64 (2): 139–143.

Tanaka S, Yajima T, Mogi A, Kuwano H. Successful management of a large bronchopleural fistula after lobectomy: Report of a case. *Surg Today.* Dec. 2011;41 (12): 1661–1664. Epub 2011 Oct. 4, 2011.

Case 36   45-year-old male with a history of bone marrow transplantation
presenting with a cough, productive of greenish sputum

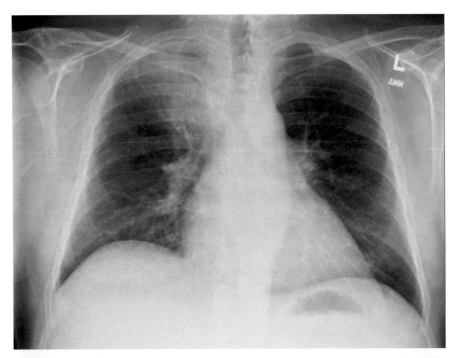

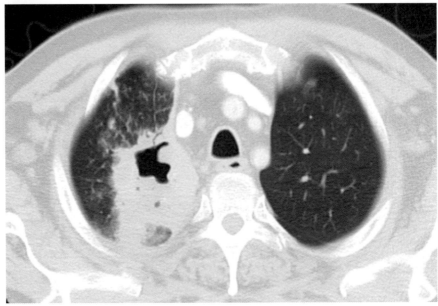

Diagnosis:
Lung abscess

PA chest radiograph shows a consolidative opacity in the right upper lobe (arrow). Axial enhanced CT scan obtained 7 days later shows a right upper lobe consolidative opacity (arrows) with central cavitation, consistent with lung abscess.

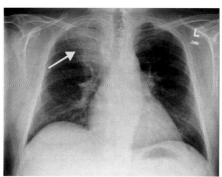 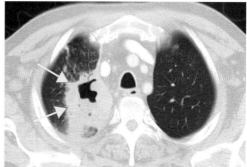

Discussion

Lung parenchymal abscess is defined by central necrosis and diameter greater than 2 cm.

- Abscesses most commonly result from aspiration or necrotizing pneumonia, and less commonly complicate infarcts or contusions.
- In aspiration, causative organisms include mixed anaerobic and aerobic gingival flora (e.g., *Bacteroides, Fusobacterium, Klebsiella, Staphylococcus, Pseudomonas*). Fungi (e.g., *Aspergillus, Candida*) and parasites (e.g., *Entamoeba*) are also sometimes implicated.

Symptoms often have a subacute onset over weeks.

- Typical, nonspecific signs and symptoms include fever, production of foul-smelling sputum, leukocytosis, and hemoptysis.
- Elderly patients and others at risk for aspiration are more vulnerable. 70 to 80 percent of affected patients are smokers.
- Immunocompromised patients are at greater risk.

Prognosis is poor without early diagnosis and treatment.

- Image-guided aspiration is avoided for lesions >4 cm in the acute phase because of risk of spillover of infected contents into normal lung.
- Treatment with antibiotics for an extended period is required; drainage is seldom needed, in contradistinction to abscesses in other organ systems.
- Interventions are generally reserved for non-resolving abscesses or when the abscess abuts the chest wall.

The typical imaging appearance is a thick-walled cavitary lesion with surrounding consolidation, containing debris or gas–fluid levels. Abscesses are more common in dependent portions of the lung.

- Chest radiography is the modality of choice for initial evaluation of any patient with a clinical presentation concerning for pulmonary infection.
- Additional uses of chest x-ray in the management of pulmonary abscess include:
  - Monitoring of response to therapy
  - Detection of important complications such as pneumothorax, empyema, bronchopleural fistula, and pulmonary hemorrhage
  - Identification of additional or alternative diagnoses
- CT may be needed for further diagnostic clarification in some cases, and to guide therapeutic interventions.

Abscess may sometimes be difficult to distinguish from empyema on chest x-ray or CT. Imaging findings that distinguish abscess from empyema are summarized in the following table:

Abscess	Empyema
Intermediately thickened (4–15 mm) walls	Thin walls
Spherical	Lenticular
Surrounded by consolidation	"Split pleura" sign (CT)
Equal-length air-fluid levels on frontal and lateral radiographs	Different-length air fluid levels on frontal and lateral radiographs
Narrow interface with chest wall (CT)	Broad contact with chest wall
Bronchovascular markings extend to abscess	Adjacent compressed lung

Clinical synopsis

Streptococcus and *Aspergillus* were cultured from the patient's sputum, and antibiotics were initiated. Life-threatening hemorrhage necessitated image-guided bronchial artery embolization. Subsequently, a drainage catheter was placed in the abscess to prevent transbronchial spread of infection. The patient's condition improved and the drainage catheter was removed prior to discharge.

Self-assessment

- *What are the most common sites for lung abscess?*

- Abscess formation is often unilateral, most commonly involving the posterior segments of the upper lobes.

- *What complication occurs when an abscess develops direct communication with the pleural space?*

- Bronchopleural fistula.

- *What is the natural history of an uncomplicated abscess?*

- If treated optimally, surrounding consolidation improves, leaving a thin-walled pneumatocele. In some cases, this pneumatocele decreases in size and completely resolves. In other cases, there is residual scarring and bronchiectasis.

Spectrum of lung abscess

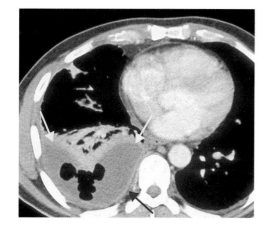

Empyema

An abscess can evolve into an empyema. Axial enhanced CT image shows right lower lobe consolidation with an adjacent empyema (yellow arrows) containing locules of gas. The pleura enhances and is slightly thickened (red arrow).

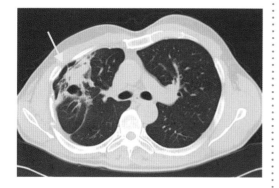

Bronchopleural fistula

A bronchopleural fistula is an abnormal communication between the pleural space and the bronchial tree, which may result from rupture of an abscess into the pleural space. These are very difficult to treat and may require a Clagett window or marsupialization of the chest cavity followed by a muscle flap for closure of the chest after the infection resolves. Axial CT image shows development of a bronchopleural fistula (arrow) in a patient with chronic *Aspergillus* infection.

Differential diagnosis of lung abscess

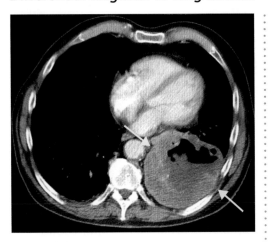

Cavitary lung cancer

Squamous cell carcinoma (SCC) is the most common histological type of lung cancer to produce cavitary lesions, followed by adenocarcinoma and large cell carcinoma. Small cell carcinoma does not tend to cavitate. Multiple cavitary lesions in primary lung cancer are rare; however, multifocal adenocarcinoma may present in this fashion. Cavitation can be seen in both benign and malignant parenchymal processes; sometimes, pathological confirmation is necessary, particularly with lack of clinical response to antibiotics. Cavities with a maximum wall thickness ≤4 mm tend to be inflammatory, while malignancy should be suspected with wall thickness >15 mm. Wall thickness between 5 and 15 mm is equivocal. Abscesses tend to have smooth internal walls, whereas the internal walls of SCC tend to be nodular or shaggy. Axial unenhanced CT shows a left upper lobe SCC (arrows) with thick, irregular walls and central, nodular cavitation.

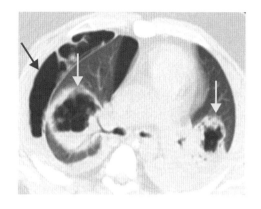

Vasculitis

Granulomatosis with polyangiitis (formerly known as Wegener's granulomatosis) and Churg–Strauss vasculitis can mimic necrotizing pneumonia. These diagnoses of exclusion may be confirmed with serological markers (c-ANCA and p-ANCA, respectively). Both of these entities can present with nodules, which undergo cavitation. Spontaneous pneumothorax may occur if the cavity ruptures into the pleural space. Unlike in cases of pulmonary abscess, fever and leukocytosis are usually absent even in the presence of extensive parenchymal abnormality. In this patient with longstanding granulomatosis with polyangiitis, axial unenhanced CT shows bilateral cavitary lesions (yellow arrows) with walls of intermediate thickness, containing a gas–fluid level on the right. There is a large, chronic hydropneumothorax (red arrow) due to rupture of the cavity into the pleural space.

Pulmonary infarct with cavitation

Parenchymal necrosis from pulmonary infarct may rarely cavitate or evolve into a pneumatocele, which is a thin-walled, gas-filled space. The diagnosis of infarct is made by demonstration of thrombus / filling defect in the vessel leading to the infarcted segment of the lung. Axial contrast-enhanced CT and axial maximum intensity projection CT images show a thin-walled pneumatocele in the posterior right upper lobe (yellow arrow) and abrupt pruning of the vascular tree (red arrow).

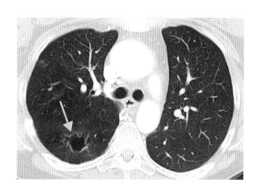

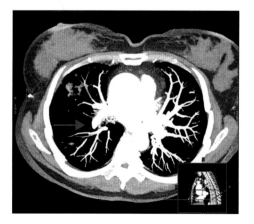

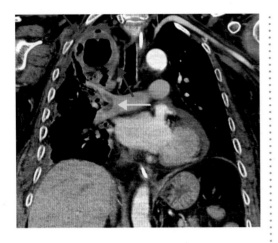

Infected infarct

A pulmonary infarct can become superinfected and evolve into an abscess or a necrotizing pneumonia. These are difficult to treat, as the blood flow to the infected area is impeded by clot and the antibiotic does not reach the infection optimally. However, these also heal to form thin-walled pneumatoceles, which eventually shrink over time and ultimately resolve. Coronal enhanced CT image shows thrombus in the right main pulmonary artery (yellow arrow) and a thick-walled parenchymal lesion in the right upper lobe (red arrow). Sputum culture was positive for *Pseudomonas aeruginosa*.

Further reading

Bartlett JG. The role of anaerobic bacteria in lung abscess. *Clin. Infect. Dis.* 2005;40 (7): 923–925.

Bartlett JG, Finegold SM. Anaerobic pleuropulmonary infections. *Medicine (Baltimore).* 1972;51 (6): 413–450.

Gaur P, Dunne R, Colson YL, Gill RR. Bronchopleural fistula and the role of contemporary imaging. *J Thorac Cardiovasc Surg.* 2014; 148(1).

Gill RR, Matsusoka S, Hatabu H. Cavities in the lung in oncology patients: imaging overview and differential diagnoses. *Applied Radiology.* June 2010; 39 (6).

Woodring JH, Fried AM. Significance of wall thickness in solitary cavities of the lung: a follow-up study. *AJR Am J Roentgenol.* 1983; 140: 473–474.

Woodring JH, Fried AM, Chuang VP. Solitary cavities of the lung: diagnostic implications of cavity wall thickness. *AJR Am J Roentgenol.* 1980; 135: 1269–1271.

Case 37   67-year-old man presenting with cough, weight loss, hoarseness, and dyspnea

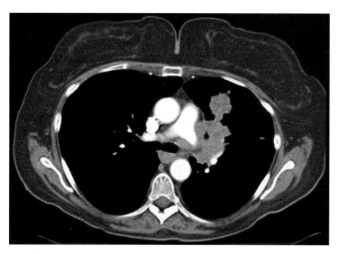

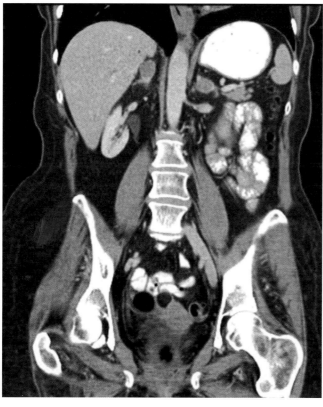

Diagnosis: **Lung cancer**	Axial (left image) and coronal (right image) contrast-enhanced CT images show a left upper lobe mass (yellow arrow) with aortopulmonary window and hilar adenopathy, and bilateral adrenal metastases (red arrows). Hoarseness was secondary to recurrent laryngeal nerve involvement. Left phrenic nerve involvement with diaphragmatic paralysis caused dyspnea.

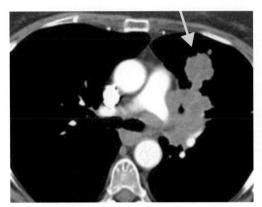 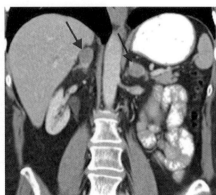

Discussion

Lung cancer is the cancer with highest mortality in the United States, accounting for 33% of cancer deaths in men and 24% of cancer deaths in women. It is only lower in incidence than skin cancer, breast cancer in women, and prostate cancer in men.

- 5-year survival is better with diagnosis in early stages (14% for all stages with breakdown as follows: stage 1A: 61%, 1B: 38%, 2A: 34%, 2B: 24%, 3A: 13%, 3B: 5% and stage 4: 1%).
- 70% of patients present with advanced stage cancers.

Primary lung tumors were most recently classified by histologic appearance in the 2004 WHO criteria.

- "Non-small-cell lung cancers" as classified as:
  - Adenocarcinoma
  - Squamous cell carcinoma
  - Large cell carcinoma
- Small cell carcinoma is considered in a different category given its different histopathological features, prognosis, and treatment considerations.

Lesions classified as "unresectable" by TNM staging are considered so because resection has not been shown to improve survival. These include:

- T4 lesions that invade the mediastinum or a vertebral body or manifest as tumor nodules in a separate ipsilateral lung lobe.

- N3 lesions (scalene, supraclavicular, or contralateral mediastinal or hilar lymph nodes greater than 1 cm in short axis).
- Metastatic lesions in the contralateral lung or distant sites.
- Effusions or lesions that may categorize disease as unresectable must be diagnostically sampled.

Metastases are a common differential consideration for primary lung cancer.

- Known non-lung primary malignancy and multiple lesions of varying shape and size favor a diagnosis of metastatic disease.
- The most common sites to which primary lung cancer metastasizes are the adrenal glands (40%), liver (30%), bones (20%), and brain (10%).
- It is important to establish histologic type and tumor receptor status (e.g., presence or absence of epidermal growth factor receptor [EGFR] mutation) to guide treatment choice.

Spectrum of lung cancer

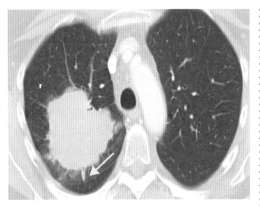

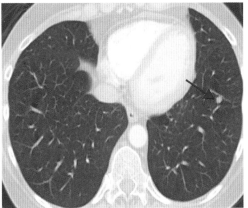

Adenocarcinoma

Adenocarcinoma is the most common type of lung cancer. Tumors tend to be peripheral and range from pure ground glass nodules (GGN), to mixed solid–GGN, to solid nodules, with a spectrum of behaviors. The nomenclature of adenocarcinomas was recently refined by histological type. The term "bronchioloalveolar carcinoma" (BAC) is being phased out. The entity previously known as "mucinous BAC" is now known as "invasive mucinous adenocarcinoma". Pure GGN may represent "pre-invasive" minimally invasive adenocarcinoma or adenocarcinoma in situ, which have 100% disease-free survival when resected. Surveillance over several years may be necessary, as many adenocarcinomas are slow-growing. Increasing solidity, even if the lesion is decreasing in size, is concerning for development of invasive malignancy. Axial contrast-enhanced CT images show an adenocarcinoma as a large, spiculated mass with linear extensions to the pleura (pleural tags; yellow arrow), and a small, contralateral metastasis (red arrow). The presence of contralateral metastasis makes this an unresectable M1 / Stage IV cancer.

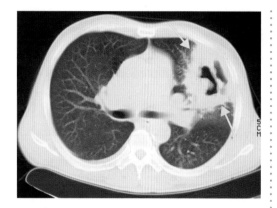

Squamous cell carcinoma (SCC)

SCC tends to be a cavitating central (75%) lesion that causes airway obstruction and obstructive atelectasis. Differential diagnosis includes necrotizing pneumonia (including tuberculosis) and pulmonary abscess. Benign infectious and inflammatory lesions tend to have surrounding consolidation and smooth, rather than "shaggy" or "nodular", internal cavitation. In this case, axial unenhanced CT shows a large, peripheral mass (arrows) with nodular internal cavitation.

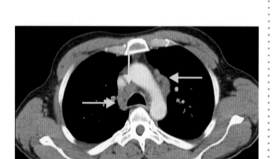

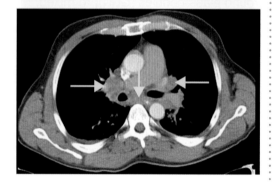

Neuroendocrine lung tumors

The spectrum of neuroendocrine tumors includes typical carcinoid, atypical carcinoid, and small cell lung cancer (SCLC), which together represent 20% of lung cancers. Typical and atypical carcinoid are often only distinguished by histological analysis. Bronchial carcinoid typically presents as a solid pulmonary nodule or an endobronchial lesion that causes distal obstructive atelectasis. Usually, prognosis is excellent with resection. SCLC may present as an extensive, bulky, poorly defined central mass, frequently causing vascular obstruction. SCLC is nearly always associated with a history of heavy tobacco use, and is presumed to be metastatic at the time of presentation. Therefore, treatment is nonsurgical and includes radiation and chemotherapy. In this case of SCLC, axial contrast-enhanced CT images show ill-defined, bulky, central masses in the subcarinal region, aortopulmonary window, right paratracheal region, and bilateral hila (arrows).

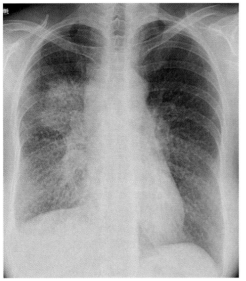

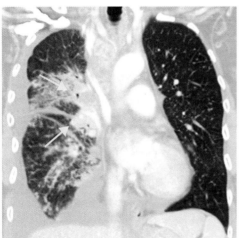

Lymphangitic carcinomatosis

In lymphangitic carcinomatosis, tumor grows into and occludes the pulmonary lymphatics, producing interstitial abnormality. Lymphangitic carcinomatosis is a less common pattern of lung cancer metastasis than angiocentric lung nodules that occur by hematogenous dissemination. The findings are commonly unilateral and nodular, which may help distinguish lymphangitic carcinomatosis from pulmonary edema. Adenocarcinoma is the most common lung cancer subtype to produce lymphangitic spread. Frontal radiograph demonstrates a right hilar mass with nodular septal thickening involving both lungs, predominantly on the right. There is a moderate right pleural effusion. Coronal CT confirms asymmetric nodular septal thickening on the right, right hilar mass (arrows), and a pleural effusion.

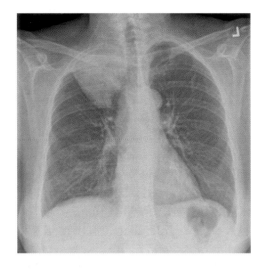

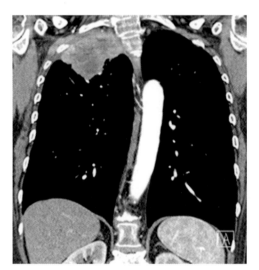

Pancoast tumor

Pancoast tumor is an apical lung cancer that produces pain radiating down the arm, Horner's syndrome due to involvement of the sympathetic ganglia (ptosis, miosis, and hemianhidrosis), destruction of ribs, and atrophy of the hand muscles due to involvement of the brachial plexus. Differential diagnosis includes metastasis, hematologic neoplasm, infection, and amyloid. Pancoast tumors are considered at least stage T3 due to chest wall invasion. Frontal chest radiograph demonstrates a right apical opacity. Coronal enhanced CT demonstrates a soft-tissue attenuation mass involving the right apical chest wall.

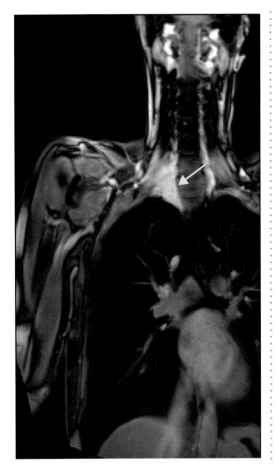

Pancoast tumor, continued.

Factors that preclude surgical resection include esophageal or tracheal invasion, involvement of the brachial plexus roots or trunks above the level of T1, invasion of more than 50% of a vertebral body, extension of the tumor into the spinal canal, and N2 ipsilateral mediastinal nodal disease. Unlike in other tumors, involvement of ipsilateral N3 supraclavicular nodes does not contraindicate resection. Coronal T1-weighted enhanced MRI with fat suppression in a different patient from above show a poorly circumscribed tumor invading the mid to lower cervical and upper thoracic neural foramina (arrow). This involvement of the brachial plexus renders the tumor unresectable.

Further reading

Aberle DR, *et al.* Reduced lung-cancer mortality with low-dose computed tomographic screening. *The New England Journal of Medicine.* 2011;365:395.

Aquino SL, Chiles C, Halford P. Distinction of consolidative bronchioloalveolar carcinoma from pneumonia: do CT criteria work? *Am J Roentgenol.* 1998; 171:359–363.

Byrd RB, Miller WE, Carr DT, Payne WS, Woolner LB. The roentgenographic appearance of squamous cell carcinoma of the bronchus. *Mayo Clinic Proceedings.* 1968;43:327–332.

Dahnert W. Chest Disorders. In: Dahnert W, ed., *Radiology Review Manual.* 3rd edn. Baltimore: Williams and Wilkins, 1996:346.

Forster BB, Muller NL, Miller RR, Nelems B, Evans KG. Neuroendocrine carcinomas of the lung: clinical, radiologic, and pathologic correlation. *Radiology.* 1989;170:441–445.

Fraser RG, Parre JAP. *Diagnosis of diseases of the chest.* 4th edn. Philadelphia, Pa.: W. B. Saunders, 1999:1142–1143.

Greaves SM, *et al.* The new staging system for lung cancer: imaging and clinical implications. *Journal of Thoracic Imaging.* 2011;26:119.

Johnson DH, *et al.* Cancer of the lung: non-small cell lung cancer and small cell lung cancer. In: Abeloff MD, *et al.*, eds. *Abeloff's Clinical Oncology.* 4th edn. Philadelphia, Pa.: Churchill Livingstone, 2008:1307.

Kazerooni EA, Bhalla M, Shepard JA, McLoud TC. Adenosquamous carcinoma of the lung: radiologic appearance. *Am J Roentgenol.* 1994;163:301–306.

Pearlberg JL, Sandler MA, Lewis JW, Jr., Beute GH, Alpern MB. Small-cell bronchogenic carcinoma: CT evaluation. *Am J Roentgenol.* 1988;150:265–268.

Travis WD, Brambilla E, Riely GJ. New pathologic classification of lung cancer: relevance for clinical practice and clinical trials. *J Clin Oncol.* 2013:331(8):992–1001.

Case 38   63-year-old male with fever and confusion

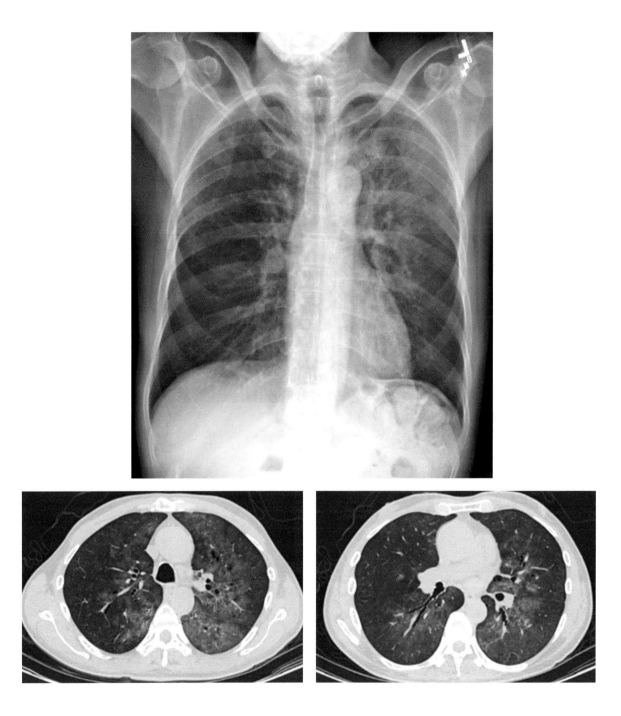

Diagnosis: PA chest radiograph demonstrates diffuse ground glass opacification (GGO) in
Pneumocystis the left upper lobe (yellow arrow). Axial CT images demonstrate bilateral
pneumonia perihilar GGO with mild bronchiectasis and cystic changes in the left upper
lobe (red arrows).

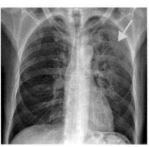 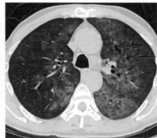 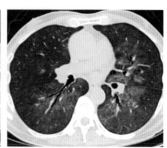

Discussion

***Pneumocystis jirovecii* pneumonia (PJP), or pneumocystosis, is a type of pneumonia that is prevalent in immunocompromised individuals.**

- The causal organism is the yeast-like fungus (previously erroneously classified as a protozoan) *Pneumocystis jirovecii*.
- Histologically, there is thickening of the interstitium and fibrous tissue of the lungs, including the alveolar septa and alveoli, which lead to compromise of gas exchange.

PJP is characterized clinically by fever, dyspnea, hypoxemia, and productive cough.

- Spontaneous pneumothorax can occur. Infection may involve extra-pulmonary sites such as liver, spleen, and skin.
- The risk of infection increases when CD4 count decreases below 200 cells/mL. Serum lactate dehydrogenase levels may be elevated and PaO_2 lower than expected for a given degree of dyspnea.

Chest radiography is the primary imaging modality in patients in whom pneumonia is suspected, including the immunocompromised. CT may be needed for further refinement of diagnosis.

- Bilateral symmetric or asymmetric perihilar GGO on both chest x-ray and CT is typical.
- Cavitation in the form of pneumatoceles without lobar predilection can be seen; with treatment, this finding resolves within 6 months.
- Pneumothorax is seen in 13% of patients.
- Lymphadenopathy, pleural effusions, and pulmonary nodules are associated findings.

Clinical ***synopsis***	The patient was found to be HIV positive, and his clinical condition improved with trimethoprim-sulfamethoxazole.

Self-assessment

- *How common is PJP in immunocompetent hosts?*

- *Name three laboratory tests that can help diagnose PJP in a patient with GGO.*

- *What is the most effective therapy for PJP?*

- *Which radionuclide scan can be used to diagnose PJP before a radiographic abnormality is detectable?*

- PJP is an opportunistic infection that is not seen in immunocompetent hosts.

- Arterial blood gas, beta-d-glucan, and serum LDH level.

- Trimethoprim-sulfamethoxazole (TMP-SMX) is the most effective therapy for PJP. Many immunocompromised individuals are treated with TMP-SMX on a prophylactic basis.

- Gallium-67 scan.

Differential diagnosis of PJP pneumonia

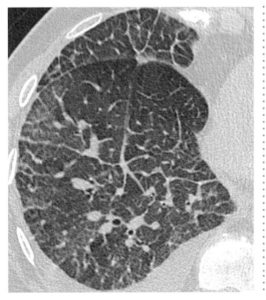

Pulmonary edema

Pulmonary edema is generally seen either due to volume overload or secondary to cardiogenic causes. Pulmonary edema manifests as smooth interlobular septal thickening with centrilobular ground glass opacification, and is usually associated with pleural effusions. Careful evaluation of serial radiographs can show fluctuation in the parenchymal opacities, which correlates with the volume status of the patient. Axial CT demonstrates smooth interlobular septal thickening, subtle ground glass attenuation peripherally, and a small dependent pleural effusion.

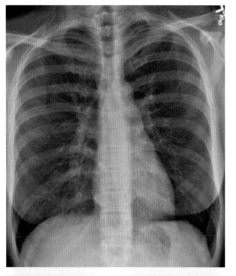

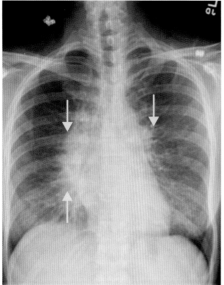

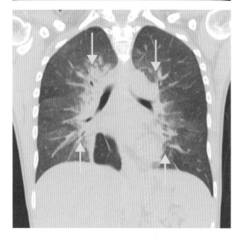

Radiation pneumonitis

Radiation pneumonitis is generally seen approximately 6 weeks after completion of radiotherapy. GGO confined to the radiation port is produced by an inflammatory response to radiation damage. Treatment is with corticosteroids. In this case, initial frontal chest x-ray (upper image) in a patient with lymphoma is normal. Six weeks following treatment with radiation therapy and methotrexate, well-demarcated consolidative and ground glass opacities on both sides of the mediastinum (arrows) are seen on both frontal chest x-ray (middle image) and coronal unenhanced CT (lower image).

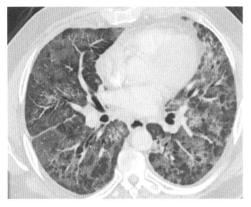

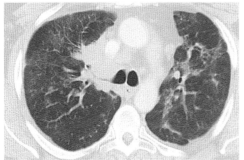

Drug reaction

Acute interstitial pneumonitis and hypersensitivity pneumonitis secondary to drug reaction can mimic *Pneumocystis* pneumonia. This diagnosis of exclusion is usually made after bronchoscopy. Treatment involves discontinuation of the offending drug and corticosteroid therapy. In this case, initial axial enhanced CT (upper image) in a patient being treated with chemotherapy shows a mosaic attenuation pattern of patchy areas of GGO and lucency. After discontinuation of the chemotherapeutic agent and treatment with high-dose corticosteroids, follow-up axial enhanced CT (lower image) shows marked improvement with some residual scarring that is more pronounced in the left lung.

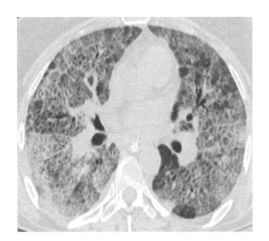

Viral pneumonia

Viral and atypical bacterial pneumonias produce an interstitial pattern, and can present as diffuse bilateral GGO with or without septal thickening. Pleural effusions are absent and consolidation is very rarely seen. In this patient with herpes simplex virus pneumonia, axial unenhanced CT shows diffuse ground glass opacification and septal thickening in a "crazy paving" pattern without pleural effusions and consolidation.

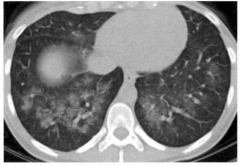

Vasculitis

Churg–Strauss vasculitis presents as hemorrhage manifested as centrilobular GGO, with mild vascular dilatation in the region of hemorrhage. This condition is generally seen in young individuals presenting with hemoptysis. p-ANCA is typically positive. Corticosteroids are the mainstay of treatment. Axial CT in a young patient with a history of smoking and hemoptysis shows alveolar GGO with mild vascular dilatation in the affected areas.

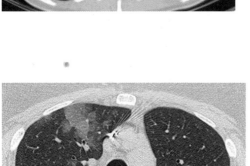

Pulmonary hemorrhage

Pulmonary hemorrhage typically appears on imaging as geographically distributed parenchymal GGO without pleural effusions. Axial CT of a patient on warfarin presenting with hemoptysis demonstrates asymmetric GGO in the right lung.

Further reading

Baughman RP. Current methods of diagnosis. In: Walzer PD, ed., *Pneumocystis carinii pneumonia*. 2nd edn. New York: Dekker, 1994:381–401.

Kovacs JA, Hiemenz JW, Macher AM, Stover D, Murray HW, Shelhamer J, *et al. Pneumocystis carinii* pneumonia: a comparison between patients with acquired immunodeficiency syndrome and patients with other immunodeficiencies. *Ann Intern Med*. 1984;100:663–671.

Metersky ML, Colt HG, Olson LK, Shanks TG. AIDS-related spontaneous pneumo-thorax: risk factors and treatment. *Chest*. 1995;108:946–951.

Opravail M, Marincek B, Fuchs WA, Weber R, Speich R, Battegay M, *et al.* Shortcom-ings of chest radiography in detecting *Pneumocystis carinii* pneumonia. *J Acquir Immune Defic Syndr*. 1994;7:39–45.

SECTION 3 OTOLARYNGOLOGY

Case 39   28-year-old woman with a history of sore throat and odynophagia
for 1 week

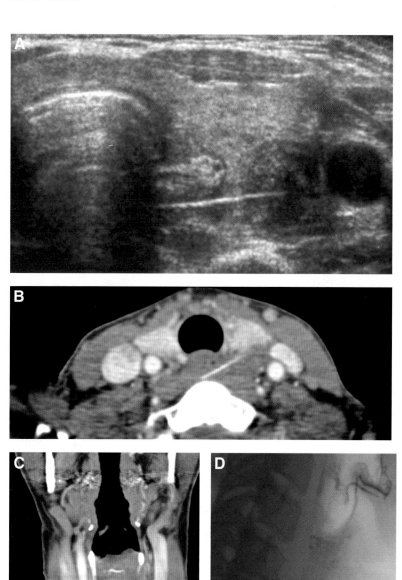

***Diagnosis:*
Paraesophageal
foreign body
(metallic bristle
from grill
brush)** Transverse grayscale ultrasound image (A) demonstrates a linear echogenic structure (yellow arrow) posterior to the thyroid gland and traversing the esophagus (red arrow). The tip of the structure is located in a hypoechoic collection (blue arrows) adjacent to the left common carotid artery. Axial (B) and coronal (C) enhanced CT images demonstrate a linear metallic-density structure (yellow arrows) embedded in the cervical esophagus and penetrating the left lobe of the thyroid, with the tip located in an ill-defined mixed-attenuation collection (blue arrow). A single lateral image from an esophagram (D) with water-soluble contrast demonstrates the linear metallic object (yellow arrow) projecting over the esophagus, with no evidence of esophageal leak.

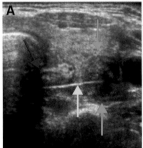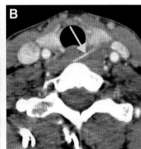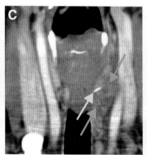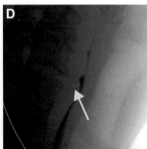

Discussion

Overview of oropharyngeal foreign bodies

- The tonsils, base of tongue, valleculae and piriform sinuses are common locations for swallowed foreign bodies to lodge, with 50% of oropharyngeal foreign bodies lodged in either the tonsils or base of tongue.
- Patients may present with dysphagia, odynophagia, sensation of foreign body, dysphonia, coughing, stridor, or hoarseness. Patients may be able to localize sharp foreign bodies above the level of the cricopharyngeus muscle better than those below it.
- Children may present with refusal to feed, drooling, or dysphonia.

Treatment of oropharyngeal foreign bodies

- Oropharyngeal foreign bodies usually require emergent removal.
- The standard of care in non-asphyxiating foreign body aspiration (passage beyond the vocal folds) is diagnostic fiberoptic bronchoscopy. If that is unsuccessful, surgery is necessary.

Imaging of oropharyngeal foreign bodies

- Plain films are limited in making the diagnosis of pharyngoesophageal and tracheobronchial foreign body aspiration, as only radiopaque foreign bodies can be clearly identified.
- Foreign bodies made of wood and some plastics as well as many food items may be radiolucent. Additionally, if the foreign body is made of clear plastic, it may also be missed on direct laryngoscopy. Because of these two problems, the diagnosis of aspirated clear plastic items may be significantly delayed.
- Foreign body aspiration is much more common in children than adults. In children, about 90% of aspirated foreign bodies are radiolucent on radiography. Of children who have a known aspirated foreign body, the chest x-ray may be normal in up to 30% of cases. In children with negative CXR and suspected foreign body aspiration, virtual bronchoscopy shows diagnostic promise with high sensitivity. If CT bronchoscopy is negative, children may be able to avoid rigid bronchoscopy. Virtual bronchoscopy has the added advantages of being able to visualize changes in the lung parenchyma, and potentially to offer an alternative diagnosis if no aspirated foreign body is seen.

Clinical synopsis

The patient recalled eating a meal of grilled steak tips the prior weekend, which immediately preceded her discomfort. Prior to cooking the meat, the grill had been cleaned with a metallic brush. Because this foreign body was felt to be in the paraesophageal soft tissues rather than the airway, the patient was taken for open (rather than endoscopic) surgical removal of foreign body. A grill brush bristle was removed after it was dissected from adjacent granulation tissue and phlegmon (the collection seen on imaging). The patient recovered well, with rare residual odynophagia and no swallowing dysfunction.

Self-assessment

- *Name three secondary signs of inflammation that may be helpful in diagnosing pharyngoesophageal foreign body on the lateral neck radiograph.*

- Prevertebral soft tissue swelling.
- Base of tongue swelling.
- Gas in atypical locations (suggestive of esophageal perforation).

- *Name three secondary signs of aspirated foreign body in the tracheobronchial tree on chest x-ray, which may indicate the presence of a radiolucent foreign body.*

- Consolidation (due to atelectasis).
- Unilateral hyperlucent lung (or other focal hyperlucency in the distribution of the tracheobronchial tree) due to air trapping.
- Mediastinal shift.

- Unilateral bronchiectasis.
- Pleural effusion.
- Pneumothorax.

- *Name three possible complications of pharyngoesophageal foreign body aspiration.*

- Mediastinitis.
- Tracheoesophageal fistula.
- Retropharyngeal abscess.
- Esophagoarterial fistula.

Differential diagnosis of paraesophageal foreign body

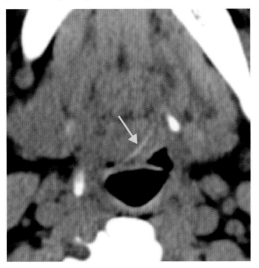

Foreign body (fish bone) in vallecula

The most commonly ingested foreign bodies in adults are fish bones, chicken bones, and coins. Fish bones are calcified, although the density of fish bones is significantly lower than human bones. Axial CT demonstrates a curvilinear, obliquely oriented high density structure (arrow) in the region of the vallecula. The vallecula is the space between the epiglottis and the glosso-epiglottic folds.

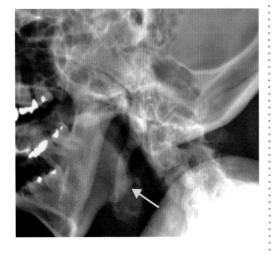

Elongated styloid process / calcified stylohyoid ligament (Eagle syndrome)

Eagle syndrome is the presence of dysphagia, foreign body sensation, and throat pain (which may be worse with head turning), caused by an elongated styloid process or calcified stylohyoid ligament. In the absence of clinical symptoms, this is an incidental finding with essentially no relevance to the patient, although it may be confused with an ingested foreign body. Treatment for those with the syndrome may be surgical or conservative, depending on the situation. Lateral neck radiograph demonstrates particularly long styloid processes of the temporal bone (arrow).

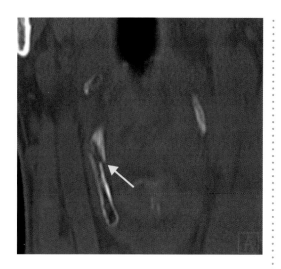

Thyroid cartilage fracture

Because the normal thyroid cartilage is radiopaque in adults, it can occasionally be difficult to distinguish a fracture of the thyroid cartilage from a radiopaque foreign body. Coronal CT demonstrates an oblique, minimally displaced fracture of the right thyroid cartilage (arrow).

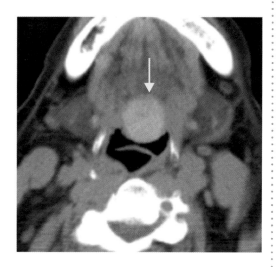

Ectopic lingual thyroid

Like a foreign body, ectopic lingual thyroid may present with globus sensation. It results from aberrant development, when thyroid tissue fails to descend from the foramen cecum (at the base of the tongue) to its typical location in the neck. On noncontrast studies, ectopic thyroid tissue at the base of the tongue (arrow) will be relatively hyperattenuating due to its iodine content, as demonstrated in this unenhanced CT. The neck should always be carefully evaluated for the presence of any normal thyroid tissue.

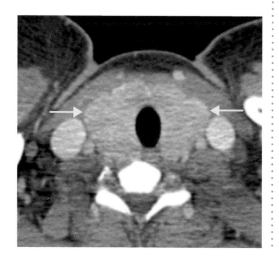

Thyroiditis

Acute thyroiditis is another cause of neck pain, which may be accompanied by fever and dysphagia. Thyroid function tests (TFTs) will be variable, depending on the phase of the disease. Initially, TFTs are elevated, but after the thyroid "burns out," T3 and T4 will be low. Axial enhanced CT demonstrates enlargement of the thyroid gland (arrows), which is abnormally low in attenuation because the follicular cells that normally concentrate iodine are damaged.

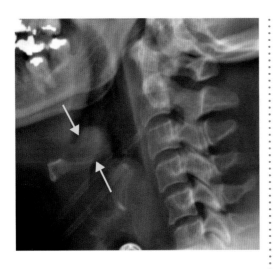

Acute epiglottitis

Acute epiglottitis is a relatively rare but potentially deadly infection most commonly found in children. Given the widespread availability of vaccination against the causative organism *Haemophilus influenzae*, the incidence of acute epiglottitis has significantly decreased in recent years; however, both child and adult immunocompromised individuals remain susceptible. A lateral neck radiograph demonstrates the classic "thumb" sign, with a markedly thickened epiglottis resembling a thumb (arrows). There may be associated narrowing of the vallecula. The treatment is IV antibiotics, airway management, and in some cases, IV corticosteroids.

Further reading

Bloom D, *et al*. Plastic laryngeal foreign bodies in children: a diagnostic challenge. *Int J Ped Otorhinolaryngology* 69:657–662 (2005).

Chawla A, *et al*. Clinics in diagnostic imaging case presentation. *Singapore Med J* 45(8):397–403 (2004).

Hajiioannou J, *et al*. Iatrogenic migration of an impacted pharyngeal foreign body of the hypopharynx to the prevertebral space. *Int J Otolaryngology* 1–4:30-34 (2011).

Haliloglu M, *et al*. CT virtual bronchoscopy in the evaluation of children with suspected foreign body aspiration. *Eur J Rad* 48:188–192 (2003).

Jhaveri K, *et al*. CT and MR imaging findings associated with subacute thyroiditis. *AJNR* 24:143–146 (2003).

Leong H, *et al*. Foreign bodies in the upper digestive tract. *Singapore Medical Journal* 28(2):162–165 (1987).

Murtagh R, *et al*. CT findings associated with Eagle syndrome. *AJNR* 22:1401–1402 (2001).

Savage J, *et al*. How I do it: fish bones in the vallecula and tongue base: removal with the rigid nasal endoscope. *J Laryngology & Otology* 116:842–843 (2002).

Schamp S, *et al*. Radiological findings in acute adult epiglottitis. *Eur Radiology* 9: 1629–1631 (1999).

Thomas G, *et al*. Ectopic lingual thyroid: a case report. *Int J Oral Maxillofac Surg* 32: 219–221 (2003).

Toso A, *et al*. Lingual thyroid causing dysphagia and dyspnoea: case reports and review of the literature. *Acta Otorhinolaryngologica Italica* 29:213–217 (2009).

Case 40   18-year-old man with odynophagia, fever, and dysphagia

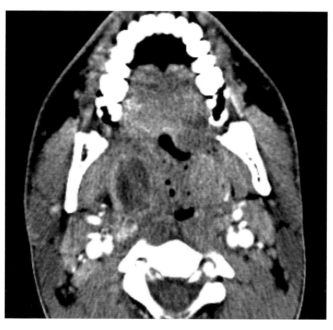

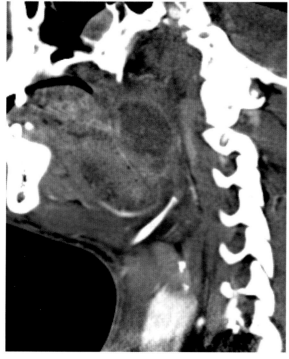

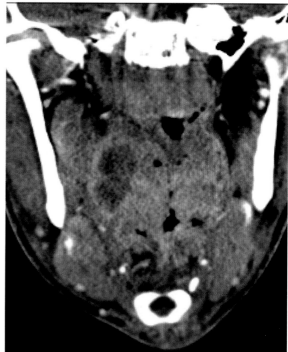

Diagnosis: **Peritonsillar abscess**	Axial (left), sagittal (middle), and coronal (right) contrast-enhanced CT images show a large, peripherally enhancing abscess in the region of the lateral right pharynx (yellow arrows) at the level of the tongue. The abscess is in the region of the right palatine tonsil at the level of the oropharynx (red arrow).

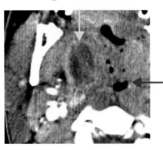 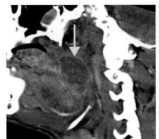 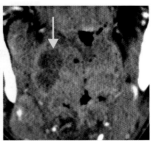

Discussion

Peritonsillar abscess is usually caused by tonsillitis and resultant suppuration, which occurs most commonly in young adults.

- Historically known as quinsy, a peritonsillar abscess may be suspected in a patient with fever, odynophagia, cervical adenopathy, and a "hot potato" (muffled) voice.
- While children have a high prevalence of pharyngotonsillitis, abscess formation is more commonly seen in young adults. Risk factors for abscess include upper respiratory infection, alcohol, smoking, recent dental procedure, and immunosuppression.
- Trismus, due to spasm of the adjacent medial pterygoid muscle, is generally not seen in tonsillitis, but is common in peritonsillar abscess. This distinction is key because tonsillitis is usually diagnosed clinically and treated with antibiotics only, while peritonsillar abscess is often diagnosed on imaging and is treated with incision and drainage in addition to antibiotics.

Anatomy of cervical fascial planes and routes of spread of infection are important to evaluate for potential complications.

- The peritonsillar space is partially encircled posteriorly and laterally by the superior pharyngeal constrictor muscle. If infection penetrates this muscle and its surrounding pharyngobasilar fascia, bacteria may spread to adjacent cervical spaces.
- The retropharyngeal space (posteromedial), carotid space (posterior), parapharyngeal space (posterolateral), and masticator space (lateral) are suprahyoid neck spaces encircled by layers of the deep cervical fascia. Any of these spaces may become secondarily involved (schematic of deep neck spaces is provided below).

Self-assessment

• *What are the most common types of bacteria to cause a peritonsillar abscess?*

• Most often, peritonsillar abscess is caused by polymicrobial bacterial flora, predominantly group A *Streptococcus* or *Staphylococcus aureus*.

• *What is the role of imaging in the work-up of suspected peritonsillar abscess?*

• Although the diagnosis of peritonsillar abscess can be made clinically, imaging is useful to distinguish peritonsillar abscess from tonsillitis in the absence of trismus, to distinguish between other deep neck infections, and to evaluate for complications.

• *What are the complications of peritonsillar abscess?*

• Complications of peritonsillar abscess can be serious and include infection of adjacent deep neck spaces, airway obstruction, suppurative jugular vein thrombophlebitis with embolism (Lemierre syndrome), carotid artery pseudo-aneurysm, and mediastinitis.

Relevant anatomy

Sagittal schematic demonstrates the anatomy of the peritonsillar space.

• The peritonsillar space is defined by loose connective tissue that surrounds the palatine tonsil, and is bounded front-to-back by the anterior tonsillar pillar (the palatoglossus muscle, connecting the soft palate to the tongue) and the posterior tonsillar pillar (the palatopharyngeus muscle, connecting the soft palate to the pharynx).

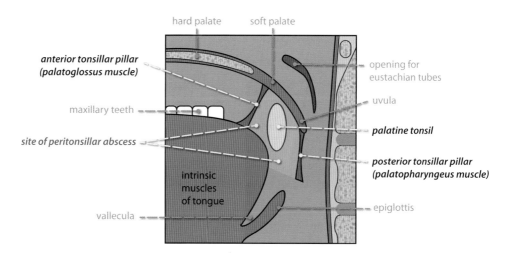

Axial schematic demonstrates the deep neck spaces adjacent to the peritonsillar space.

- The peritonsillar space is adjacent to the parapharyngeal space, carotid space, retropharyngeal space, and masticator space. If infection spreads to the posterior retropharyngeal space, mediastinitis may result via the *danger* space if the alar fascia is violated.

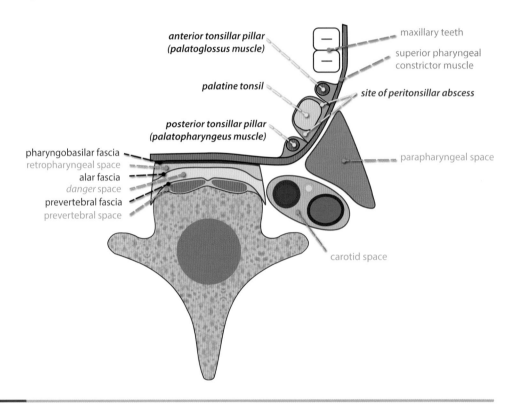

Clinical synopsis	This 18-year-old male with peritonsillar abscess underwent incision and drainage and received a course of intravenous antibiotics. He did well after the procedure.

Complications of peritonsillar abscess

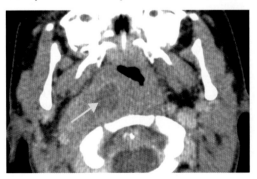

Retropharyngeal abscess

The retropharyngeal space is a potential space directly posterior to the pharynx. Infections of the retropharyngeal space may be secondary to direct extension from tonsillitis. Other locations in the head and neck drain to retropharyngeal lymph nodes, including the oral cavity, the pharynx, and the external ear. Axial enhanced CT shows an abscess (arrow) posterior to the pharynx.

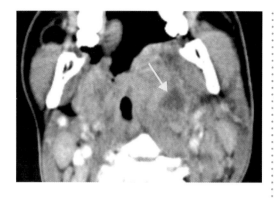

Parapharyngeal abscess

Primary processes involving the parapharyngeal space are rare, because it normally only contains fat, and occasionally, ectopic minor salivary gland tissue; however, secondary involvement of the parapharyngeal space by direct extension of a peritonsillar abscess may occur. Axial enhanced CT demonstrates a heterogeneous, centrally low-attenuation collection in the parapharyngeal space (arrow).

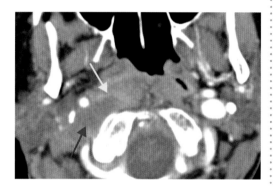

Lemierre syndrome

Lemierre syndrome is an uncommon but potentially deadly complication of oropharyngeal infection that tends to affect otherwise healthy young adults, characterized by rapidly progressive thrombophlebitis that spreads to the internal jugular veins and causes septic emboli. Enhanced CT demonstrates a retropharyngeal fluid collection (yellow arrow) and adjacent thrombosis of the right internal jugular vein (red arrow).

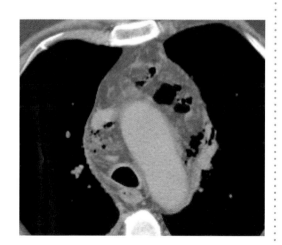

Mediastinitis

Descending necrotizing mediastinitis is a clinical emergency caused by spread of infection to the mediastinum via the *danger* space, which extends caudally to the diaphragm. The *danger* space of the neck is a potential space located directly posterior to the retropharyngeal space and anterior to the prevertebral space. The *danger* space is separated from these spaces by the alar fascia anteriorly and the prevertebral fascia posteriorly. Axial enhanced CT in a patient with esophageal perforation and mediastinitis demonstrates diffuse mediastinal fat stranding and multiple gas collections.

Internal carotid pseudoaneurysm

Carotid artery involvement is an extremely rare, but important-to-recognize complication of deep neck space infection. Carotid artery pseudoaneurysm, arteritis, and rupture have been reported. If a retropharyngeal abscess extends into the carotid space, careful assessment for vascular complications should be undertaken.

Differential diagnosis of peritonsillar abscess

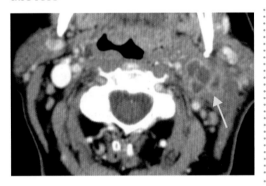

Cystic malignant adenopathy

Papillary thyroid cancer and squamous cell carcinoma of the base of the tongue may cause metastatic cystic adenopathy. In particular, a papillary thyroid cancer metastasis may appear cystic. This case demonstrates a peripherally enhancing, lobulated cystic mass (arrow), that represented a nodal squamous cell carcinoma metastasis.

Branchial cleft cyst

Most branchial cleft anomalies are second branchial cleft cysts, which can appear anywhere in a line from the tonsillar fossa superiorly to the supraclavicular region inferiorly. Axial enhanced CT demonstrates the most common location for a second branchial cleft cyst (arrow), at the angle of the mandible, anterior to the sternocleidomastoid and posterior to the submandibular gland. *Image courtesy Mary Beth Cunnane, MD.*

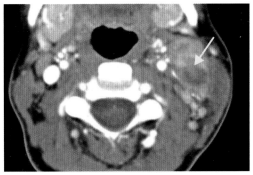

Histiocytic necrotizing lymphadenitis

Otherwise known as Kikuchi disease, histiocytic necrotizing lymphadenitis is a rare inflammatory cause of cervical lymphadenitis with central necrosis that can mimic infection. Kikuchi disease occurs most commonly in adolescents. It is usually a self-limited clinical syndrome, best treated supportively. Axial enhanced CT demonstrates an ill-defined, centrally necrotic lymph node in the left neck (arrow).

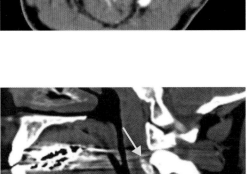

Calcific tendinitis

Acute calcific tendinitis of the longus colli, caused by hydroxyapatite deposition and resultant inflammatory response, may cause a prevertebral effusion than can mimic an abscess. In the case of calcific tendinitis, however, the pathognomonic finding is a calcific density in the prevertebral tissues. Sagittal unenhanced CT demonstrates globular mineralization in the prevertebral tissues (yellow arrow) with an adjacent effusion (red arrow).

Further reading

Baldassari, C. M., Howell, R., Amorn, M., Budacki, R., Choi, S., & Pena, M. (2011). Complications in pediatric deep neck space abscesses. *Otolaryngology – head and neck surgery: official journal of American Academy of Otolaryngology – Head and Neck Surgery*, 144(4), 592–595.

Capps, E., Kinsella, J., Gupta, M., Bhatki, A., & Opatowsky, M. (2010). Emergency imaging asessment of acute, nontraumatic conditions of the head and neck. *Radiographics*, 30(5), 1335–1353.

Vieira, F., Allen, S. M., Stocks, R. M. S., & Thompson, J. W. (2008). Deep neck infection. *Otolaryngologic clinics of North America*, 41(3), 459–483.

Wald, E. R. (2011). Peritonsillar cellulitis and abscess. On UpToDate, Post TW (ed.), UpToDate, Waltham, MA (accessed June 29, 2015).

Case 41   48-year-old male with recurrent left facial swelling and pain with eating

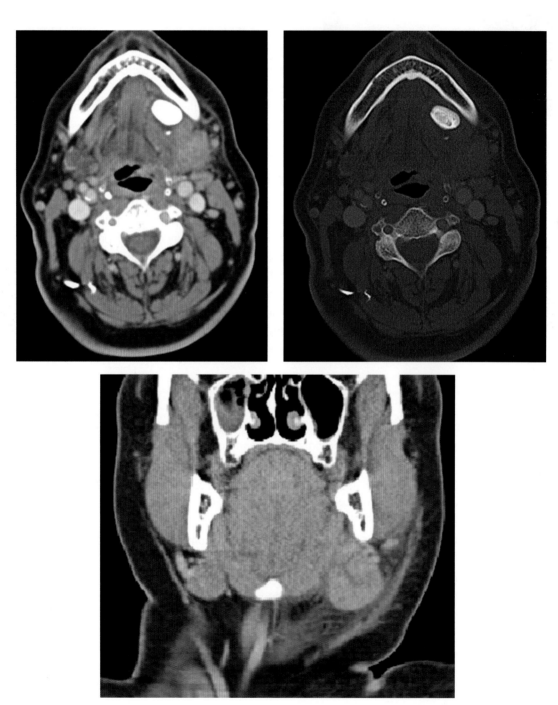

Diagnosis:
Submandibular duct sialolithiasis with sialadenitis

Noncontrast axial CT in soft tissue (left image) and bone windows (middle image) demonstrates a 2.1 cm radiopaque Wharton's duct calculus (yellow arrows) in the left sublingual space between the extrinsic tongue musculature and left mylohyoid muscle with inflammation and effacement of adjacent fat. A smaller punctate calculus is seen within the more proximal aspect of the duct (red arrows). The left submandibular gland is enlarged and inflamed (blue arrows).

On coronal noncontrast CT (right image), the left submandibular gland is enlarged with internal dilated linear hypodensities representing dilated excretory ducts (green arrow). The right submandibular gland is normal. There is extensive inflammatory reticulation of the fat surrounding the submandibular gland and thickening of the platysma (white arrow).

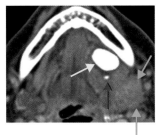 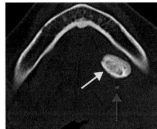 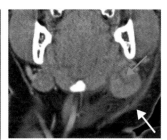

Discussion

Overview of sialolithiasis

- Sialolithiasis is the most common pathological condition affecting the salivary glands.
- 80 to 90 percent of cases involve the submandibular gland or duct (Wharton's duct) while most remaining cases involve the parotid gland or duct (Stensen's duct). Sublingual gland stones have been reported to occur rarely, in 1–7% of cases. In 25% of cases, stones are multiple.
- This disease process most commonly affects adults in the 4th to 7th decades of life with a slight male predilection. Gout predisposes to the formation of uric acid stones that may not be seen on radiography but are clearly evident on CT.
- The submandibular duct is thought to be the most common site of stones due to its long anatomical course, the narrow caliber of its orifice in comparison to the rest of the duct, and its relatively high salivary alkalinity and hydroxyapatite content. About 85% of submandibular stones are seen within Wharton's duct and 15% are seen within the gland itself.

Clinical presentation and complications of sialolithiasis

- Patients classically present with a history of recurrent facial swelling superficial to the affected gland that is worse with eating or gustatory stimulation.
- Salivary transit is obstructed at the level of the stone resulting in proximal dilatation, stasis, and eventual glandular infection.
- Abscess formation and deep cervical infection are known complications. Chronic obstruction may lead to duct strictures and fatty atrophy of the gland.
- Rarely, an obstructing stone can cause salivary duct rupture and formation of an extravasating mucocele.

Anatomy of the salivary ducts

- Detailed knowledge of the courses of the submandibular (Wharton's) and parotid (Stensen's) ducts is critical in evaluating for ductal calculi.
- The submandibular (Wharton's) duct courses through the sublingual space which is located between the mylohyoid muscle sling and extrinsic musculature of the tongue.

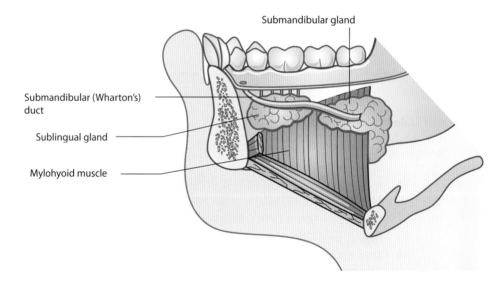

Submandibular gland

Submandibular (Wharton's) duct

Sublingual gland

Mylohyoid muscle

- The parotid (Stensen's) duct extends anteriorly from the parotid gland, running parallel to the masseter muscle within the buccal space. Along the anterior aspect of the masseter muscle, the duct courses medially, pierces the buccinator muscle and enters the oral cavity opposite the second upper premolar.

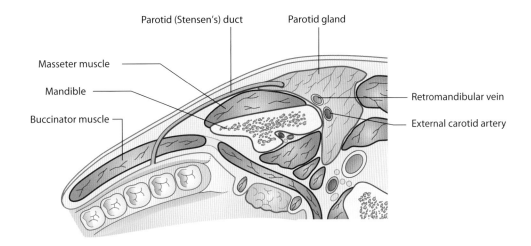

Parotid (Stensen's) duct   Parotid gland

Masseter muscle

Mandible

Buccinator muscle

Retromandibular vein

External carotid artery

- A calcific density along the course of either duct is a definitive sign of sialolithiasis.

Imaging of salivary gland stones

- Most salivary gland stones are readily apparent on CT as they are composed of various radiographically dense calcium salts. On contrast-enhanced studies, small vessels in the sublingual space may mimic small calculi. With a severe enough degree of obstruction, the dilated duct may be seen as a tubular centrally hypodense structure.
- In the setting of ductal infection, the fatty fascia surrounding the duct will appear infiltrated. Enlargement of the gland with surrounding inflammatory changes is typical of glandular infection. Peripherally enhancing, centrally hypodense areas within the gland or around the duct are suspicious for abscess formation.
- MRI findings parallel those of CT. On T2-weighted images, stones appear as low-signal filling defects within the salivary duct, which is otherwise filled with high-signal saliva. The proximal duct may be dilated. An acutely inflamed or infected gland will exhibit high signal on T2-weighted images with fat suppression and low signal on T1-weighted images. In the setting of chronic obstruction, fatty infiltration of the gland appears as high signal intensity on T1-weighted and low signal intensity on T2-weighted images.
- Although ultrasound may be useful to evaluate for sialolithiasis, image quality is highly operator-dependent and may be affected by the patient's physical characteristics. High frequency transducers via an intra-oral approach have been found to be most effective with stones appearing as echogenic foci with posterior acoustic shadowing. If the duct is dilated, it typically appears as a

tubular, anechoic structure proximal to the stone. In cases of severe obstruction, excretory ducts within the gland may also be dilated.

Treatment of salivary gland stones

- Treatment of sialolithiasis includes hydration, NSAID therapy, and application of warm compresses. Occasionally, sour candies are used to increase salivary production in order to expel stones. If these non-invasive measures fail, surgery may be necessary.

Self-assessment

- *Put the major salivary glands (parotid, submandibular, sublingual) in order of likelihood of being affected by sialo-lithiasis. What factors predispose the gland most frequently affected?*

- Submandibular (Wharton's duct) > Parotid (Stensen's duct) > Sublingual. Wharton's duct of the submandibular gland is most commonly involved because of its long anatomical course, the narrow caliber of its orifice in comparison to the rest of the duct, and its relatively high salivary alkalinity and hydroxyapatite content.

- *Describe the courses of the submandibular and parotid ducts.*

- The submandibular duct courses through the sublingual space which is located between the mylohyoid muscle sling and extrinsic muscula-ture of the tongue. The parotid duct extends anteriorly from the parotid gland running parallel to the masseter muscle within the buccal space. Along the anterior aspect of the masseter muscle, the duct courses medially, pierces the buccinator muscle, and enters the oral cavity opposite the second maxillary premolar.

- *Name three potential complications of sialolithiasis.*

- Glandular infection may occur and may lead to abscess formation. Chronic obstruction may lead to duct strictures and fatty atrophy of the gland. Rarely, an obstructing stone can cause salivary duct rupture and formation of an extravasating mucocele.

Spectrum of sialolithiasis

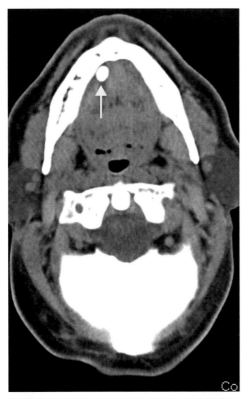

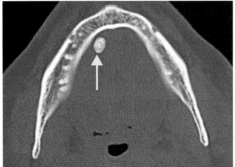

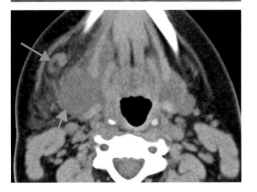

Submandibular duct sialolithiasis with sialadenitis

The submandibular gland and duct are most commonly affected by sialolithiasis, as illustrated by this case and the index case. In this patient with right-sided facial pain, axial enhanced CT in soft tissue (upper image) and bone windows (middle) shows an 8 mm calculus in the anterior right sublingual space near the orifice of the right submandibular duct (yellow arrows). At a lower level (lower image) the right submandibular gland is enlarged (blue arrow) with surrounding inflammatory changes. There is also a reactive lymph node anterior to the gland (green arrow).

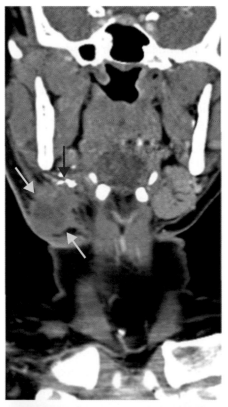

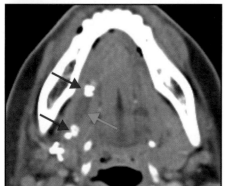

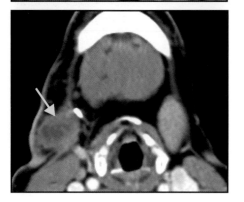

Submandibular sialolithiasis with abscess

Abscess formation is a potential complication of sialolithiasis. Coronal contrast-enhanced CT (upper image) demonstrates a peripherally enhancing, centrally low-attenuating abscess centered within the right submandibular gland (yellow arrows). Superior to the abscess are several small calculi (red arrow). An axial image (middle image) demonstrates that these calculi (red arrows) are within the dilated submandibular duct (blue arrow, between the extrinsic tongue muscles medially and the mylohyoid laterally). Axial CT at a lower level (lower image) again shows the submandibular abscess (yellow arrow).

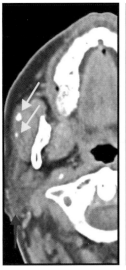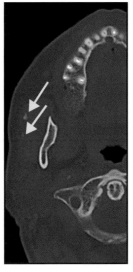

Parotid duct sialolithiasis

Axial CT in soft tissue (left image) and bone (right image) windows depicts two punctate calculi along the course of the right parotid duct (yellow arrows). The duct is dilated and can be seen along the lateral surface of the masseter muscle. The right parotid gland (red arrow) is normal.

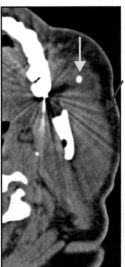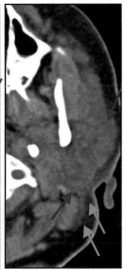

Parotid sialadenitis secondary to sialolithiasis

Axial unenhanced CT shows a punctate calculus (yellow arrow) along the horizontal segment of the left parotid duct just before it pierces the buccinator muscle. The superficial and deep lobes of the gland are enlarged and hypodense due to inflammation (red arrows). There is mild inflammatory stranding along the lateral aspect of the left parotid gland (blue arrows).

Further reading

Bialek EJ, Jakubowski W, Zajkowski P, *et al*. US of the major salivary glands: anatomy and spatial relationships, pathologic conditions, and pitfalls. *Radiographics.* 2006; 26 (3): 745-763.

Gritzmann N. Sonography of the salivary glands. *AJR Am J Roentgenol*. 1989; 153 (1): 161-166.

Som PM, Curtin HD. *Head and Neck Imaging*. 4th edn. St. Louis, MO: Mosby, 2003.

Sumi M, Izumi M, Yonetsu K, *et al*. The MR imaging assessment of submandibular gland sialoadenitis secondary to sialolithiasis: correlation with CT and histopathologic findings. *AJNR Am J Neuroradiol*. 1999; 20 (9): 1737-1743.

Witt RL. *Salivary Gland Diseases, Surgical and Medical Management*. New York; Thieme Medical Pub., 2006.

Case 42   78-year-old male with a 6-month history of failure to thrive from severe malnutrition, a remote history of plasma cell dyscrasia, and multiple recent episodes of Herpes zoster infection presented with left greater than right ptosis, left eye pain, diplopia, and facial numbness

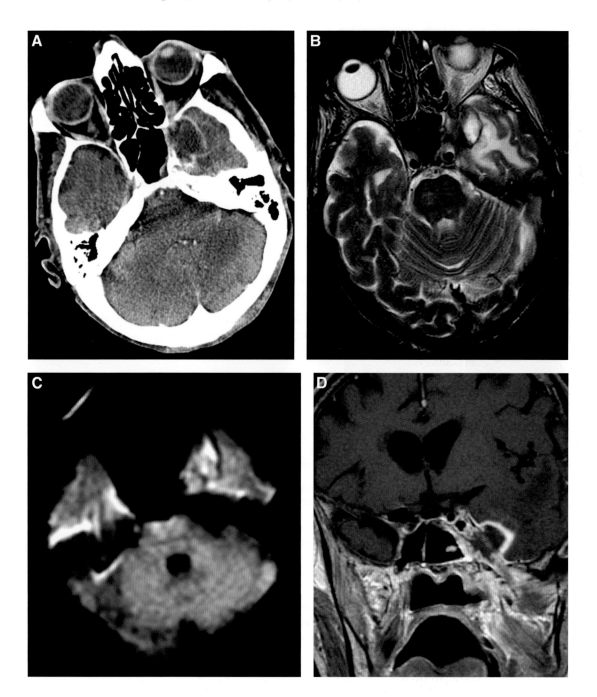

Diagnosis: **Intracranial abscess due to sinusitis**

Axial contrast-enhanced CT (A) shows partial opacification in the left sphenoid sinus (yellow arrow) and a ring-enhancing abscess (red arrows) in the left middle cranial fossa. On axial T2-weighted (B), axial diffusion-weighted imaging (DWI; C), and coronal contrast-enhanced T1-weighted MR (D), the rim of the abscess demonstrates T2 shortening and enhancement (red arrows). Internal contents show abnormal signal on DWI (blue arrow). Low signal in the left cavernous sinus on T2-weighted imaging is suggestive of fungal invasion (green arrow).

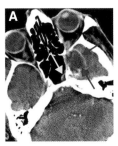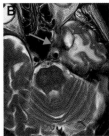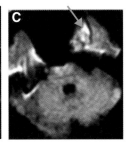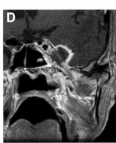

Discussion

Overview of sinusitis

- Sinusitis or rhinosinusitis is a common disease that affects 30–37 million patients annually in the US. It is the fifth most common reason for antibiotic prescription.
- Sinusitis is caused by the inflammation of the lining of the sinuses due to blockage of mucous drainage. Patients are predisposed by upper respiratory infection, allergies, polyps, and deviation of the nasal septum. Risk factors for sinusitis include immunocompromise, autoimmune disease, cystic fibrosis, and exposure to second-hand cigarette smoke. The majority of cases of acute sinusitis (70–80%) are caused by viral infection. Bacterial infection (30% of cases) is caused by organisms such as *Haemophilus influenzae*, *Streptococcus pneumoniae* and *Moraxella catarrhalis*.
- Symptoms of sinusitis include facial pain/pressure, congestion, nasal discharge, headache, cough, toothache, anosmia, and halitosis. Bending over or lying down may exacerbate symptoms. Maxillary sinusitis is often due to odontogenic etiology.
- Acute sinusitis is defined as infection lasting up to 4 weeks.
- Subacute infection lasts 4–12 weeks, and chronic, greater than 12 weeks.
- Patients with recurrent sinusitis have 4 or more separate episodes of acute sinusitis within one year.
- Sinusitis due to viral respiratory infection is usually self-limited, lasting 7–10 days, while bacterial infections last for more than 10 days.

Fungal sinusitis

- Fungal sinusitis is a more serious illness often encountered in immunocompromised patients with conditions such as AIDS, stem cell or organ transplant, and diabetes.
- Allergic non-invasive fungal sinus disease is more prevalent in patients with asthma and nasal polyposis.

Complications of sinusitis

- Untreated or aggressive sinusitis can progress to involve the frontal bone (otherwise known as Pott's puffy tumor – a condition characterized by osteomyelitis and subperiosteal abscess in children) or orbits.
- Intracranial involvement of aggressive sinusitis includes meningitis, epi- or subdural empyema, intracranial abscess, and occasionally cavernous sinus thrombosis either by direct infectious extension or via emissary and diploic veins.
- About 10% of intracranial abscesses are due to sinus infection, occurring most commonly in young men. Infectious organisms travel either by direct extension or via the valveless venous system that connects sinus mucosal veins to dural venous sinuses and eventually to subdural and cerebral veins. Patients may present with seizures, hemiparesis, or nonspecific symptoms such as headache (70%), altered mental status, fever, and nausea and vomiting. Papilledema may be found on clinical exam if there is elevated intracranial pressure. Even with antibiotics, the mortality rate of brain abscess is 5–15%, reaching up to 80% if there is abscess rupture.

Imaging of sinusitis-associated complications

- CT and MR contribute to the decrease of mortality of sinusitis-associated brain abscess by facilitating timely diagnosis, surgical drainage, and administration of antibiotics.
- CT is useful in evaluating sinus disease and associated osseous findings such as sinus wall erosion or sclerosis.
- Abnormal diffusion signal within the abscess cavity on DWI, bright T1 and dark T2 rim from free radicals in macrophages, and predominantly thin, smooth enhancement of the abscess wall differentiate abscess from other ring-enhancing lesions such as tumor or demyelinating disease.
- Occasionally MR spectroscopy may be used to differentiate among causal organisms, with bacterial agents characterized by elevated amino acid (0.9 ppm) and lactate (1.3 ppm) peaks, fungal agents by trehalose (3.6; 3.8 ppm) peaks and toxoplasmosis and tuberculosis by lipid (1.3 ppm) peaks.

Treatment of sinusitis-associated complications

- Treatment of sinusitis-associated brain abscess requires surgical drainage (for both diagnostic and therapeutic purposes) and antibiotics, often with concurrent sinus surgery.

Clinical synopsis   Surgical drainage was performed and microbiological analysis of drained fluid showed *Mucor* organisms. The patient improved after surgery and was discharged with continued antifungal therapy and planned follow-up in the infectious disease clinic.

Self-assessment

- *Name five underlying conditions or physical characteristics that predispose to sinusitis.*

- Upper respiratory infection, allergies, polyps, deviation of the nasal septum, immunocompromise, autoimmune disease, cystic fibrosis, and exposure to second-hand smoke.

- *Briefly describe the pathophysiology and course of sinusitis-associated intracranial abscess including route of spread.*

- Infectious organisms travel from the paranasal sinuses either by direct extension or via the valveless venous system that connects sinus mucosal veins to dural venous sinuses and eventually to subdural and cerebral veins. Patients may present with seizures, hemiparesis or nonspecific symptoms such as headache (70%), altered mental status, fever, and nausea and vomiting. Papilledema may be found on clinical exam if there is elevated intracranial pressure. Abscess is treated with drainage and antibiotics.

- *Describe the MR imaging features of brain abscess.*

- Abnormal diffusion signal within the abscess cavity on DWI, bright T1 and dark T2 rim with predominantly thin, smooth enhancement of the abscess wall.

Spectrum of complications of sinusitis

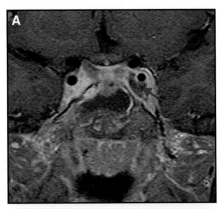

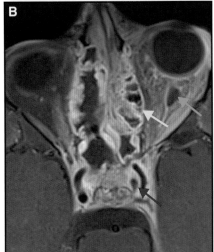

Sinusitis with cavernous sinus thrombosis

Sinusitis extending to the cavernous sinus can result in venous thrombosis and associated cranial nerve palsies involving III, IV, V, and VI. Coronal (A, C, and D) and axial (B) T1-weighted gadolinium-enhanced images with fat saturation show bilateral ethmoid and right maxillary sinus disease (yellow arrows) causing thrombophlebitis with filling defects of the left cavernous sinus (red arrows), left inferior ophthalmic vein (blue arrow), and left internal jugular vein (green arrow).

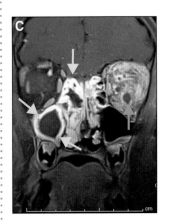

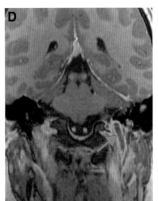

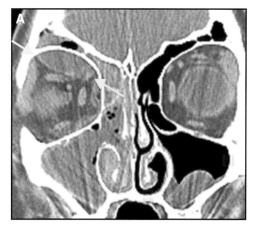

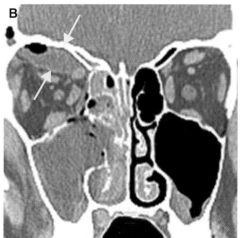

Sinusitis with orbital abscess

Orbital abscess is a surgical emergency due to risk of blindness from elevated intraocular pressure. Coronal (A and B) and axial (C and D) post-contrast CT images show right frontal, ethmoid, and maxillary sinus opacification in this patient with right eye swelling. There is an extraconal, peripherally enhancing air and fluid collection along the right superior orbital wall (yellow arrows), consistent with orbital abscess. Infiltration of the right medial orbital fat (red arrows) suggests sub-periosteal (underneath the periosteum) cellulitis and phlegmon.

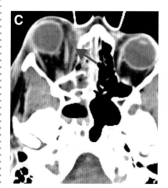

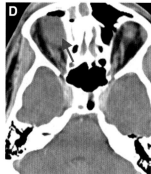

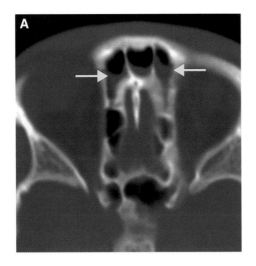

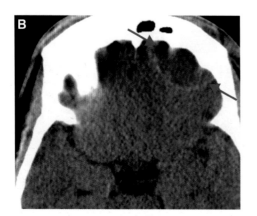

Sinusitis with epidural empyema

Epidural empyema is infection in the epidural space, superficial to the dura. Similar to epidural hematoma, epidural empyema is typically lentiform in shape and does not cross the cranial sutures. This patient with sickle-cell disease presented with a 2-week history of headache, left-sided ptosis and ecchymosis. Axial noncontrast CT images (A and B) show air fluid levels within the frontal sinus (yellow arrows) and an epidural collection just above the left orbit (red arrows). Axial T2-weighted (C) and axial contrast-enhanced T1-weighted (D) MR images confirm the presence of a lenticular rim-enhancing epidural collection (red arrows).

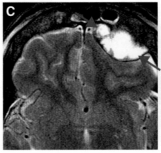 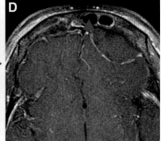

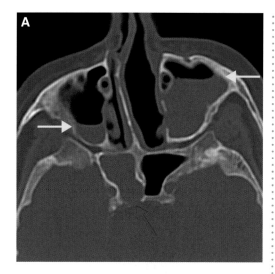

Sinusitis with subdural empyema

Subdural empyema is infection subjacent to the dura. Like subdural hematoma, subdural empyema can cross the cranial sutures. Axial CT in bone window (A) shows air-fluid levels within the bilateral maxillary sinuses (yellow arrows) in this elderly patient with slurred speech and headache. There is a bony defect of the posterior wall of the right sphenoid sinus (red arrow). Axial enhanced CT (B), Fluid attenuated inversion recovery (FLAIR, C) and DWI (D) MR sequences show a proteinaceous left subdural empyema with internal high signal on DWI (blue arrows).

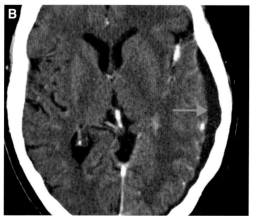

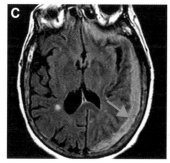

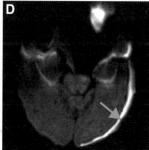

Differential diagnosis of complications of sinusitis

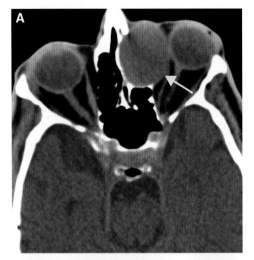

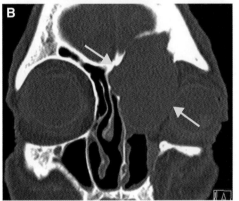

Mucocele

A mucocele is an expanded sinus caused by obstruction of the sinus ostia and resulting in remodeling of the sinus walls. Mucocele most commonly occurs secondary to inflammatory sinus disease. Axial and coronal unenhanced CT (A and B) shows a well-defined fluid-attenuation lesion (arrows) in the left frontal and ethmoid sinuses with smooth sinus wall thinning. High signal intensity on axial T2-weighted (arrow; C) and sagittal T1-weighted (arrow; D) images are consistent with proteinaceous material within a large left frontoethmoid mucocele.

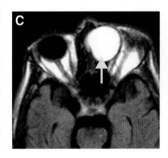

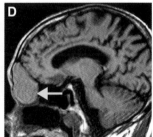

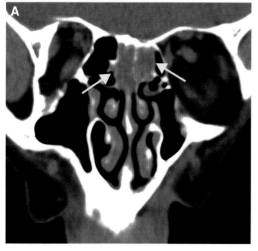

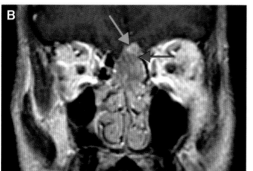

Esthesioneuroblastoma

Esthesioneuroblastoma, also known as olfactory neuroblastoma, is a malignant neural crest tumor that arises from olfactory epithelium. Coronal unenhanced CT (A) demonstrates soft tissue (yellow arrows) in the ethmoid sinus abutting the cribiform plate with relative absence of other sinus disease. Coronal and axial T1-weighted post-contrast (B and C) and axial T2-weighted (D) MR of the anterior skull base shows enhancing soft tissue within the ethmoid sinuses traversing the cribiform plate (red arrow) with left frontal intracranial extension (blue arrows).

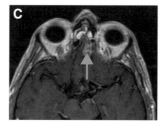 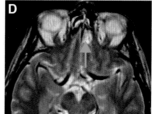

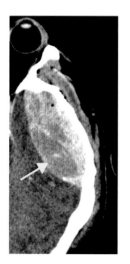 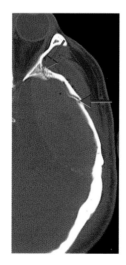

Epidural hematoma

An epidural hematoma is an extra-axial collection of blood superficial to the dura classically caused by fracture of the squamous portion of the temporal bone with injury of the middle meningeal artery. Axial noncontrast head CT (left image) demonstrates a large, heterogeneous, lenticular left epidural hematoma (yellow arrow). Axial CT in bone window at the same level (right image) reveals the associated minimally displaced fractures of the left sphenoid wing (red arrows).

Further
reading

Brock I. Microbiology and antimicrobial treatment of orbital and intracranial complications of sinusitis in children and their management. *Int J Pediatr Otorhinolaryngol* Sept. 2009; 73(9):1183–1186.

Brock I. Microbiology of intracranial abscesses and their associated sinusitis. *Arch Otolaryngol Head Neck Surg* Nov. 2005; 131(11):1017–1019.

Luthra G *et al.* Comparative evaluation of fungal, tubercular and pyogenic brain abscesses with conventional and diffusional MR imaging and proton MR spectroscopy. *AJNR* Aug. 2007; 28:1332–1338.

Muzumdar D *et al.* Brain abscess: an overview. *Int J Surgery* 2011; 9(2):136–144.

43-year-old woman presented with new onset neck pain and odynophagia

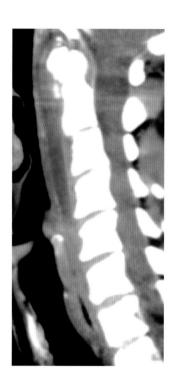

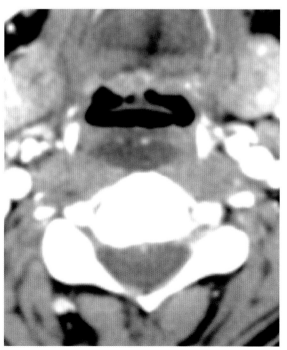
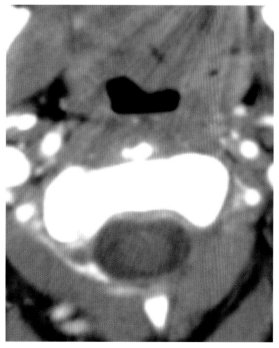

Diagnosis: **Longus colli calcific tendinitis (acute calcific prevertebral tendinitis)**

Sagittal (left image) and axial (middle and right images) contrast-enhanced CT images reveal a non-enhancing, hypodense prevertebral collection (yellow arrows) extending from C1 through C4–C5. Axial CT at the level of the dens shows prevertebral calcification (red arrow) in the location of the longus colli tendon. The fluid collection produces minimal mass effect.

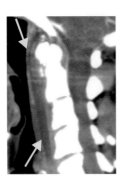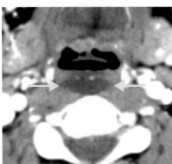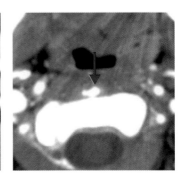

Discussion

Overview and clinical presentation of calcific prevertebral tendinitis

- Acute calcific prevertebral tendinitis is a benign, self-limited, acute inflammatory condition of the longus colli tendon. Like calcific tendinitis elsewhere in the body, it is characterized by intra-tendinous calcium hydroxyapatite deposition.
- The typical presentation is acute onset of neck pain, sore throat, and dysphagia. Patients are usually in minimal distress and have, at most, low grade fever. Laboratory analysis may show mild leukocytosis and elevated erythrocyte sedimentation rate. Whereas retropharyngeal abscess is seen in children, immunosuppressed patients, and following penetrating trauma, longus colli tendinitis tends to affect healthy adults.

Imaging of calcific prevertebral tendinitis

- Imaging findings include a prevertebral/retropharyngeal effusion that typically extends from C1 to C4–C5 or C5–C6. A calcium deposit at the C1–C2 level is seen on cross-sectional imaging.
- Diffuse enhancement may occur; however, rim enhancement, a more typical feature of abscess, is absent. There are no associated suppurative lymph nodes or jugular venous thrombi.

Treatment and differential diagnosis

- Treatment of calcific prevertebral tendinitis is non-operative, and includes NSAIDs and observation.
- The differential diagnosis includes retropharyngeal abscess, jugular venous thrombophlebitis resulting in retropharyngeal edema or effusion, cellulitis, soft tissue mass (such as a suppurative lymph node), and foreign body. The most important distinction is between infected and non-infected collections, as management differs in these two entities.

Clinical synopsis

This 43-year-old woman was treated conservatively with NSAIDs and recovered uneventfully.

Self-assessment

- *Describe the clinical presentations of longus colli calcific tendinitis and retropharyngeal abscess, stressing the differences.*

- The typical clinical scenario for longus colli tendinitis is a previously healthy adult patient who presents with acute onset neck or throat pain and dysphagia, and minimal constitutional symptoms and lab abnormalities. The clinical course is benign. In contrast, retropharyngeal abscess presents with sepsis in children, immunocompromised patients, and victims of penetrating trauma, and requires aggressive intervention.

- *Describe the differences in imaging appearances between longus colli tendinitis and retropharyngeal abscess.*

- Retropharyngeal/prevertebral fluid collections are common to both entities. Abscesses typically have enhancing walls and may be associated with suppurative lymphadenitis. Calcifications are an important feature that distinguishes longus colli tendinitis from abscess.

Spectrum of longus colli calcific tendinitis

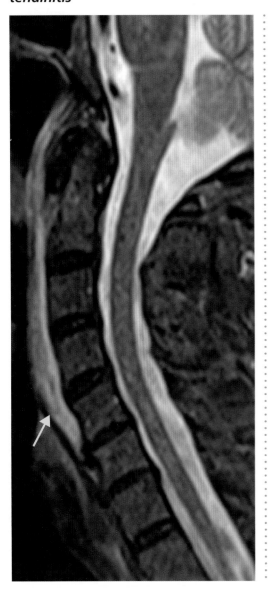

Longus colli calcific tendinitis (MRI and CT)

This 76-year-old man presented with neck pain and difficulty swallowing. Sagittal STIR (left image) and axial T2-weighted MRI (middle image) reveal a hyperintense prevertebral collection (yellow arrows) extending to C6. Axial CT image from the C2 level (right image) shows calcification of the left longus colli tendon (red arrow).

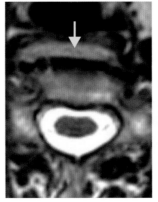
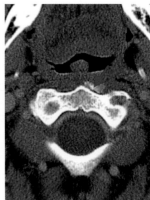

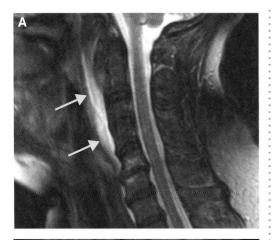

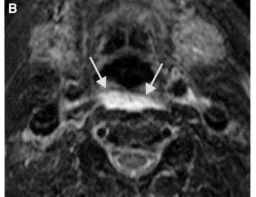

Longus colli calcific tendinitis (MR with contrast)

This 49-year-old woman presented with neck pain and swelling. She was afebrile and did not have leukocytosis. Sagittal (A) and axial (B) T2-weighted images with fat suppression reveal a hyperintense prevertebral collection extending to the level of C5–C6 (yellow arrows). Sagittal (C) and axial (D) post-gadolinium images with fat suppression show diffuse enhancement of the collection (yellow arrow) and a low signal intensity calcification of the right longus colli tendon (red arrow). Conservative management led to uneventful resolution.

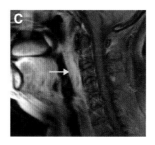

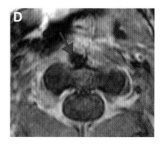

Differential diagnosis of longus colli calcific tendinitis

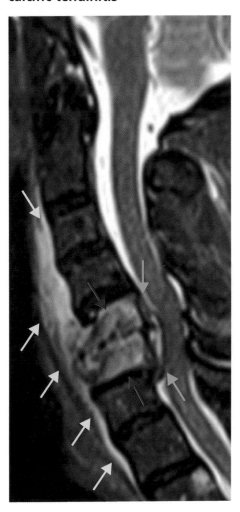

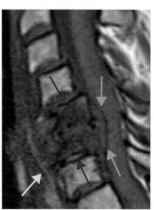

Prevertebral abscess secondary to discitis and osteomyelitis

This 87-year-old woman presented with 2 weeks of neck pain, and was found to have leukocytosis and an elevated erythrocyte sedimentation rate. Sagittal T2-weighted (left image) and T1-weighted (right image) MR show a fluid collection (yellow arrows) tracking anterior to the spine from C2 through T1. This abscess is associated with C5–C6 discitis, osteomyelitis (red arrows), and epidural phlegmon (blue arrows). In contrast to longus colli tendinitis, retropharyngeal abscess is a peripherally enhancing prevertebral collection that lacks calcification and may track inferiorly to the danger space. Rarely, gas is present within the collection. Mass effect tends to be greater than in longus colli tendinitis or effusion of another etiology. Patients with retropharyngeal abscess or cellulitis tend to be more systemically ill than those with longus colli tendinitis. Distinction from sterile fluid collection is vital, as antibiotics and drainage or debridement are key to management. On imaging interpretation, source of infection should be sought. History of recent surgery or penetrating trauma, or the presence of suppurative lymphadenopathy, adjacent spinal infection, or foreign body may provide clues to the underlying etiology.

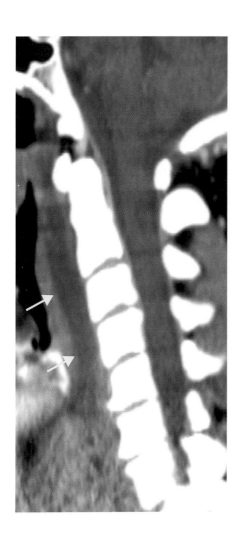

Retropharyngeal edema or effusion

This 48-year-old man presented with a neck mass. Sagittal enhanced CT (left image) shows a retropharyngeal effusion (yellow arrows). Axial CT (middle and right images) shows the effusion (yellow arrow) and avidly enhancing right neck lymphadenopathy (red arrows). A large right neck mass (blue arrows) compresses the right internal jugular vein (green arrow). Retropharyngeal edema or effusion may be seen in longus colli tendinitis or other conditions including jugular vein thrombophlebitis or obstruction. These conditions produce lymphatic leakage into the retropharyngeal space. As opposed to retropharyngeal abscess, retropharyngeal edema tends to be bow-tie shaped, ovoid, or rectangular, with tapered edges and only mild mass effect. The internal jugular vein should be examined for obstruction or thrombosis when effusion is present. Foreign bodies may cause reactive sterile or infected fluid collections to form.

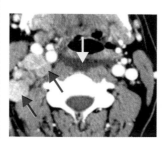 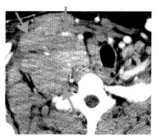

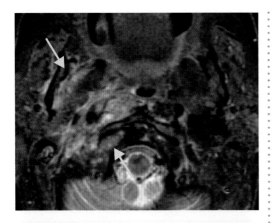

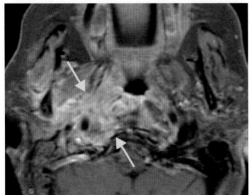

Prevertebral cellulitis

Axial T2-weighted (upper image) and post-gadolinium T1-weighted (lower image) MR images with fat suppression in an 82-year-old diabetic woman with right ear pain and leukocytosis show extensive T2 prolongation and enhancement involving the right prevertebral, parapharyngeal, and masticator spaces (arrows). Biopsy showed *Pseudomonas* infection. Retropharyngeal cellulitis or phlegmon, as opposed to abscess or effusion, tends to be asymmetric and ill-defined, with soft tissue swelling crossing anatomic spaces. Patients with this condition tend to be systemically ill.

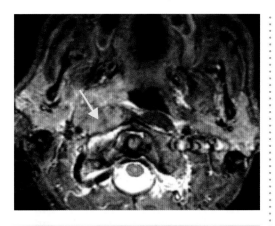

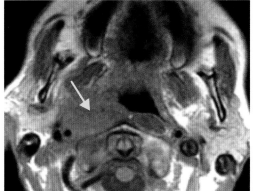

Nasopharyngeal carcinoma

Axial T2-weighted (upper image) and T1-weighted (lower image) MR images from a 58-year-old male with difficulty swallowing show a large nasopharyngeal carcinoma arising from the right nasopharynx, extending into the longus colli muscle (arrows) and parapharyngeal space. In contrast to retropharyngeal abscess or effusion, nasopharyngeal carcinoma is usually unilateral and arises from the nasopharyngeal space, effacing the normal nasopharyngeal recesses such as the opening of the eustachian tube and fossa of Rosenmüller. Nasopharyngeal carcinoma is a solid mass without calcification that may extend into the prevertebral space.

Further reading

Eastwood JD, Hudgins PA, Malone D. Retropharyngeal effusion in acute calcific prevertebral tendinitis: diagnosis with CT and MR imaging. *AJNR* 1998; 19:1789-1792.

Hoang JK, Branstetter IV BF, Eastwood JD, Glastonbury CM. Multiplanar CT and MRI of collections in the retropharyngeal space: is it an abscess? *AJR* 2011; 196: W426–W432.

SECTION 4 NEUROLOGY

Case 44   77-year-old male with a history of hypertension and atrial fibrillation
presented at an outside hospital with sudden onset of left facial droop,
left arm and leg weakness

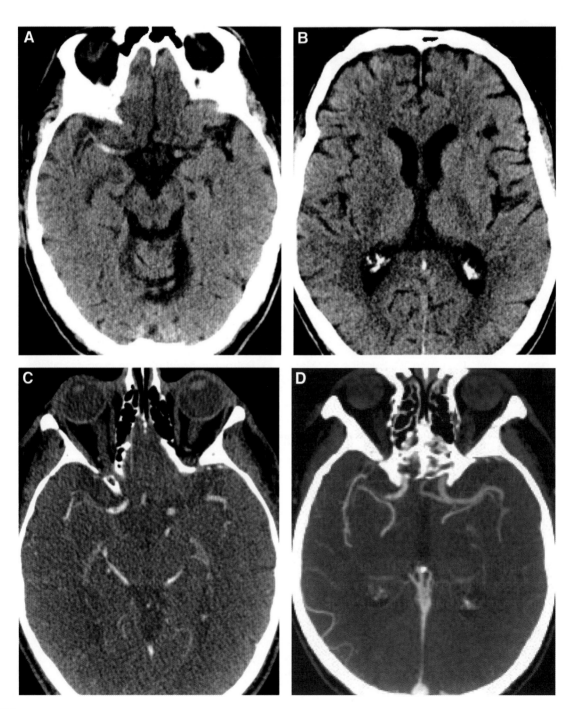

Diagnosis:
Acute stroke

Axial noncontrast CT images of the brain (A, B) show a dense right middle cerebral artery (MCA) sign (yellow arrow, A) and subtle loss of definition in the right basal ganglia (red arrows, B) without hemorrhage. On contrast-enhanced CT angiogram (C, D), there is a cutoff at the proximal right M1 segment (blue arrows) on both the axial source (C) and axial maximum intensity projection (D) images.

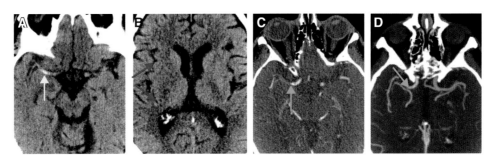

Serial cerebral angiogram images of a right internal carotid artery (ICA) injection in the same patient demonstrate cut-off at the proximal right M1 segment (E) followed by deployment of a MERCI clot retrieval device at the inferior division of M2 (yellow arrow, F) with restoration of this branch, though there is remaining thrombus of the superior division (red arrow, G). More thrombus was removed as the device entered the superior division (H) with resultant improved flow on the final injection (I). *Case courtesy Ajit Puri, MD.*

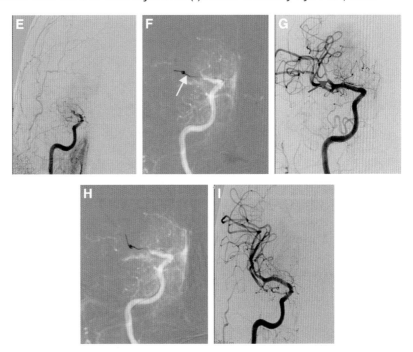

Discussion

Overview of stroke

- Stroke is defined as cerebral tissue injury due to hemorrhage or ischemia, and is clinically characterized by focal or global neurological symptoms that last longer than 24 hours. Silent stroke without overt symptoms is uncommon, but has been recognized as a risk factor for future transient ischemic attacks (TIA) and stroke.
- Stroke is the second most common cause of death worldwide and the third most common in the United States. It is the primary cause of adult disability, with an estimated cost of more than $50 billion per year. Approximately 5-700,000 people suffer strokes each year, with 17–34% dying within one month. 15 percent also suffer a second stroke within 5 years.

Risk factors and etiology of stroke

- Risk factors for stroke include advanced age, hypertension, prior stroke or TIA, diabetes, hyperlipidemia, smoking, and atrial fibrillation.
- Cerebral vascular ischemia accounts for approximately 80% of all strokes. Common causes include arterial compromise (thrombosis, atherosclerosis), embolism from cardiac causes, microvascular disease associated with conditions such as diabetes or hypertension, cerebral venous occlusion, and trauma-associated vascular injury such as dissection.
- Other causes of stroke include vasculitis, patent foramen ovale (especially in younger patients), sickle cell disease, Moyamoya disease, and global hypoperfusion from events such as cardiac arrest. About 30–40% of the time, no clear etiology can be determined.

Clinical diagnosis of stroke

- Patients with stroke often present with sudden rather than progressive symptoms. The constellation of presenting symptoms is highly dependent on the territory of infarction. Common symptoms of infarction include facial weakness, arm drift, and speech impairment.
- Cranial neuropathy may be a prominent feature in brainstem stroke, while nausea and vomiting may indicate cerebellar stroke.
- Only about a quarter of patients with stroke will have headaches.
- Symptoms are scored using the National Institutes of Health Stroke Scale (NIHSS) which assigns a numerical value according to severity.
- In approximately 13% of cases, non-ischemic conditions such as infection, seizure, syncope, metabolic disturbance, subdural collection, demyelinating disease, and tumor are mistaken for stroke.

- Hemorrhage is more commonly seen in patients presenting with coma, vomiting, or headache and in patients who are hypertensive, hyperglycemic, or coagulopathic. About 15–20% of infarcts show hemorrhagic transformation at one week. Large infarcts and those that involve the brainstem are particularly prone to hemorrhagic transformation.

Physiology of stroke

- Normal blood perfusion in tissue measures 50–55 mL/100 g/min.
- Oligemia is defined as 30% of normal perfusion.
- Cell death occurs at <12 mL/100 g/min. Unless timely and adequate reperfusion occurs, neurons become permanently depolarized and infarction ensues over minutes to hours.
- The severity and time course of injury depend on the duration and degree of hypoperfusion and the integrity of compensation mechanisms such as cerebral autoregulation and collateral circulation.
- Stroke is a dynamic process with imaging findings that evolve over time in a predictable manner. These findings correlate with underlying tissue pathology.

CT imaging of stroke

- CT is not sensitive in the hyperacute period (within hours), and in about half of cases the brain appears normal. This is especially true of small infarcts and those occurring in the posterior fossa. In the acute period (hours to days), there is cytotoxic edema due to disrupted membrane protein function resulting in influx of sodium and extracellular water that leads to subsequent cell swelling. This usually appears as regional low attenuation, loss of gray–white matter differentiation, and sulcal effacement on CT.
- In MCA strokes, the insular ribbon and basal ganglia are common sites for loss of gray–white differentiation. Hyperdense thrombus lodged in the M1 segment of the MCA is called the "dense MCA" sign.
- A key role of CT in the hyperacute period is to assess efficiently for potential contraindications to thrombolysis, such as hemorrhage and infarct affecting more than one-third of the MCA territory. In the acute period, hypodensity, sulcal effacement, and loss of gray–white differentiation in the area of infarction become better defined.

MR imaging of stroke

- DWI is the current gold standard for diagnosis of early or small acute ischemic changes, as it is often the only sequence that shows abnormality in the hyperacute to acute period. Decreased diffusivity from restricted Brownian motion of water molecules in infarcted tissue is seen as high signal on DWI and low signal on the apparent diffusion coefficient (ADC) map. Note that high signal on *both* DWI and the ADC map suggests "shine through" of T2 prolongation on DWI, as the diffusion-weighted image is inherently T2-weighted.

- On FLAIR imaging, increased parenchymal signal typically appears hours after stroke onset. In addition, thrombus within an intracranial vessel may exhibit high signal on FLAIR and increased susceptibility on gradient echo imaging.
- In large territory infarcts, gradient-recalled echo (GRE) and susceptibility weighted imaging (SWI) are sensitive in detecting small or petechial hemorrhage.
- Gyriform enhancement due to slow vascular flow and endothelial damage with resultant capillary leakage (breakdown of the blood–brain barrier) occurs in the subacute period (days to weeks following stroke) and may last from weeks to months. The mass effect that characterizes the acute period disappears once enhancement begins.
- "Luxury perfusion", defined as return of cerebral blood flow to normal or higher-than-normal levels due to loss of autoregulation may also occur.
- In the chronic period (after weeks to months), the infarct appears as an area of cerebrospinal fluid (CSF) signal intensity. Volume loss indicates encephalomalacia, and surrounding high FLAIR signal intensity reflects gliosis. Cortical laminar necrosis in the chronic stage appears as gyriform hyperintensity on T1-weighted imaging due to fatty necrosis or sometimes mineralization.

Clinical role of imaging in evaluation of suspected stroke

- Unenhanced head CT is usually the first study ordered for stroke patients in the emergency setting. This is often followed by CT angiography (CTA) of the head and neck. If CT studies are negative or equivocal, patients may undergo MRI and MR angiography (MRA), with or without MR perfusion imaging. Selection of imaging studies is often determined by the availability of local resources and regional practice variation.
- In patients with stroke resulting from systemic hypotension, one should look for watershed infarcts between vascular territories (e.g., between the anterior cerebral arterial (ACA) and MCA territories, or between superficial and deep medullary arterial territories). Embolic infarcts are often multi-territorial, peripheral, and small. In metabolic (e.g., hypoglycemic) or hypoxic scenarios, abnormalities are seen at sites that are vulnerable due to high metabolic demands, such as the cortical ribbon, hippocampus, and basal ganglia.

Treatment of stroke

- Similar to the experiences of management of myocardial infarction, improved prognosis of stroke results from expeditious treatment. The variability and often subtle nature of stroke symptoms have made it difficult to establish guidelines for treatment of stroke patients beyond the 3–4.5-hour window from time of ictus.
- The therapeutic window for intravenous tissue plasminogen activator (IV tPA) is 3–4.5 hours. For consideration of interventional options such as intra-arterial (IA) tPA and mechanical thrombolysis, the patient must present within 6 hours of the onset of symptoms. In vertebrobasilar territory infarcts, which are associated with 70–80% mortality, there is no time limit for intra-arterial thrombolysis as recanalization is associated with 55–75% survival, compared to 0–10% in the untreated population.

Clinical synopsis

Initially, the NIHSS score of the patient presented in the index case was 14, indicating a moderate severity stroke. After CT showed no evidence of intracranial hemorrhage, the patient was given IV tPA (at about 3 hours after the onset of symptoms). CTA of the head and neck demonstrated occlusion of the right M1 segment, which was confirmed by conventional angiogram. Administration of intra-arterial tPA with a MERCI clot retrieval device was successful in re-establishing cerebral blood flow to the MCA territory within 6 hours after the onset of symptoms. The patient did well and was discharged to a rehabilitation center a week later.

Self-assessment

- *Name various risk factors for stroke.*

- Advanced age, hypertension, prior stroke or TIA, diabetes, hyperlipidemia, smoking, and atrial fibrillation.

- *Briefly describe common CT and MRI imaging findings in the hyperacute, acute, subacute, and chronic stages of stroke.*

- Hyperacute (hours): CT may be normal or show subtle hypodensity, sulcal effacement, or loss of gray–white differentiation. "Dense MCA" sign is occasionally seen. MR DWI shows hyperintense signal with low signal on ADC map.
- Acute (hours to days): low diffusivity on DWI/ADC (bright on DWI, dark on ADC), with increasing mass effect and hyperintensity on T2-weighted images. CT shows progressive decrease in attenuation and more obvious territorial demarcation.

- Subacute (days to weeks): gyral enhancement due to breakdown of the blood–brain barrier.
- Chronic (weeks to months): normalization of DWI/ADC, encephalomalacia, cortical laminar necrosis, and gliosis (T2 hyperintensity).

- *What is the therapeutic window after the onset of symptoms for the various major treatments for stroke?*

- Intravenous tPA: 3–4.5 hrs.
- Intra-arterial tPA, clot retrieval, and mechanical thrombolysis (anterior circulation): 6 hours.

Spectrum of infarction

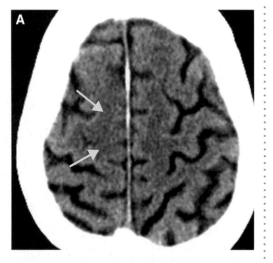

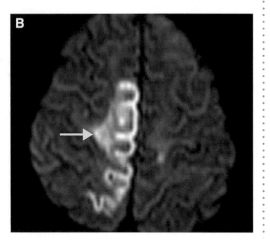

Anterior cerebral artery infarction

An important clue to the diagnosis of infarction is involvement of a vascular territory. In this ACA infarction, subtle loss of gray–white differentiation and effacement of sulci in the right medial frontal lobe is seen on unenhanced CT (yellow arrows, A) corresponding to high signal on the DWI image (yellow arrow, B). Coronal CTA maximum intensity projection (MIP, C) shows a cut-off at the proximal right A2 segment (red arrow). Follow-up noncontrast CT (D) reveals a better-defined lower attenuation subacute infarct of the right ACA territory (blue arrow).

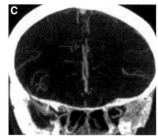

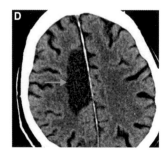

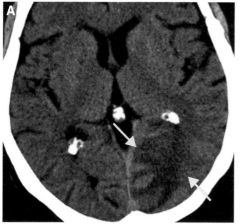

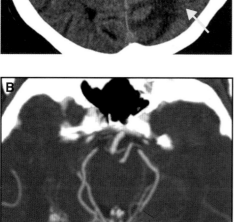

Hemorrhagic transformation of posterior cerebral artery (PCA) infarct

Up to 20% of infarcts may undergo hemorrhagic conversion. Axial noncontrast CT (A) shows a left PCA territory infarct (yellow arrows) with a cut-off at the distal left PCA on CTA (red arrow, B) that underwent hemorrhagic transformation. This is seen as an area of susceptibility signal loss on inherently T2-weighted DWI (blue arrow, C) and high signal on noncontrast T1-weighted imaging (green arrow, D).

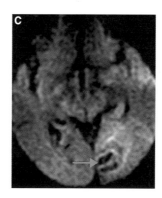

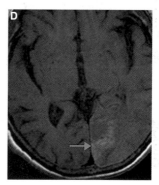

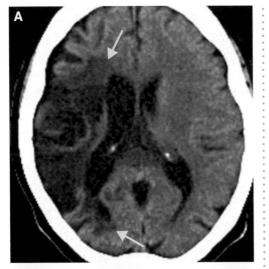

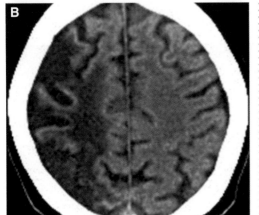

Chronic infarct

The chronic phase of an infarct is characterized by removal of cellular debris and dead brain tissue by macrophages resulting in encephalomalacia. Occasionally (not in this case), cortical laminar necrosis, in which lipid-laden macrophages produce hyperintensity on both T1 and T2-weighted sequences, may develop. Axial images from non-contrast CT (A and B), DWI (C) and T1-weighted MR (D) show an old right MCA territory infarct (arrows) with volume loss and ex-vacuo dilatation of the right lateral ventricle without associated diffusion signal abnormality.

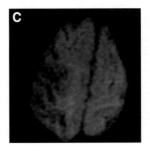

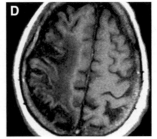

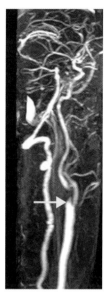
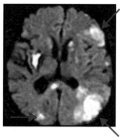
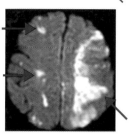

Watershed infarcts

A watershed infarct occurs between vascular territories due to systemic hypoperfusion. Coronal–oblique maximum intensity projection image from a time-of-flight MRA (left image) shows moderate-to-severe stenosis of the proximal left internal carotid artery (yellow arrow). Axial DWI (right images) shows watershed infarcts at the left ACA–MCA, MCA–PCA, and bilateral deep and superficial borderzones (red arrows).

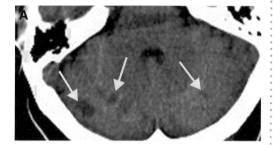
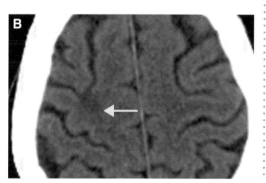

Embolic infarcts

Embolic infarcts are caused by showering of emboli from an extracranial source, most commonly the left atrium in the setting of atrial fibrillation. Echocardiogram should be obtained if embolic infarcts are suspected. Axial noncontrast CT (A and B) and MR DWI (C and D) show multiple, small, peripheral foci of infarction in multiple territories bilaterally (arrows), consistent with embolism.

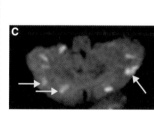
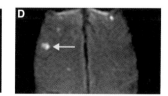

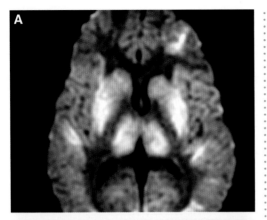

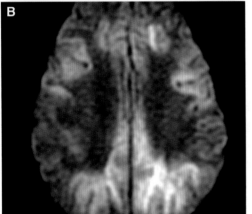

Global metabolic insult

Severe prolonged systemic hypotension or a global metabolic insult produce ischemic changes of the bilateral basal ganglia, thalamus, and cortex. Axial DWI (A and B) demonstrate global abnormality involving the deep gray matter (basal ganglia and thalami) and cortex due to metabolic injury from drug overdose. The ADC map (C) shows corresponding low signal, while the T2-weighted image (D) demonstrates slight hyperintensity.

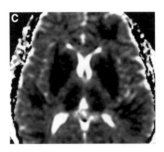

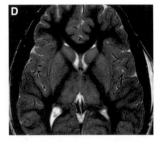

Differential diagnosis of infarct

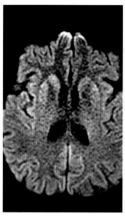
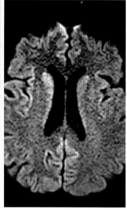

Creutzfeldt-Jakob disease

Creutzfeldt–Jakob disease (CJD) is a rare prion-related neurodegenerative disease. Diffusion abnormality of the cortex and the deep gray matter on MR DWI are seen in CJD, as in the case of this patient who presented after several months of altered mental status. History is crucial for differentiating this condition from hypoxic, anoxic, and metabolic insults. In contrast to infarction, DWI signal abnormality in CJD is irreversible and progressive.

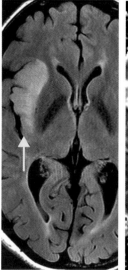
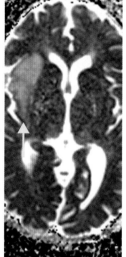

Low-grade glioma

A low-grade glioma can mimic infarct on some MR sequences. Axial FLAIR (left image) demonstrates a focal region of T2 prolongation in the right insular and subinsular region involving both gray and white matter (arrow). This is not associated with low diffusivity, as the lesion is high rather than low signal on ADC (arrow; right image). Low-grade gliomas often do not enhance. History and the lack of change in imaging appearance over time are helpful in establishing the diagnosis.

Further reading

Blackham KA *et al.* Endovascular therapy of acute ischemic stroke: report of the Standards of Practice Committee of the Society of Neurointerventional Surgery. *J Neurointerventional Surgery* 2012; 4: 87–93

Del Zoppo GJ *et al.* Expansion of the time window for treatment of acute ischemic stroke with intravenous tissue plasminogen activator: a science advisory from the American Heart Association/American Stroke Association. *Stroke* 2009; 40: 1–4

Nagar, VA, McKinney AM, Karagulle AT, Truwit CL. Reperfusion phenomenon masking acute and subacute infarcts at dynamic perfusion CT: confirmation by fusion of CT and diffusion-weighted MR images. *AJNR* 2009; 193(6): 1629–1638

Srinivasan A *et al.* State-of-the-art imaging of acute stroke. *Radiographics* 2006; 26: 575–595

Case 45   54-year-old woman who fell while at work

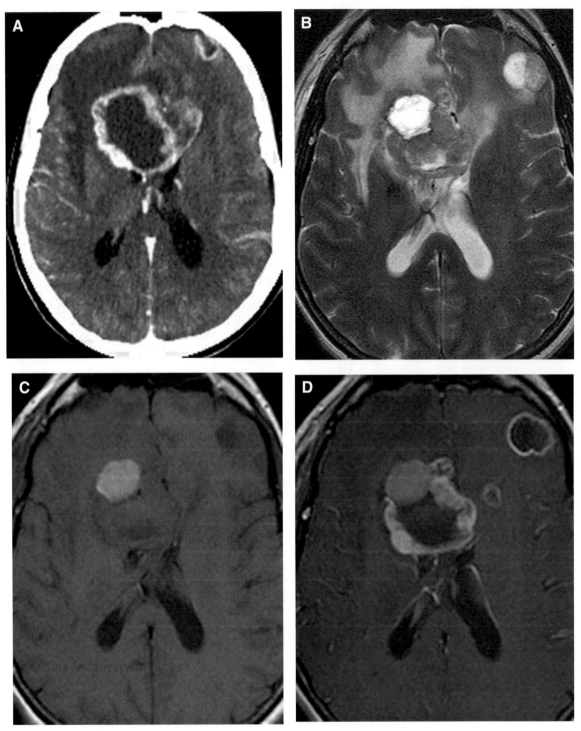

Diagnosis:
**Glioblastoma
multiforme**

Contrast-enhanced CT (A) reveals an irregular, peripherally enhancing, centrally necrotic transcallosal mass (yellow arrows). Peritumoral low attenuation within the right frontal white matter (red arrow) represents a combination of infiltrative tumor and vasogenic edema. A second peripherally enhancing lesion is seen within the anterior left frontal lobe (blue arrows), consistent with multicentric disease.

Axial T2-weighted (B), T1-weighted (C) and T1-weighted post-gadolinium (D) MR sequences show multiple enhancing foci, some with high signal on T1- and T2-weighted imaging (white arrows) due to hemorrhagic or proteinaceous contents. Hypercellular components (green arrows) are hypointense on T2-weighted imaging and enhance after administration of gadolinium. Right greater than left nonenhancing white matter abnormality (red arrows) represents combination of vasogenic edema and tumor infiltration.

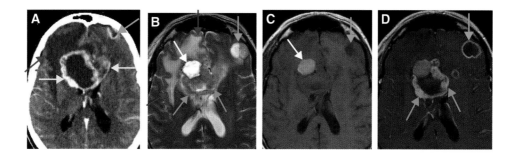

Discussion

Overview of glioblastoma multiforme

- Glioblastoma multiforme (GBM, WHO grade IV glioma) is the most common aggressive primary brain tumor, comprising about 12–15% of all intracranial tumors and 50–60% of all glial tumors. The incidence of GBM is approximately 2–3 per 100,000 people per year. GBM can be primary, arising de novo (60%), or secondary (40%), developing from pre-existing low grade (WHO Grade II) or anaplastic (WHO Grade III) astrocytomas. These are thought to represent distinct disease processes that evolve via different genetic pathways. The average age in primary GBM is older (62 years) than in secondary GBM (45 years). Treatment response tends to be poorer in primary GBM. GBM occurs slightly more often in Caucasians, with a male-to-female ratio of 3:2.
- GBM is an infiltrative tumor that travels along white matter tracts. GBM may be focal or multicentric, with half involving more than one lobe or both

hemispheres. Approximately 2–7% truly arise in multiple independent sites, with the rest of apparently "multicentric" disease representing diffuse infiltration. Temporal lobe involvement is the most common, followed closely by the parietal and frontal lobes. Occipital lobe disease is the least common. Occasionally, tumor extends to the ventricular system, leading to CSF spread with leptomeningeal disease and drop metastases.

Clinical presentation of glioblastoma

- The most common clinical presentation is headache, with other symptoms such as motor weakness and nausea and vomiting resulting from increased intracranial pressure. In approximately one-fifth of cases, patients present with seizures.

Pathology of glioblastoma

- Histologically, GBM is differentiated from lower-grade gliomas by necrotic tissue surrounded by poorly differentiated pleomorphic astrocytes and microvascular proliferation.
- Grossly, GBM is poorly circumscribed, with central yellowish tissue from myelin breakdown amid blood products of varying age.
- Glioblastomas are also distinguished from other gliomas by greater genetic alterations, with mutations in genes such as p53 and EGFR. Extracranial GBM metastasis is rare, though has been described.
- Gliosarcoma represents approximately 2.1% of GBM and is histologically distinguished by both glial and sarcomatous components. Gliosarcoma also has a greater propensity for extracranial metastasis.

Imaging of glioblastoma

- Heterogeneous imaging appearances of GBM reflect the complexity of its molecular and histological features. MR is superior to CT in evaluating GBM, especially in the detection of leptomeningeal disease.
- The spectrum of imaging findings ranges from small and homogeneously enhancing foci to large and heterogeneously enhancing masses.
- The classic imaging appearance is a necrotic "butterfly" lesion straddling the corpus callosum to involve both cerebral hemispheres.
- T2 prolongation surrounding tumor represents a combination of vasogenic edema and tumor infiltration. This is in contrast to brain metastases, where the abnormal T2 prolongation usually reflects vasogenic edema without tumor cells. It is important to note that GBM is known to extend microscopically beyond the margins of signal abnormality seen on MR.

Post-treatment imaging of glioblastoma

- Differentiating tumor from post-treatment changes can be difficult. Modalities such as MR perfusion (elevated cerebral blood volume and vascular permeability due to tumoral neovascularity), PET (increased metabolism in tumor) and MR spectroscopy (elevated choline and lactate and decreased N-acetyl aspartate [NAA] peaks) are generally reserved for follow-up assessment of treatment response and tumor recurrence.

Prognosis and treatment of glioblastoma

- Prognosis for patients with GBM remains very poor despite therapeutic and diagnostic advances; median survival is approximately 3 months without treatment and 12 months with treatment. Fewer than 25% of patients survive at 2 years and fewer than 10% survive by 5 years. Slightly more favorable prognosis is conferred by age less than 50 at presentation, higher Karnofsky score (measure of ability for daily tasks in cancer patients), and at least 98% surgical tumor resection.
- Treatment goals for GBM are aimed primarily at prolongation of survival and palliation rather than at cure. Initial treatment strategies combine surgery, radiation, and chemotherapy (mainly temozolomide, which sensitizes tumor cells to radiation). Bevacizumab (an anti-angiogenic agent) is generally reserved for progression or recurrence.

Clinical synopsis

This patient was transferred from an outside hospital with altered mental status and hyponatremia. CT and MRI showed a large necrotic GBM. The patient underwent biopsy followed by subtotal resection and radiation, but died within a year.

Self-assessment

- *Name several imaging characteristics that indicate high grade and aggressiveness in gliomas.*

- Enhancing, solid, hypercellular components that show reduced diffusion on DWI.
- Necrotic components.
- Hemorrhage seen as susceptibility effect on T2*-weighted sequences.
- Elevated cerebral blood volume (CBV) on perfusion imaging.
- Elevated choline and lactate and decreased NAA on MR spectroscopy.
- Leptomeningeal spread.

- *What are three current tools used to help differentiate recurrent disease from treatment changes?*

- MR spectroscopy.
- Perfusion imaging.
- Longitudinal assessment (enhancing or solid foci that increase in size over time).
- PET.

- *What are three factors that confer a slight advantage over the usually poor prognosis of GBM?*

- High Karnofsky score.
- Patient age less than 50.
- Removal of >98% of tumor at resection.

Spectrum of glioblastoma multiforme

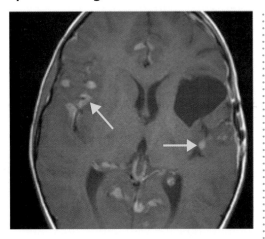

CSF seeding

One year after resection of a left frontal GBM, axial T1-weighted post-contrast MR image demonstrates extensive nodular enhancement within the subarachnoid space and leptomeninges, most prominently along the sylvian fissures (arrows).

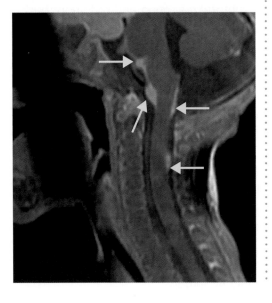

Spinal drop metastases

CSF spread can result in drop metastases to the brainstem and spinal cord. Sagittal T1-weighted post-contrast MR demonstrates multiple enhancing nodules seeded along the dorsal and ventral aspect of the brain stem and cervical spinal cord (arrows). Linear leptomeningeal enhancement along the spinal cord produces a "sugar coating" or "zuckerguss" appearance on imaging. Other primary CNS neoplasms with a propensity to produce drop metastases include ependymoma, medulloblastoma, lymphoma, and oligodendroglioma.

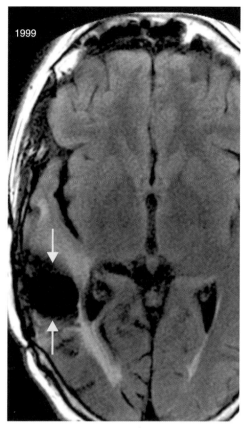

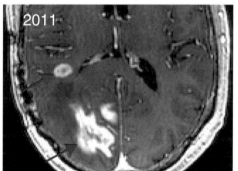

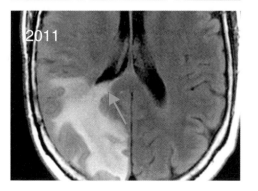

Secondary glioblastoma

Secondary GBM is defined as a low-grade glioma (in this case oligodendroglioma) that undergoes malignant transformation to a higher-grade tumor. This patient underwent resection of a right posterior temporal lobe oligodendroglioma in 1999 (upper image, yellow arrows indicate resection cavity in this FLAIR image). In 2011, axial T1-weighted post-contrast MR (middle image) shows new, multifocal, irregular enhancement within the right posterior temporal and occipital lobes (red arrows) reflecting higher-grade tumor progression. Signal abnormality within the surrounding white matter on FLAIR (lower image) in 2011, involving the splenium of the corpus callosum (blue arrow), is compatible with infiltrative tumor progression.

Differential diagnosis of glioblastoma

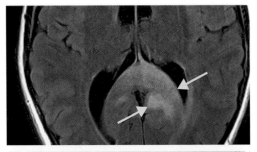

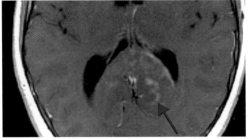

Tumefactive multiple sclerosis

Tumefactive multiple sclerosis (MS) is a subtype of multiple sclerosis that presents as a solitary enhancing parenchymal mass. The corpus callosum may be involved. Unique features that distinguish tumefactive MS from primary CNS neoplasms such as GBM include an incomplete enhancing ring, concentric T2 dark and/or enhancing bands of demyelination giving an "onion skin" appearance, and a relative paucity of surrounding edema. If demyelination is suspected, a steroid trial with follow-up imaging showing interval improvement is helpful. Axial FLAIR (upper image) and T1-weighted post-contrast MRI (lower image) demonstrate expansile signal abnormality (yellow arrows) involving the splenium of the corpus callosum with incomplete ring enhancement (red arrow).

Lymphoma

Primary CNS lymphoma (most commonly large B-cell non-Hodgkin's lymphoma) can appear similar to GBM, particularly in immunocompromised (e.g., HIV-infected) patients in whom tumoral hemorrhage and necrosis are common. Both lymphoma and GBM can involve the corpus callosum. The imaging appearance of CNS lymphoma typically reflects its hypercellularity, with hyperdensity on CT and low signal on T2-weighted images, although the MR appearance can be variable. Lymphoma typically involves the periventricular white matter along ependymal surfaces and the basal ganglia. Leptomeningeal dissemination is seen in 30–40 percent of cases. In this case of primary CNS lymphoma, axial T2-weighted (left) and post-contrast T1-weighted MR (right) images show multiple T2-isointense (to cortex), enhancing lesions within the corpus callosum (yellow arrows) as well as the periventricular white matter (red arrow).

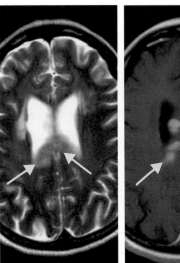
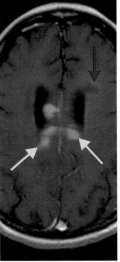

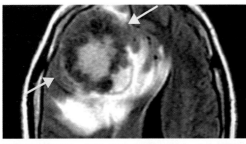

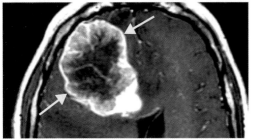

Metastasis

One-third of intracranial metastatic lesions are solitary and can mimic GBM, as in this case. Features such as irregular enhancement, central necrosis, surrounding non-enhancing signal abnormality, and hemorrhage can be seen in both entities. Metastatic lesions may also involve the corpus callosum. Biopsy samples obtained beyond the margins of the lesion will be abnormal in GBM due to its infiltrative nature, while samples from beyond the margins of metastatic lesions will not contain tumor cells. Axial FLAIR (upper image) and post-contrast T1-weighted (lower image) MR images demonstrate a heterogeneous, peripherally enhancing right frontal lesion (arrows) with mass effect, involvement of the corpus callosum, and extensive peritumoral vasogenic edema.

Meningioma

Meningiomas are readily distinguished from GBM by their dural-based extra-axial location. Gray matter buckling, CSF signal intensity cleft, and dural tail are signs that a mass is extra-axial. Typical meningiomas are intermediate in signal intensity on T2-weighted imaging and exhibit avid homogeneous enhancement. Vasogenic edema may be seen within the brain parenchyma adjacent to a meningioma. Calcification on CT and adjacent bony hyperostosis are additional helpful imaging findings. Axial unenhanced CT (left image) and T1-weighted post-contrast MR (right image) demonstrate a calcified, avidly enhancing falcine mass (yellow arrows) with a dural tail (red arrow) posterior to the splenium of the corpus callosum.

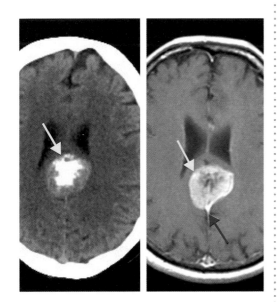

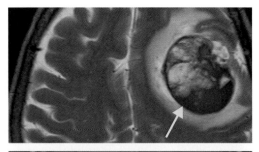

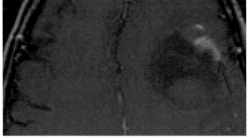

Hemorrhagic neoplasm

Hemorrhagic neoplasms (e.g., GBM, oligodendro-glioma, metastatic disease) may result in apparent spontaneous hemorrhage. Common hemorrhagic metastases include renal and thyroid carcinoma, melanoma, and choriocarcinoma. Contrast-enhanced MRI can assess for abnormal enhancement in the setting of hemorrhage to uncover an underlying neoplastic etiology. This patient presented with a large left frontal lobe hemorrhage. Axial T2-weighted MR (upper image) demonstrates blood products of various ages in the left frontal lobe (yellow arrow) surrounded by vasogenic edema. There is irregular nodular enhancement along the anterosuperior margin of the mass on the T1-weighted enhanced MR (red arrow, lower image). Biopsy showed metastatic breast carcinoma.

Further reading

Lantos PL *et al*. Tumors of the nervous system. In Graham DI, Lantos PL, eds. *Greenfield's neuropathology*. 7th edn. Boca Raton, Fla.: CRC Press, 2002, 789-798

Wen PY, Kesari S. Malignant gliomas in adults. *NEJM* July 2008; 359(5): 492-507

Lacroix M *et al*. A multivariate analysis of 416 patients with glioblastoma multiforme: prognosis, extent of resection, and survival. *J Neurosurgery* Aug. 2001; 95(2): 190-198

Ryken TC *et al*. Surgical management of newly diagnosed glioblastoma in adults: role of cytoreductive surgery. *J Neurooncology* Sept. 2008; 89(3): 271-286

Case 46 74-year-old woman presents with rapidly deteriorating mental status over 3 months

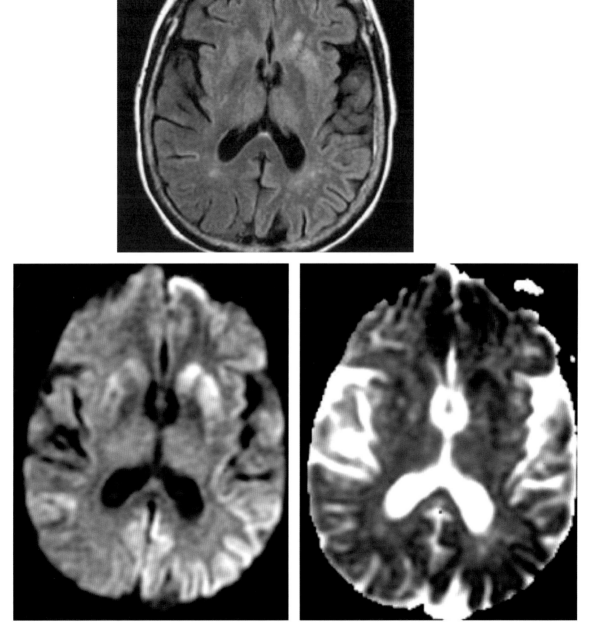

Diagnosis:
Sporadic
Creutzfeldt–
Jakob
disease (sCJD)

Axial FLAIR (left image) reveals mild putaminal and caudate hyperintensity (yellow arrows), and subtle hyperintensity of the left parietal cortical ribbon (red arrow). Axial DWI (middle image) reveals hyperintensity of the putamina and caudate heads (yellow arrows), and patchy areas of cortical hyperintensity most pronounced in the left parietal lobe (red arrows). ADC map (right image) reveals corresponding hypointensity indicating that signal abnormality on the diffusion-weighted image represents reduced diffusion rather than T2 "shine through."

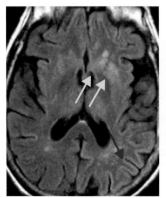 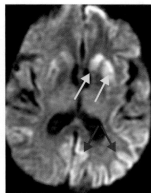 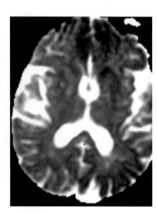

Discussion

Overview of Creutzfeldt–Jakob disease

- Creutzfeldt–Jakob disease (CJD) is a prion disease that is classified as a transmissible spongiform encephalopathy. It may be sporadic, familial, or iatrogenically spread via contaminated surgical instruments, human growth hormone therapy, cadaveric dural grafts, and corneal implants.
- The term "variant CJD" refers to bovine spongiform encephalopathy ("mad cow disease"). This entity characteristically involves the pulvinar nuclei of the posterior thalami, and thus, has a different appearance from "non-variant" etiologies. Signal abnormality in the pulvinar and dorsomedial thalami seen in variant CJD characteristically produces the "hockey stick" sign on FLAIR imaging.

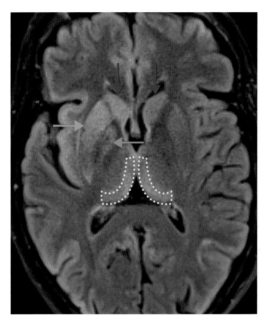

Axial FLAIR MR in a patient with variant CJD demonstrates symmetrical dorsomedial thalamic and pulvinar hyperintense signal bilaterally, producing the "hockey-stick" sign (yellow dashed outlines). There is also hyperintense signal in the cortex, bilateral caudate (red arrows), right putamen (blue arrow), and right globus pallidus (green arrow).

Clinical presentation of CJD

- Patients are most commonly between 50 and 75 years of age, and typically present with myoclonus, akinetic mutism, and dementia that is rapidly progressive over several months.
- Occasionally, clinical presentation is atypical, with dementia that has a protracted but progressive course, worsening over several years.
- Later in the disease course, EEG may show "periodic sharp wave" complexes.
- Cerebrospinal fluid analysis may reveal the presence of 14–3–3 protein, but this finding is neither sensitive nor specific. Some cases are diagnosed by brain biopsy or autopsy.
- Virtually all cases are fatal within 1 year of diagnosis.

Imaging findings of CJD

- CJD is distinguished from other neurodegenerative diseases by the characteristic appearance of restricted diffusion in the cortex and basal ganglia on diffusion-weighted MRI.
- Involvement of the brain may be patchy and asymmetric.

Imaging differential diagnosis of CJD

- On imaging, CJD may appear similar to various conditions, such as arterial or venous infarction, toxic encephalopathy (e.g., from methanol poisoning), mitochondrial disease, paraneoplastic syndrome, and viral encephalitis.
- Specific clinical and imaging findings may be used to differentiate among these entities.

Clinical differential diagnosis of CJD

- Rapidly progressive dementia may occur from neurodegenerative diseases, toxic or metabolic conditions, infections, autoimmune diseases including Hashimoto's encephalopathy, and paraneoplastic phenomena.

Clinical management of CJD

- As no curative or life-prolonging therapy is currently available, treatment is supportive.

Clinical synopsis   This 74-year-old woman with sporadic CJD and rapidly progressive dementia died several months after diagnosis.

Self-assessment

- *Which imaging technique is most specific for identifying CJD?*

- *Which area of the brain is most commonly abnormal on brain MRI?*

- *True or false: the JC virus is the infectious agent in CJD.*

- Diffusion-weighted brain MRI.

- The cortex is more commonly involved than the basal ganglia.

- False: CJD is a prion disease. JC virus is the causative agent of progressive multifocal leukoencephalopathy (PML), a disease that affects immunocompromised patients.

Spectrum of CJD

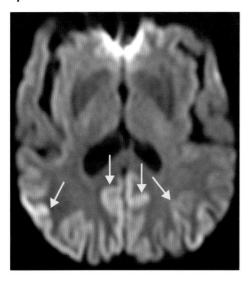

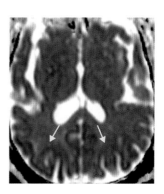

CJD with cortical involvement only

This 56-year-old male presented with subtle cognitive decline that progressed over 7 months. DWI (left images) reveals areas of cortical hyperintensity in the occipital and frontal lobes (arrows). The basal ganglia are not involved. ADC map (right image) obtained at same level as the upper left image confirms reduced diffusion in the cortex (hypointensity, arrows). While CJD typically presents with rapidly progressive dementia, some cases have a more protracted course. At this time, it is not known whether the patient's cognitive reserve plays a role in the clinical outcome. It has been posited that subtype of CJD may have bearing on clinical outcome, but phenotypes for specific subtypes of CJD are not currently established. The index case is an example of CJD with both cortical and basal ganglia involvement.

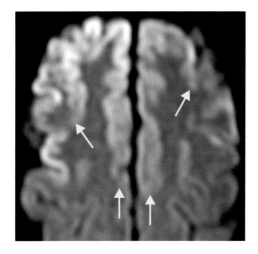

Differential diagnosis of CJD

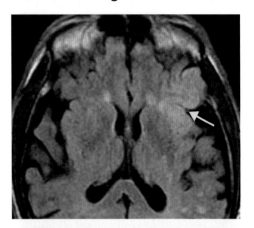

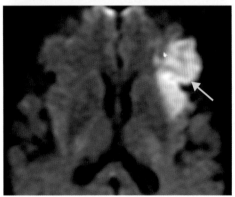

Arterial infarction

In this 75-year-old man with acute onset of slurred speech, axial FLAIR image (upper image) shows subtle hyperintensity and swelling in the left inferior frontal cortex (arrow). Axial DWI (lower image) shows reduced diffusion (arrow) indicating acute infarction within the territory of the anterior division of the left middle cerebral artery (Broca's area). The acute clinical presentation of stroke syndrome and confinement of abnormality to an established arterial territory are consistent with arterial infarction rather than CJD. In contrast, the diffusion abnormality in CJD does not correspond to an arterial territory, and the typical presentation is subacute onset of progressive cognitive decline. Unlike in CJD, diffusion abnormalities evolve over time in cerebral infarction.

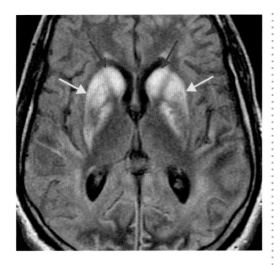

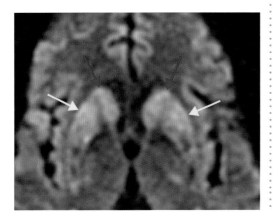

Hypoxic ischemic encephalopathy

This 44-year-old man underwent cardiac arrest due to drug overdose. Axial FLAIR image (upper image) shows hyperintensity within the putamina (yellow arrows) and caudate heads (red arrows), with corresponding hyperintensity on DWI (lower image). The acute clinical presentation typically differentiates hypoxic ischemic encephalopathy (HIE) from CJD. Mild HIE may only affect the watershed areas, while more severe HIE can affect gray matter structures including the cerebral cortex, basal ganglia, and hippocampi. CT imaging of HIE (not shown) typically shows diffuse edema of the affected structures, leading to decreased attenuation of the cortical gray matter and diffuse loss of normal gray–white differentiation. The CT "reversal" sign refers to relative hyperattenuation of the white matter, which is typically spared. Similarly, the "white cerebellum" sign is caused by diffuse supratentorial damage resulting in lower attenuation of the cerebral cortex in comparison with the spared cerebellum and brainstem.

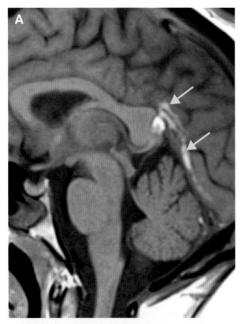

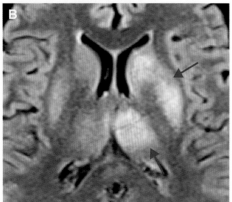

Venous infarction

This 27-year-old woman on oral contraceptives presented after 1 week of headache, vomiting, and somnolence. Sagittal T1-weighted MR (A) reveals hyperintense thrombus within the straight sinus and vein of Galen (yellow arrows). Axial FLAIR image (B) shows hyperintensity within the basal ganglia, predominantly on the left (red arrows). Axial DWI (C) and corresponding ADC map (D) demonstrate reduced diffusion in the areas of FLAIR abnormality. Within 30 days, the patient's symptoms had resolved. Follow-up MRI (not shown) showed resolution of imaging abnormalities. Venous infarction is differentiated from CJD in this case by patient age, clinical presentation and course, identification of causal venous thrombus, and transience of MRI signal abnormalities.

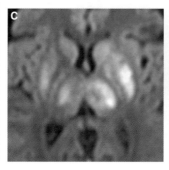

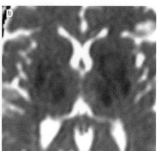

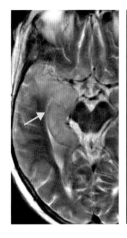 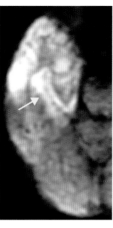

Viral encephalitis

This 79-year-old woman presented with progressive deterioration of mental status over 1 week and was found to have *Herpes simplex* encephalitis. Axial T2-weighted image (left image) and DWI (right image) show T2 hyperintensity, edema, and reduced diffusion in the right temporal lobe (arrows). Viral encephalitis is distinguished from CJD by reduced diffusion in the deep gray nuclei and white matter rather than the cortex. Presentation is acute or subacute, and patients often have constitutional symptoms. Polymerase chain reaction of CSF is usually needed to identify the causal agent.

Progressive multifocal leukoencephalopathy

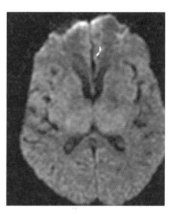

This 45-year-old woman with HIV infection presented with seizures and gait disturbance. Axial FLAIR image (left image) reveals extensive thalamic and putaminal hyperintensity. DWI (right image) is normal. Progressive multifocal leukoencephalopathy (PML), which is caused by the JC virus, involves the deep white matter and gray nuclei, typically occurs in immunocompromised patients, and usually does not cause reduced diffusion in the cortex.

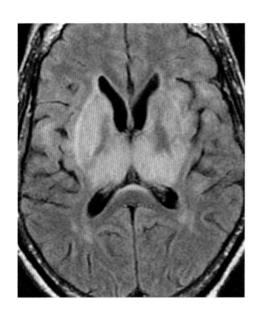

Other conditions

Methanol poisoning causes putaminal infarction without cortical involvement and is usually seen in younger patients than those affected by CJD. Mitochondrial disease tends to occur in younger patients, and has greater cortical swelling than CJD. Lactate is elevated on MR spectroscopy. Paraneoplastic disease produces hyperintensity of deep gray nuclei on FLAIR imaging without reduced diffusion, and primary malignancy is present.

Further reading

Hegde A N, Mohan S, Lath N, Lim C. Differential diagnosis for bilateral abnormalities of the basal ganglia and thalamus. *Radiographics* 2011; 31(1): 5.

Schaefer PW, Grant PE, Gonzalez RG. Diffusion-weighted MR imaging of the brain. *Radiology* 2000; 217: 331–345.

Ukisu R, Kushihashi T, Kitanosono T, *et al*. Serial diffusion-weighted MRI of Creutzfeldt–Jakob disease. *AJR* 2005; 184: 560–566.

Ukisu R, Kushihashi T, Tanaka E, *et al*. Diffusion-weighted imaging of early-stage Creutzfeldt–Jakob disease: typical and atypical manifestations. *Radiographics* 2006; 26 (suppl 1): S191–S204.

Vitali P, Maccagnano E, Caverzasi E, *et al*. Diffusion-weighted MRI hyperintensity patterns differentiate CJD from other rapid dementias. *Neurology* 2011; 76: 1711–1719.

Case 47   62-year-old man presented with orthostatic headache

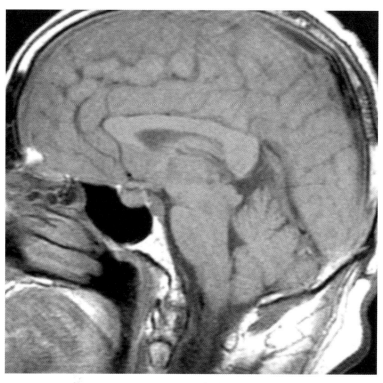

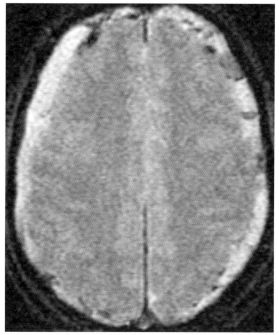

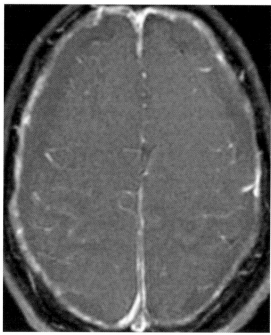

Diagnosis: **Intracranial hypotension with subdural hematomas**

Sagittal T1-weighted image (left) shows downward sagging of the brainstem (yellow arrow). Axial gradient echo image (middle) shows bilateral subdural collections (red arrows) with areas of loculation and dark susceptibility effect (blue arrows) indicating blood products, consistent with chronic subdural hematomas. Gadolinium-enhanced axial T1-weighted image (right) reveals diffuse pachymeningeal thickening and enhancement (green arrows) with subjacent non-enhancing, intermediate intensity subdural collections (red arrows).

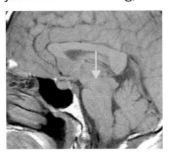 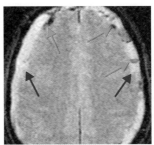 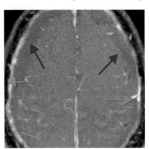

Discussion

Overview and physiology of intracranial hypotension

- Intracranial hypotension is caused by iatrogenic or spontaneous cerebrospinal fluid (CSF) leak.
- Clinical presentation includes orthostatic headache (worse in the upright position), dizziness, tinnitus, and abducens palsy. Headache may be absent.
- When CSF volume is lost, intracranial volume is usually maintained by venous expansion. On imaging, this appears as pachymeningeal thickening and enhancement due to venous engorgement, with enlargement of the venous sinuses, pituitary gland, and cervical spine epidural plexus. Less frequently, cranial or spinal hygromas or hematomas form in the spinal or intracranial epidural or subdural spaces. Hematomas form as a consequence of tearing of subdural bridging veins. Loss of CSF volume results in loss of buoyant force, which results in brainstem sagging, descent of the cerebellar tonsils, downward tilt of the optic chiasm, and enlargement of the pituitary gland. Findings may be seen in isolation or combination.

Treatment of intracranial hypotension

- Spontaneous CSF leaks can often be managed conservatively with bed rest, hydration, and caffeine or theophylline, but refractory cases may require epidural blood patch placement.
- In the setting of intracranial hypotension, subdural hematomas are generally not evacuated due to risk of downward herniation and cerebellar hemorrhage. Instead, the cause of the CSF leak is addressed.

- If an intraventricular shunt is present, the shunt pressure should be adjusted.
- If there was recent spinal surgery, post-operative drains may need to be removed.

Clinical synopsis	This 62-year-old man with intracranial hypotension and chronic subdural hematomas was treated conservatively and made a full recovery.

Self-assessment

- *What is the typical clinical presentation of intracranial hypotension?*

- *Describe compensatory mechanisms for low intracranial pressure and list three associated imaging findings.*

- *True or false: in the setting of intracranial hypotension, subdural hematomas should be emergently evacuated.*

- Orthostatic headache, often associated with tinnitus and sixth nerve palsy.

- Intracranial volume must be maintained. This is accomplished by venous engorgement and formation of extra-axial fluid collections. Findings include pachymeningeal enhancement, formation of epidural or subdural collections, downward descent of the cerebellar tonsils, and downward tilt of the optic chiasm.

- False: evacuation can result in downward brain herniation. Instead, the cause of the CSF leak should be treated.

Spectrum of intracranial hypotension

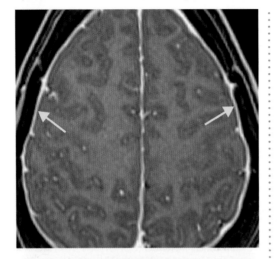

Intracranial hypotension

This 18-year-old woman presented with persistent postural headache several months following spinal surgery. Axial post-gadolinium T1-weighted images (left images) show diffuse pachymeningeal enhancement (yellow arrows) and venous sinus dilation (red arrow). Sagittal T1-weighted image (bottom right image) shows brainstem sagging manifested by downward displacement of the cerebellar tonsils (blue arrow), pituitary enlargement (green arrow), and downward tilting of the optic chiasm (white arrow).

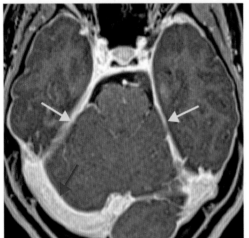

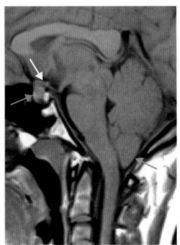

Differential diagnosis of intracranial hypotension

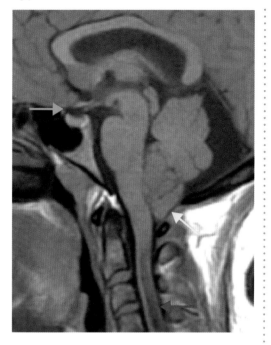

Arnold–Chiari malformation

This 27-year-old woman presented with occipital headache and visual blurring. Sagittal T1-weighted image shows downward descent of the cerebellar tonsils (yellow arrow) and a cervical syrinx (red arrow). The pituitary is normal in size and there is no downward chiasmatic tilt (blue arrow). In Chiari I malformation, as opposed to intracranial hypotension, the pituitary is normal in size, there is no downward tilt of the optic chiasm, and there is no brainstem sagging. A cervical syrinx may be present. Headache associated with Chiari I malformation is not typically orthostatic, although it may be positional.

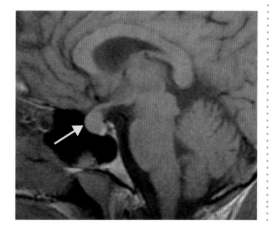

Pituitary adenoma

Sagittal T1-weighted image in a 19-year-old woman with visual blurring and dull headache reveals pituitary enlargement due to the presence of a macroadenoma (yellow arrow). There is no downward tilting of the optic chiasm and no downward descent of the cerebellar tonsils. As opposed to pituitary enlargement in intracranial hypotension, pituitary adenoma does not present with orthostatic headache and is not associated with brainstem sagging.

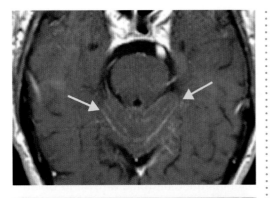

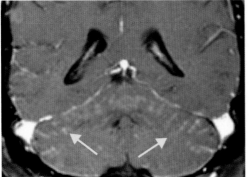

Carcinomatous meningitis

Axial (upper image) and coronal (lower image) gadolinium-enhanced T1-weighted images from two separate patients with carcinomatous meningitis from lung carcinoma show leptomeningeal enhancement extending into cerebellar folia (arrows). This case highlights an important distinction between carcinomatous meningitis and intracranial hypotension. In carcinomatous meningitis, there is no thick, peripheral, pachymeningeal (dural) enhancement, as seen in intracranial hypotension. Instead, carcinomatous meningitis involves the leptomeninges (arachnoid and pia). It is notable, however, that the dura may be separately involved by metastatic disease, as highlighted by the next example.

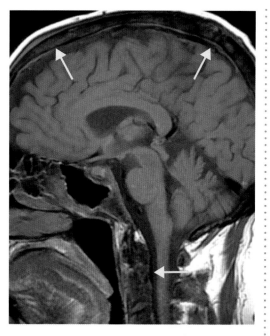

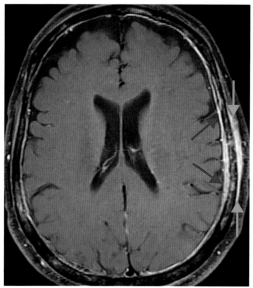

Dural metastases

A 66-year-old man with metastatic prostate carcinoma presented with vertigo and ptosis. Sagittal T1-weighted image (upper image) reveals diffuse hypointensity of the calvarial and cervical spinal marrow due to infiltrative metastatic involvement (yellow arrows). Post-gadolinium axial T1-weighted image (lower image) shows relatively diffuse pachymeningeal enhancement. In the left inferior frontal region, pachymeningeal thickening (red arrows) is more pronounced subjacent to an area of bony and subgaleal enhancement (blue arrows) corresponding to a bone metastasis. The pachymeninges are more commonly involved directly by overlying bone metastasis than by hematogenous implantation of tumor.

Further reading

Schievink WI. Spontaneous spinal cerebrospinal fluid leaks and intracranial hypotension. *JAMA* 2006; 295: 2286-2296.

Schievink WI, Maya MM, Louy C, *et al.* Diagnostic criteria for spontaneous spinal CSF leaks and intracranial hypotension. *AJNR* 2008; 29: 853-856.

Smirniotopoulos JG, Murphy FM, Rushing EJ, Rees JH, Schroeder JW. From the Archives of the AFIP: patterns of contrast enhancement in the brain and meninges. *Radiographics* 2007; 27: 525-551.

Case 48   79-year-old woman with progressive deterioration in mental status over the course of 1 week

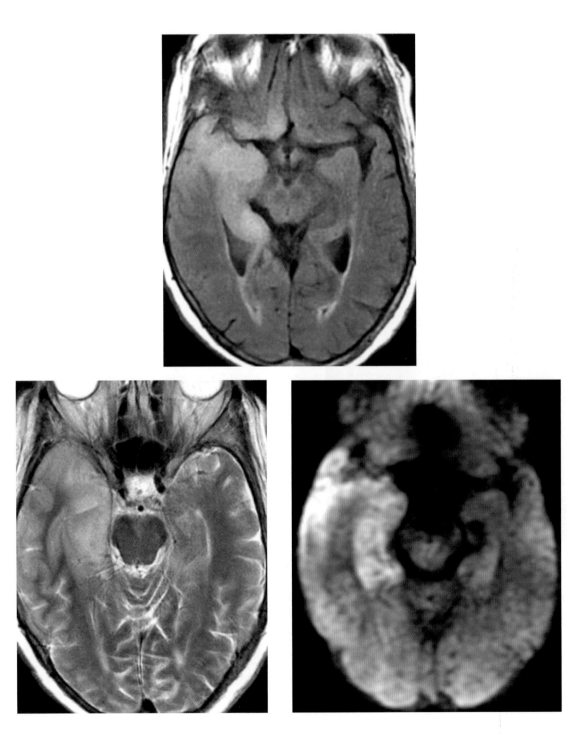

Diagnosis: Axial FLAIR (left image) and T2-weighted (middle image) MR images show
Herpes simplex edema and swelling of the right temporal lobe (arrows) with minimal mass
encephalitis effect upon the cerebral peduncle. DWI (right image) reveals corresponding
restricted diffusion.

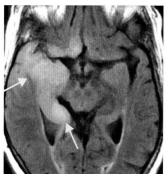
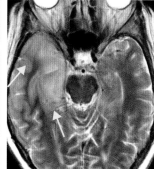
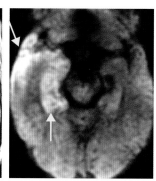

Discussion

HSE is the most common cause of acute viral inflammation of the brain and meninges.

- The clinical presentation of Herpes simplex encephalitis (HSV) typically involves deterioration of mental status, fever, headache, and seizures, often progressing over several days.
- Other causes of viral encephalitis may have overlapping imaging and clinical manifestations and include Eastern Equine Encephalitis (EEE), influenza, and HIV. EEE is caused by an arbovirus infection, typically in late summer or autumn, with neurological deterioration progressing to coma within 1–3 days. HIV encephalitis is a chronic, indolent process that presents with cognitive decline.

Imaging findings of viral encephalitis

- Whereas HSE typically involves one or both temporal lobes with putaminal sparing, EEE typically involves deep nuclear gray matter structures and the brainstem. HIV causes diffuse leukoencephalopathy. Influenza may involve the thalami, brainstem, and corpus callosum, but lobar and putaminal involvement is not typical. West Nile virus can produce various brain findings, but lacks a characteristic pattern.
- CT is useful in uncooperative patients, as it can evaluate for other causes of mental status deterioration such as hemorrhage and tumor, and may show areas of brain swelling.

- MRI is more accurate in characterizing sites and extent of brain involvement. Diffusion is often mildly restricted, but may be normal. Hemorrhage may accompany HSE, but is usually absent in EEE.
- While MRI findings may suggest a specific etiology, diagnosis is established by serum or CSF analysis. Other processes involving the temporal lobe include tumor, middle cerebral artery territory stroke, and post-ictal change. Tumor has a more insidious onset than HSE. Tumor enhancement, if present, may aid in diagnosis. MR spectroscopy shows elevated choline in higher-grade neoplasms. Acute stroke presents with acute onset neurological symptoms, involves a vascular territory, and may involve the putamen. Post-ictal change may be indistinguishable from HSE on imaging. This condition is characterized by restricted diffusion in the temporal lobe, which corresponds to depolarization and glutamate-mediated hyperexcitation.

Clinical management of viral encephalitis

- When there is clinical suspicion for HSE, empiric antiviral treatment with acyclovir should begin immediately. The diagnosis may later be confirmed by CSF analysis, including *Herpes simplex* virus (HSV) polymerase chain reaction. Treatment for EEE is supportive, as no currently existing antiviral agent has been proven effective.

Clinical synopsis
This 79-year-old woman with HSE was treated with acyclovir and made a moderate recovery with residual memory loss.

Self-assessment

- *Which parts of the brain are differentially affected in HSE and EEE?*

  - HSE primarily affects the temporal lobes, sparing the putamina. EEE involves the deep gray nuclei and brainstem.

- *What features can be used to differentiate between HSE and temporal lobe neoplasm?*

  - HSE exerts mild mass effect and shows minimal to no enhancement. Tumor often has prominent mass effect, enhancement, and elevated choline on MR spectroscopy.

- *True or False: antiviral treatment should begin only after the diagnosis of HSE is confirmed due to risk of drug toxicity.*

  - False: empiric antiviral treatment with acyclovir should begin as soon as the diagnosis of HSE is clinically suspected.

Spectrum of Herpes simplex encephalitis

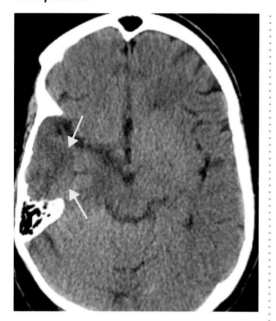

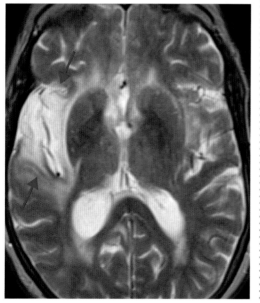

Early HSE

In the same patient who was discussed in the index case, CT (upper image) reveals subtle right temporal lobe hypodensity (yellow arrows). Axial T2-weighted MR (lower image) at the level of basal ganglia performed 4 months later reveals evolving encephalomalacia (red arrows). The putamen is characteristically spared.

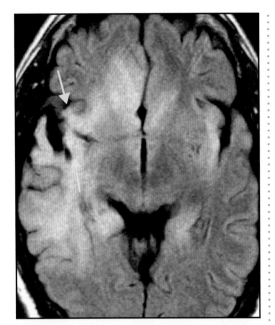

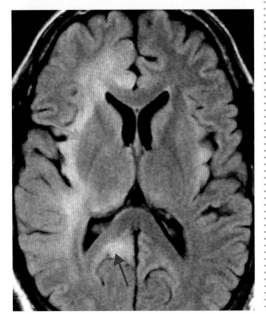

Advanced HSE

This 44-year-old man with HSE presented with progressive memory loss. Axial MR FLAIR images reveal right temporal lobe hyperintensity with additional involvement of the insula (yellow arrows) and cingulate gyrus (red arrow), as well as mild left insular hyperintensity. Note sparing of the putamen (blue arrow).

Differential diagnosis of Herpes simplex encephalitis

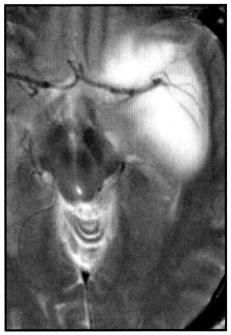

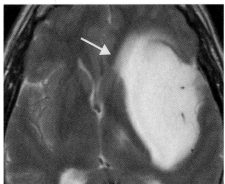

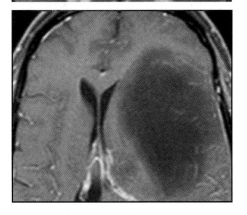

Temporal lobe glioma

This 46-year-old man presented with progressive memory loss and seizure. Axial T2-weighted images (upper and middle) reveal confluent left temporal lobe hyperintensity with considerable mass effect upon the putamen and internal capsule (arrow). There is no enhancement on the post-gadolinium T1-weighted image (lower). Higher-grade gliomas are more likely to enhance.

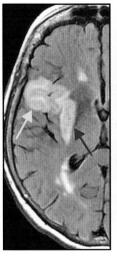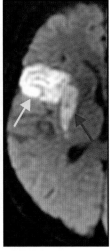

Acute MCA territory infarct

This 85-year-old woman presented with acute-onset left hemiparesis. Axial MR FLAIR image (left image) shows right temporal lobe hyperintensity and cortical swelling (yellow arrow). There is also T2 prolongation in the putamen (red arrow). DWI (right image) reveals corresponding high signal. Corresponding low signal was seen on the ADC map (not shown), consistent with reduced diffusivity. The acute presentation, signal abnormality corresponding to a vascular territory, and putaminal involvement favor acute infarction over HSE.

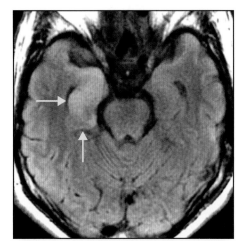

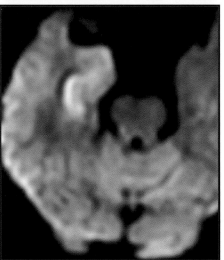

Post-ictal change

This 67-year-old man presented with protracted seizures. Axial FLAIR image (upper) shows hyperintensity in the right hippocampal formation (arrows). DWI (lower image) shows corresponding restricted diffusion. HSE cannot be excluded solely on the basis of these imaging findings.

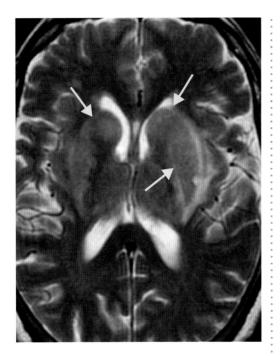

Eastern Equine Encephalitis (EEE)

This 73-year-old man presented with rapid deterioration of mental status and fever progressing to coma over 24 hours. Axial T2-weighted MR (upper image) shows edema and swelling of the putamina and heads of the caudate nuclei (arrows). There is T2 prolongation of the midbrain (middle image). There is no restricted diffusion on DWI (lower image).

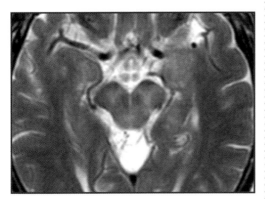

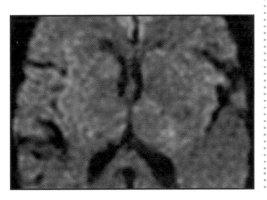

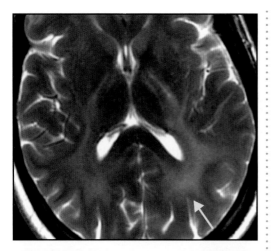

HIV encephalitis

This 34-year-old man with known HIV infection presented with chronic cognitive decline and ataxia. Axial T2-weighted MR images reveal diffuse leukoencephalopathy characterized by white matter hyperintensity (arrows).

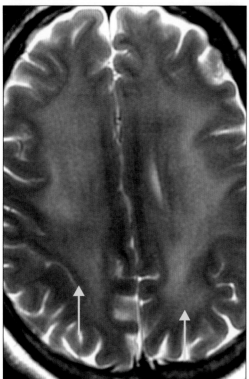

Further reading

Chaudhuri A, Kennedy PGE. Diagnosis and treatment of viral encephalitis. *Postgrad Med J* 2002; 78:575–583.

Deresiewicz RL, Thaler SJ, Hsu L, Zamani AA. Clinical and neuroradiological manifestations of eastern equine encephalitis. *NEJM* 1997; 26:1867–1874.

Kennedy PGE. Viral encephalitis: causes, differential diagnosis, and management. *J Neurol Neurosurg Psychiatry* 2004; 75:i10–15.

Case 49 72-year-old female with a 2-day history of progressively worsening headache, nausea, and vomiting

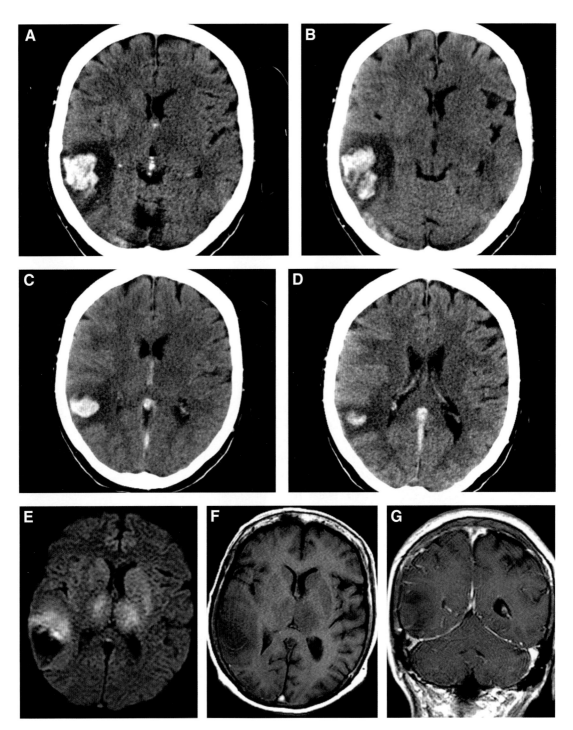

Diagnosis:
Dural venous sinus thrombosis and hemorrhagic infarctions

Axial unenhanced CT images (A, C, D; image B is not shown in these annotated images) show a right posterior temporal hemorrhage and left larger than right thalamic and left basal ganglia venous infarcts (seen as subtle asymmetrical hypoattenuation) due to thrombosis (high attenuation) of the right transverse sinus (yellow arrow, A); internal cerebral veins (red arrow, C), vein of Galen (blue arrow, C) and straight sinus (green arrow, D).

MR images (E–G) demonstrate similar findings: DWI (E) shows signal abnormality in the left greater than right thalamus, basal ganglia, and posterior right temporal lobe consistent with infarction. The right temporal lobe infarct is hemorrhagic. Thrombus in the superior sagittal sinus is hyperintense on T1-weighted imaging (white arrow, F). Post-contrast T1-weighted image (G) shows filling defects within the superior sagittal (white arrow) and right transverse (yellow arrow) sinuses.

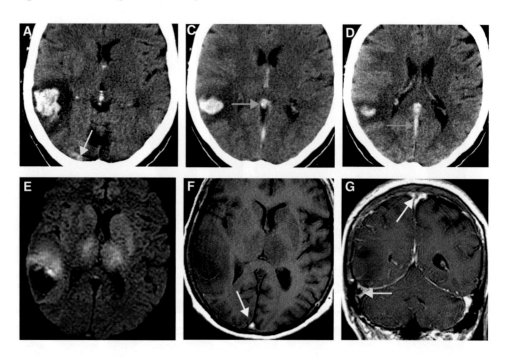

Discussion

Overview and risk factors for intracranial venous thrombosis

- Intracranial venous thrombosis is thrombosis of cortical veins or deep venous sinuses and is one of the more common causes of stroke in young patients.

- Intracranial venous thrombosis more commonly affects females, with a female-to-male ratio of approximately 3:1. Women in their thirties are often affected due to usage of oral contraceptive pills and pregnancy, as both conditions promote a hypercoagulable state.
- Neonates who have undergone complicated deliveries are also at relatively increased risk for venous thrombosis due to dehydration and shock. The incidence of peripartum and postpartum venous sinus thrombosis is approximately 12 cases per 100,000 deliveries.
- Other predisposing conditions include thrombophilias, head and neck infections including sinusitis, trauma, neoplasms, medical instrumentation, renal insufficiency, and inflammatory diseases such as Behçet's.

Clinical presentation of intracranial venous thrombosis

- Intracranial venous thrombosis is an uncommon, at times diagnostically challenging, condition that presents with nonspecific symptoms.
- Patients with intracranial venous thrombosis most commonly present with headaches (in more than 90% of cases). Headaches tend to progress slowly, from mild to severe, differentiating them from the "worst headache of life" typical of subarachnoid hemorrhage from aneurysm rupture.
- Other presenting symptoms include visual changes (with the clinical exam finding of papilledema from increased intracranial pressure), stroke-like syndrome, and seizures. In the elderly, symptoms can be even less specific (e.g., mental status change).

Physiology of intracranial venous thrombosis

- The pathophysiology of venous infarct differs from that of arterial infarct. Occlusion of the major intracranial venous sinuses results in venous congestion, impaired CSF absorption, and ultimately, increased intracranial pressure.
- Elevated intracranial pressure may sometimes be the only sequela of venous sinus thrombosis. In the setting of robust collateral drainage (pre-existing or developed in response to venous thrombosis) or recanalization of the thrombosed vein, parenchymal damage may be absent or completely reversible. If venous pressure exceeds arterial perfusion pressure, infarction and hemorrhage may occur.
- Cavernous sinus thrombosis is an uncommon condition due to retrograde extension of sinonasal or orbital infection, although the incidence of this condition has decreased since the advent of antibiotics. Immunocompromised patients are at higher risk. The typical presentation is sinusitis with cranial neuropathy that progresses from unilateral to bilateral over a relatively short period of time.

Intracranial venous anatomy

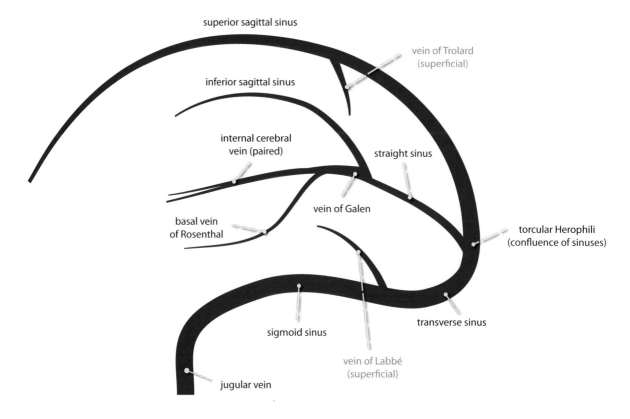

Imaging of intracranial venous thrombosis

- The appearance of venous sinus thrombus on unenhanced CT is variable depending on the age of the clot and the patient's hydration status. Noncontrast CT may show high-attenuation thrombus within a superficial or deep venous sinus (often, the superior sagittal sinus), with or without associated venous infarction that may or may not have hemorrhaged.
- In cortical vein thrombosis, linear, irregular, high-attenuation material within the vein is known as the "cord" sign. The triangular hyperdensity associated with superior sagittal sinus thrombosis is referred to as the "delta" sign.
- Venous sinus thrombosis should always be considered in the setting of a peripheral hemorrhage or infarct that does not correspond to a typical arterial distribution.
- Deep system thrombosis (involving the paired internal cerebral veins, vein of Galen, or straight sinus) should be included in the differential diagnosis of bilateral thalamic infarction in addition to occlusion of the artery of Percheron.
- In comparison to unenhanced CT, contrast CT venography (CTV) is superior for delineation of the site and extent of sinus thrombosis. If thrombus is present

within the superior sagittal sinus, axial images will demonstrate a central filling defect outlined by a rim of enhancement (the "empty delta" sign).

- There are several potential challenges in interpreting CTV. Venous sinus filling defects from normal arachnoid granulations may create false positives. Conversely, hyperdense clot may simulate a patent sinus, resulting in a false negative study. Thus, it is imperative to compare CTV images with noncontrast CT images. Appropriate timing of the contrast bolus (ideally a 45–50-second delay) is also an important technical consideration.
- On MR imaging, thrombus demonstrates increased signal on T1-weighted images and loss of normal flow void on T2-weighted sequences and time-of flight MR venogram (MRV).
- False positives on MRV can be caused by slow flow. In addition, T1 shine-through from methemoglobin-containing thrombus may mimic flow, leading to false negatives. Comparison between contrast-enhanced and noncontrast T1-weighted images is therefore useful in resolving these potential pitfalls.
- The signal characteristics of thrombus vary over time. Subacute thrombus exhibits high signal intensity on T1-weighted images, while acute and chronic clots tend to be isointense to venous blood. Arachnoid granulations present as filling defects within the dural venous sinuses, though often assume a more discrete lobulated round appearance as compared to thrombus.
- Gradient echo images are useful to detect susceptibility "blooming" effect associated with paramagnetic components within blood products.

Treatment of venous sinus thrombosis

- Timely treatment is essential for minimizing morbidity and mortality in cerebral venous thrombosis. Treatment includes correcting underlying causes (hydration, stopping oral contraceptives, treating infection, etc.) and alleviating elevated intracranial pressure. Anticoagulation with thrombectomy or thrombolysis is generally reserved for severe or refractory cases.
- More than half of patients with intracranial venous thrombosis will have full recovery after treatment. Approximately a third will have mild residual symptoms, while 2–3% of patients may experience moderate to severe residual symptoms.
- Mortality is approximately 8% at 16-month follow-up. Male sex, age greater than 37 years, coma, hemorrhage, infection, cancer, and involvement of the deep venous system all confer poorer prognosis.

Clinical synopsis

The patient was admitted to the neurological ICU and treated with IV heparin for 5 days and was transitioned to warfarin on discharge. Work-up was positive for lupus anticoagulant. The patient's condition has returned to baseline at 1-year follow-up.

Self-assessment

- *Describe three CT or MR findings associated with cerebral venous thrombosis.*

- The "delta" sign is hyperdense thrombus in superior sagittal sinus or the torcular Herophili on noncontrast CT.
- The "empty delta" sign is rim enhancement surrounding a thrombus on CT venography.
- Absence of flow void is seen on T2-weighted MR or MR venography, with increased signal on non-contrast T1-weighted imaging. It is important to use information from all MR sequences to improve accuracy of diagnosis on MR venography.

- *What veins are included in the deep and superficial intracranial venous systems?*

- The superficial venous system includes the superior sagittal sinus, transverse sinuses, and sigmoid sinuses.
- Cortical veins such as the veins of Labbé and Trolard are also considered superficial.
- The deep system includes the paired internal cerebral veins, the vein of Galen, and the straight sinus.

- *Name several risk factors for venous thrombosis.*

- Risk factors overlap with those for extracranial venous thromboses, and include:
  - Dehydration
  - Oral contraceptive use
  - Pregnancy
  - Infection
  - Malignancy
  - Inflammatory diseases
  - Renal insufficiency
  - Recent surgery

Spectrum of intracranial venous thrombosis

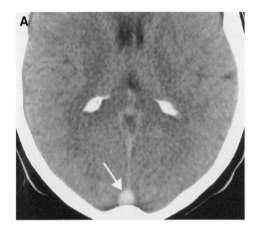

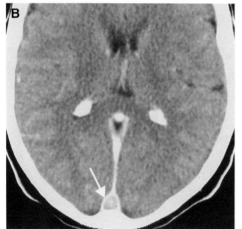

Superior sagittal sinus thrombosis

Pre- (A) and post-contrast (B) CT of a patient with superior sagittal sinus thrombosis show classic delta and empty delta sign (arrows). Noncontrast sagittal T1-weighted MR image (C) demonstrates high signal intensity thrombus (arrows) with corresponding MRV (D) showing loss of normal flow signal. This patient had a history of lower extremity DVT.

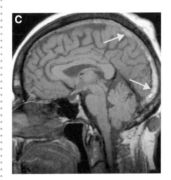
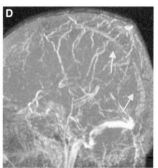

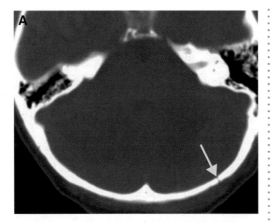

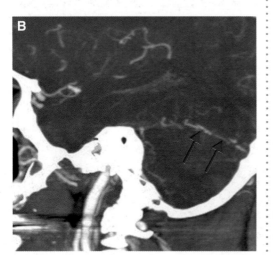

Sinus injury due to trauma

This patient suffered a fall while intoxicated. Axial CT in bone window (A) shows a non-displaced left occipital fracture (yellow arrow). Sagittal maximum intensity projection image from a CT angiogram (B) shows decreased caliber of the left transverse sinus (red arrows). Axial CTA source images (C and D) confirm reduced caliber of the left transverse sinus (red arrows) and also demonstrate right anterior temporal and left frontal contusions (blue arrows). Trauma is an uncommon cause of venous sinus injury and thrombosis.

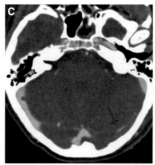

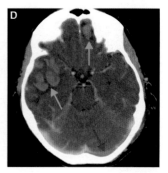

Differential diagnosis of venous thrombosis

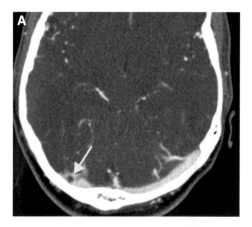

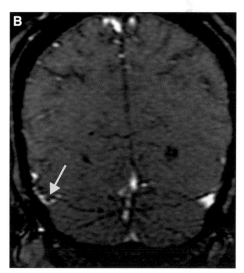

Arachnoid granulation

Not all filling defects within dural venous sinuses represent thrombus. Arachnoid granulations are the most common cause of filling defects, especially in the transverse and superior sagittal sinuses. They can appear multi-lobulated and are often found at the confluences of draining cortical veins and sinuses. Axial enhanced CT (A) shows a small filling defect (arrow) within the right transverse sinus at its confluence with draining cortical veins. Coronal T1-weighted enhanced source MRV images (B) demonstrate an arachnoid granulation in the right transverse sinus (arrow). Corresponding axial images show the granulations as foci of high signal intensity on T2-weighted imaging (arrow, C) and filling defects on post-contrast T1-weighted imaging (arrow, D).

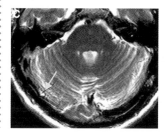

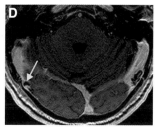

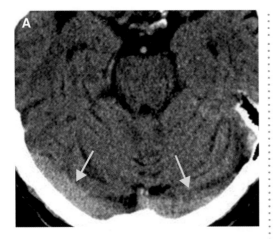

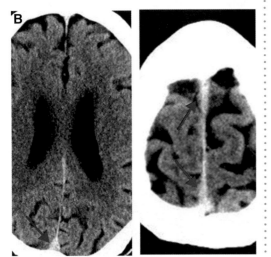

Dehydration or elevated hematocrit

Dehydration or other causes of high hematocrit can cause high attenuation within blood vessels on unenhanced CT as seen in this patient presenting with urosepsis. Axial unenhanced CT images (A and B) demonstrate relative increased attenuation of the transverse (yellow arrows) and superior sagittal (red arrows) sinuses. CT angiogram performed subsequently (C and D) does not show corresponding filling defects.

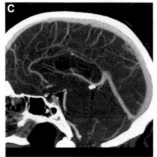

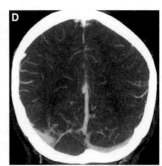

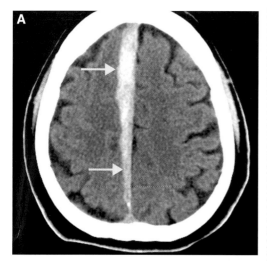

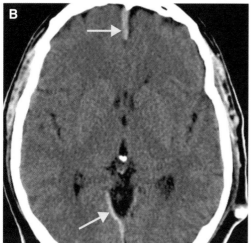

Subdural hematoma

Sometimes, diffuse subdural hemorrhage along the falx and tentorium mimics sinus thrombosis, as in this patient who suffered a fall. Axial unenhanced CT (A and B) shows subdural hematoma along the entire falx and tentorium (arrows). Irregularity of margins, uneven thickness, and localization of the collection to one side of the dura indicate that this hyperdensity is not within the dural venous sinuses. Subsequent MRI showed this acute to subacute subdural hematoma (arrows) as iso- to hyperintense signal on T1-weighted MR (C) and hypointense signal on T2-weighted MR (D).

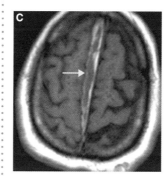

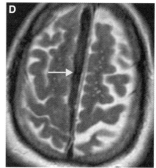

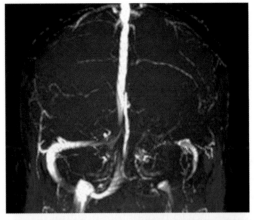

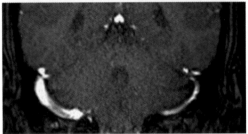

Normal variant asymmetry of the transverse sinuses

Coronal MR venogram (upper image) and coronal contrast-enhanced T1-weighted MRI (lower image) illustrate asymmetry of the transverse sinuses, right larger than left. Asymmetry of the transverse sinuses is considered a normal anatomic variant – in one angiographic study, 49% of cases had asymmetric transverse sinuses. The right transverse sinus was larger than the left in the majority of cases. A study using MR venography showed hypoplasia of the left transverse sinus in 39% and atresia in 20% of cases. The importance of interpreting MRV in the context of supporting findings from other sequences is re-emphasized, as normal variant asymmetry of the transverse sinuses may mimic thrombosis. The presence of susceptibility effect on GRE imaging and the presence of hyperintense methemoglobin on T1-weighted imaging would support the diagnosis of thrombus and decrease diagnostic uncertainty.

Further reading

Dentali F *et al*. Natural history of cerebral vein thrombosis: a systemic review. *Blood* 2006; 108(4):1129-1134

Ferro JM *et al*. Prognosis of cerebral vein and dural sinus thrombosis: results of the International Study on Cerebral Vein and Dural Sinus Thrombosis. *Stroke* 2004; 35(3):664-670

Martinelli I *et al*. How I treat rare venous thromboses. *Blood* 2008; 112(13): 4818-4823

Stam J. Thrombosis of the cerebral veins and sinuses. *NEJM* 2005; 352(17): 1791-1798

55-year-old female with sudden onset of the "worst headache of her life"

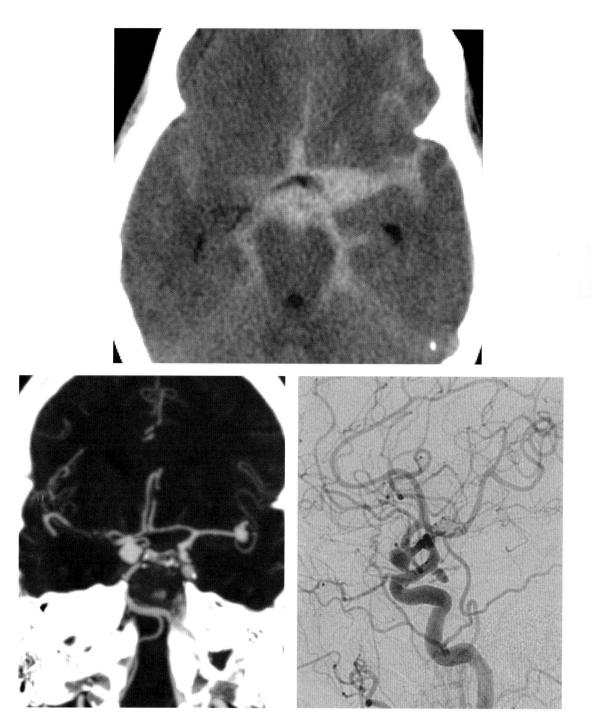

Diagnosis: **Aneurysmal** **subarachnoid** **hemorrhage**	Noncontrast head CT (left image) shows diffuse subarachnoid hemorrhage, more prominent on the left (yellow arrow). Coronal CTA MIP reconstruction (middle image) and lateral view of a cerebral angiogram of left internal carotid artery injection (right image) show multiple aneurysms of both posterior communicating arteries (Pcom; red arrows) and the left MCA bifurcation (blue arrow).

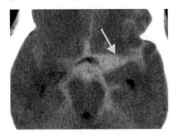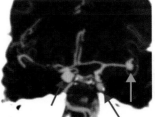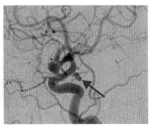

Discussion
- Diffuse subarachnoid hemorrhage (SAH) secondary to aneurysm rupture classically presents as rapid onset of the worst headache of a patient's life. Associated symptoms may include retro-orbital pain, double vision, seizures, cognitive impairment, and vomiting.
- The Hunt and Hess scale is a clinical scoring system that was developed in 1968 to classify the severity of a subarachnoid hemorrhage in order to predict patient prognosis.

Grade	Description	Survival
0	No deficit or discomfort	
I	Headache but no neurological impairment	70%
II	Cognitive impairment or difficulty in arousal	60%
III	Cognitive/arousal deficit and limb deficit (power, tone, and/or sensation)	50%
IV	Unconscious with marked changes in limb tone, power	20%
V	Unresponsive	10%
****	Add one grade if major concurrent heart, lung, liver, renal pathology.	

Risk factors for aneurysm rupture
- The usual cause of aneurysmal subarachnoid hemorrhage is rupture of a "berry" or saccular aneurysm at the circle of Willis or its branches that has

formed as a result of weakness of the vessel wall. Most commonly, aneurysms form at the anterior communicating artery (ACom, ~30%), posterior communicating artery (PCom, ~30%), MCA bifurcation (MCA, ~30%), and posterior circulation (~10%, with the basilar tip constituting ~90% of this group).

- Aneurysms more than 1 cm in diameter are more likely to bleed than those <5 mm. Larger aneurysms are much less common than smaller aneurysms. Although larger aneurysms are more prone to rupture, smaller aneurysms are implicated in the majority of cases of SAH. Intracranial aneurysms are multiple in about one-third of patients.
- Intracranial aneurysms tend to affect patients from 35 to 60 years of age with a female-to-male ratio of 3:2. Other risk factors for aneurysmal SAH include black race, hypertension, autosomal dominant polycystic kidney disease, smoking, heavy alcohol use, first-degree relative with SAH, and disorders of abnormal connective tissue.
- Fusiform aneurysms may arise from atherosclerotic or traumatic etiologies, while smaller, peripherally located mycotic aneurysms are seen in patients with endocarditis or other infectious causes.
- Intracranial aneurysms affect approximately 1–5% of the population. Overall, 0.2–3% of the population suffers from intracranial aneurysm rupture each year. 10 to 15% of patients die before reaching the hospital, and 40–50% of patients die within 30 days.
- The risk of recurrent aneurysmal hemorrhage on the first day is 4%, with an additional 1.2% risk each subsequent day for the first 2 weeks. Subarachnoid hemorrhage places the patient at risk for communicating hydrocephalus by causing blockage of the arachnoid granulations, which perform fluid exchange between the CSF and venous sinuses. Evaluation and monitoring of ventricular size is essential early on.

Vasospasm

- Delayed cerebral ischemia as a result of vasospasm is a common complication of SAH that may double the mortality rate. Vasospasm occurs in approximately 50–70% of patients with SAH and delayed cerebral ischemia occurs in approximately 19–46%. Vasospasm is thought to account for up to 23% of disability and death related to SAH.
- Vasospasm tends to occur between days 5 and 10 after SAH with the onset of new neurological symptoms. Transcranial Doppler and cerebral angiography are sometimes used to complement clinical surveillance for this complication. Calcium channel blockers (nimodipine, verapamil) and "HHT" (hypervolemic hypertensive therapy) are established treatments for vasospasm.

- The **Fisher CT grading scale**, which identified vasospasm as a major cause of morbidity due to delayed ischemia in patients with SAH, was developed in 1980. This scale, among others, is used to estimate the risk for vasospasm based on the amount of subarachnoid hemorrhage.

Grade	Amount of subarachnoid hemorrhage
1	None evident
2	Less than 1 mm thick
3	More than 1 mm thick
4	Any thickness with intraventricular or parenchymal hemorrhage

Treatment of aneurysms

- Treatment of aneurysms includes medical therapy (only if non-ruptured, including hypertension control and smoking cessation), surgery (aneurysm clipping), as well as endovascular options (coil embolization and flow diversion).

Clinical synopsis

This patient presented with Hunt and Hess Grade II and Fisher Grade III. At the time of initial angiography, the left PCom aneurysm was deemed the origin of SAH. This and the unruptured MCA aneurysm were both clipped. The patient's 21-day hospital course was complicated by vasospasm that was successfully treated with verapamil. The non-ruptured right PCom aneurysm was successfully clipped 6 months later.

Self-assessment

- *Describe typical imaging patterns of SAH.*

- SAH may be focal or diffuse, depending on delay between rupture and imaging and the location, size, and shape of the aneurysm. Multilobed or irregular contour of the aneurysm suggests recent hemorrhage. Aneurysms at certain characteristic locations may produce hemorrhage at typical sites:

Site of aneurysm	Typical site of focal hemorrhage
Anterior communicating artery (ACom)	Interhemispheric fissure, callosal sulcus
Middle cerebral artery (MCA)	Sylvian fissure
Posterior communicating artery (PCom)	Suprasellar cistern, medial temporal lobe
Basilar tip	Perimesencephalic cistern

- Name other causes of SAH besides aneurysm rupture.

- Trauma, coagulopathy, cortical vein thrombosis, idiopathic (perimesencephalic subarachnoid hemorrhage: PMSAH).

- Name two important clinical complications that may occur following SAH from aneurysm rupture. What is the time frame in which each may be anticipated?

- Vasospasm: 5–10 days after initial SAH.
- Recurrent hemorrhage: risk is 4% the day of initial SAH, and 1.2% each subsequent day up to day 14.

- Name several risk factors for aneurysmal SAH.

- Female sex, black race, hypertension, smoking, heavy alcohol use, first-degree relative with SAH, and disorders characterized by abnormal connective tissue.

Spectrum of aneurysmal subarachnoid hemorrhage

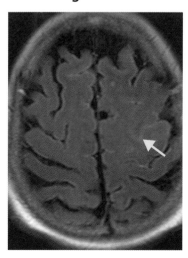

MRI of subarachnoid hemorrhage

Fluid attenuated inversion recovery (FLAIR) and gradient-recalled echo (GRE) MRI sequences can detect trace amounts of SAH. On FLAIR imaging, acute subarachnoid blood appears as increased signal within the involved sulci (arrow). Other etiologies of high signal within the cerebral sulci on FLAIR imaging include meningitis, cortical vein thrombosis, oxygen administration, anesthesia agents, and recent gadolinium administration (especially in patients with renal failure). On GRE imaging, blood products and mineralization appear as dark signal secondary to susceptibility effects.

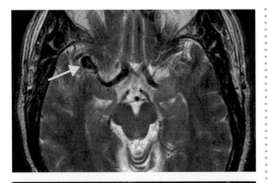

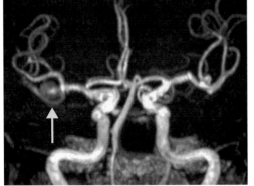

Unruptured intracranial aneurysm

Typically, CT is the initial imaging modality of choice in cases of suspected ruptured intracranial aneurysm. This is often followed by CTA or conventional cerebral angiography. MRI and MRA are more often used for screening of high-risk populations or surveillance of non-ruptured aneurysms, especially those that are less than 1 cm in diameter or located at the skull base. Aneurysms often exhibit pulsation artifact in the phase-encoding direction. Axial T2-weighted image (upper image) and MRA (lower image) show an unruptured right MCA aneurysm (arrows) in a patient with a family history of polycystic kidney disease.

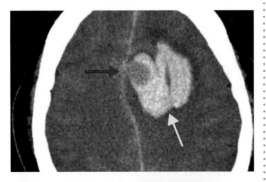

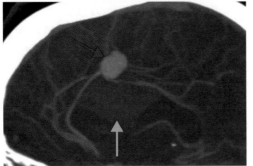

Anterior cerebral artery aneurysm rupture

Axial noncontrast CT (upper image) demonstrates a large left-sided parafalcine parenchymal hemorrhage (yellow arrow). The relatively hypodense ruptured aneurysm (red arrow) is outlined by high-attenuation parenchymal blood on the noncontrast CT. Sagittal reconstructed MIP CTA shows SAH along the callosal sulcus (blue arrow) due to a ruptured distal A2 aneurysm (red arrow).

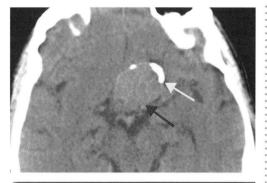

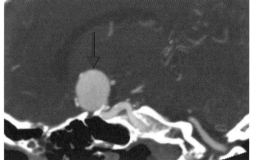

Giant aneurysm

Giant aneurysms are larger than 2 cm in diameter and are often partially thrombosed at presentation. 25% of patients with giant aneurysms will present with SAH, with the remaining 75% having symptoms related to mass effect. These aneurysms are difficult to treat by either surgical or endovascular intervention because perforating vessels often arise from their walls. Peripheral linear calcifications (yellow arrow) are seen along the anterolateral wall of this giant aneurysm (red arrows) on axial noncontrast CT (upper image) and sagittal reconstructed CTA (lower image). The aneurysm extends into the suprasellar cistern.

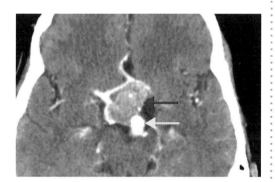

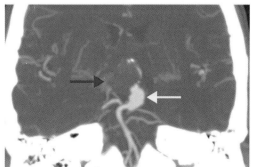

Basilar tip aneurysm

Axial CTA (upper image) and coronal reconstructed CTA (lower image) demonstrate a giant, partially thrombosed, lobulated basilar tip aneurysm extending into the suprasellar cistern. The aneurysm fills with contrast laterally (yellow arrows) with a large thrombus (red arrows) medially.

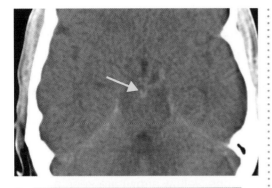

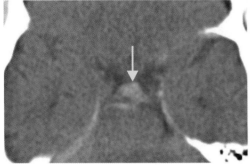

Perimesencephalic subarachnoid hemorrhage

No definitive source of bleeding can be identified in approximately 15% of SAH patients. In nontraumatic non-aneurysmal perimesencephalic subarachnoid hemorrhage (PMSAH), bleeding is typically confined to the interpeduncular, perimesencephalic, and prepontine cisterns, as demonstrated in this case by two axial noncontrast CT images. The yellow arrows localize blood in the interpeduncular (upper image) and prepontine (lower image) cisterns. In the US, incidence of PMSAH is about 0.5 cases per 100,000 persons age >18. Patients with PMSAH tend to be younger and present with very mild symptoms regardless of the amount of hemorrhage. Clinical outcome is also generally much better than for SAH from other causes. CT or conventional angiography should always be performed to exclude aneurysmal hemorrhage.

Differential diagnosis of aneurysmal subarachnoid hemorrhage

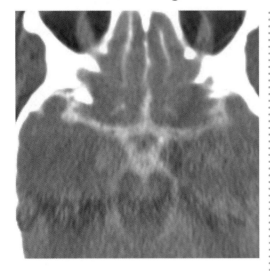

Intrathecal contrast administration

For cerebral cisternogram, typically used for evaluation of occult or overt CSF leak, contrast is administered intrathecally following a lumbar puncture. One should be aware that iodinated contrast within the subarachnoid space may mimic SAH, though the density will usually be slightly higher than hemorrhage as on this non-contrast axial CT image. On MRI, patients with renal failure may retain gadolinium contrast agents within the CSF spaces due to impaired or delayed renal clearance, resulting in high sulcal FLAIR signal that may mimic SAH. In both of these scenarios, correlation with patient history is critical.

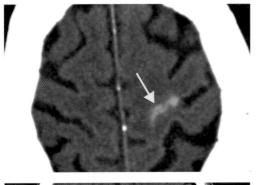

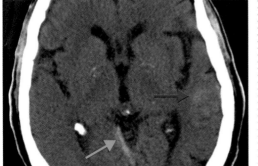

Traumatic subarachnoid hemorrhage

Noncontrast CT images in a case of traumatic SAH show hyperdense material in a sulcus along the left frontal high convexity (yellow arrow). Additional findings that suggest a traumatic etiology include inferior left temporal hemorrhagic contusion (red arrow) and subdural hematoma layering along the right tentorium (blue arrow).

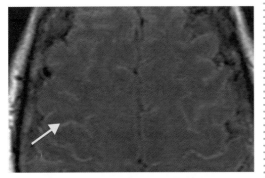

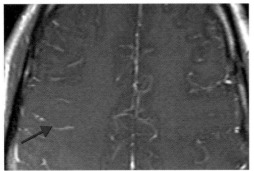

Meningitis

While MRI and CT (not pictured) appearance of meningitis may mimic SAH, these processes can usually be distinguished on clinical grounds. Both meningitis and SAH may present with hyperdense material throughout the subarachnoid spaces on CT and signal hyperintensity on FLAIR MRI (yellow arrow). In meningitis, linear leptomeningeal enhancement is typical (red arrow). Unless it is hemorrhagic, meningitis will not produce susceptibility artifact on GRE pulse sequences.

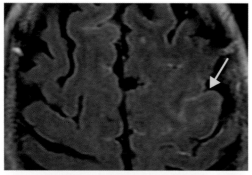

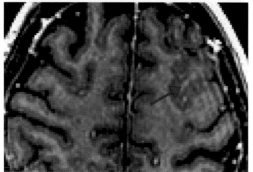

Carcinomatosis

Leptomeningeal carcinomatosis represents spread of malignant cells to the subarachnoid space, and can present with focal or diffuse abnormal signal on MR imaging. Contrast-enhanced T1-weighted images are reported to have greater sensitivity than FLAIR. Axial FLAIR MR (upper image) demonstrates focal abnormal signal within the subarachnoid space of the left frontal lobe (yellow arrow). Axial contrast-enhanced T1-weighted 3D MPRAGE image (lower image) shows nodular enhancement in the subarachnoid space (red arrow).

Further reading

Fisher C, Kistler J, Davis J. Relation of cerebral vasospasm to subarachnoid hemorrhage visualized by computerized tomographic scanning. *Neurosurgery* 1980; 6(1): 1–9

Flaherty ML *et al.* Perimesencephalic subarachnoid hemorrhage: incidence, risk factors and outcome. *J Stroke Cerebrovasc Dis* 2005; 14(6): 267–271

Hunt WE, Hess RM. Surgical risk as related to time of intervention in the repair of intracranial aneurysms. *Journal of Neurosurgery* 1968; 28(1): 14–20

Keyrouz SG, Diringer MN. Clinical review: prevention and therapy of vasospasm in subarachnoid hemorrhage. *Critical Care* 2007; 11(4): 220

Le Roux P, Winn R, Newell D. *Management of cerebral aneurysms*. Philadelphia, PA: Saunders 1st edn. 2003

Molyneux A, *et al.* International subarachnoid aneurysm trial (ISAT) of neurosurgical clipping vs endovascular clipping of 2143 patients with ruptured intracranial aneurysms: a randomized trial. *Lancet* 2002; 360: 1267–1274

Molyneux A, *et al.* ISAT trial: coiling or clipping of intracranial aneurysm. *Lancet* 2005; 366: 783–785

Osborn AG. *Diagnostic cerebral angiography*. Philadelphia, PA: Lippincott Williams and Wilkins, 2nd edn. 1998

van Gijn J, Kerr RS, Rinkel GJ. Subarachnoid haemorrhage. *Lancet* 2007; 369(9558): 306–318

Case 51   90-year-old male with elevated blood pressure and change
in mental status. No history of trauma

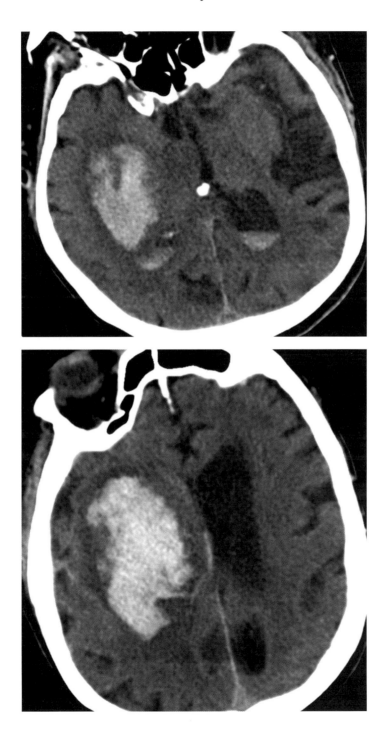

Diagnosis:
Nontraumatic intraparen-chymal hematoma (due to hypertension)

Axial unenhanced head CT shows a large right basal ganglia hematoma (yellow arrows), with layering blood in the lateral ventricles (red arrows). There is moderate mass effect from the hematoma.

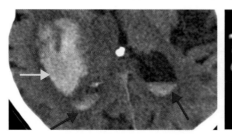 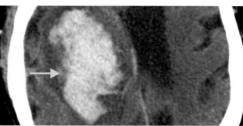

Discussion

Overview of nontraumatic intraparenchymal hemorrhage (IPH)

- Nontraumatic intraparenchymal hemorrhage (IPH) is the cause of 10% of first strokes and is a major cause of death and permanent disability. Clinically, IPH may manifest as a new neurologic deficit (mimicking ischemic stroke), seizure, headache, or altered consciousness.
- Nontraumatic IPH is most commonly due to longstanding hypertension in elderly individuals. Chronic smooth muscle hyperplasia leads to replacement of smooth muscle with collagen, which predisposes to vascular ectasia and hemorrhage. The risk of hemorrhage, even without underlying hypertension, is increased in patients receiving anticoagulation therapy.
- Less common causes of IPH include amyloid angiopathy, arteriovenous malformation (AVM), intracranial aneurysm, venous sinus thrombosis, cavernoma, hemorrhagic neoplasm, dural arterial–venous fistula (dAVF), hemorrhagic conversion of infarct, vasculitis, and cocaine use.

Imaging of nontraumatic intraparenchymal hemorrhage

- Noncontrast CT is typically the first study performed in the emergent setting in a patient with a suspected intracranial hemorrhage.
- Patterns of hemorrhage on initial noncontrast head CT, combined with clinical attributes such as age, presence of pre-existing hypertension, and treatment with anticoagulant medications, may suggest a specific etiology, but often, more advanced imaging (MR or CT angiography) is necessary to arrive at a specific diagnosis.
- CTA is generally considered to be equivalent to invasive angiography for evaluation of vascular causes of intraparenchymal hemorrhage, such as AVM, dAVF, ruptured aneurysm, and venous thrombosis.

- MR is better for evaluation of cavernoma, amyloid angiopathy, hypertensive encephalopathy, diffuse axonal injury, and hemorrhagic conversion of infarct all of which may present with multiple foci of susceptibility on gradient-recalled echo (GRE) MRI.
- The MR imaging appearance of hemorrhage is dependent on the signal characteristics of blood degradation products, which progress in a predictable manner, allowing "dating". This progression depends on intra-axial location and macrophage breakdown of blood products, which follows a predictable time-course. Extra-axial hemorrhage such as subdural hematoma cannot be dated in the same way.

Clinical synopsis

This 90-year-old male with a large basal ganglia hematoma due to hypertension was emergently intubated for hypoxic respiratory failure. He was unable to open his eyes, but was able to move his right thumb. Due to his poor prognosis, he was treated conservatively and died the following day.

Evolution of IPH

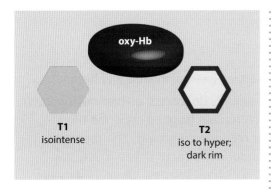

Hyperacute hematoma (oxyhemoglobin; 0–6 hours)

Up to a few hours after the ictus, the blood located centrally within a hyperacute hematoma contains intracellular oxyhemoglobin, which is isointense to brain on T1-weighted imaging and isointense to slightly hyperintense on T2-weighted imaging. T2-weighting characteristically features a hypointense peripheral rim, which is thought to be caused by peripheral deoxygenation.

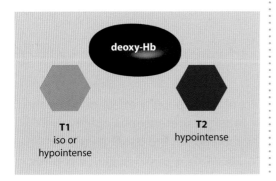

Acute hematoma (deoxyhemoglobin; 6–72 hours)

As the blood within the entire hematoma begins to deoxygenate, the appearance on T2-weighted imaging becomes uniformly hypointense due to predomination of deoxyhemoglobin. The appearance on T1-weighted imaging is iso- or hypointense to brain.

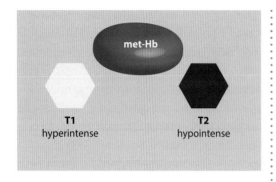

Early subacute hematoma (intracellular methemoglobin; 3 days – 1 week)

At this stage of hematoma evolution, the intracellular hemoglobin has been converted to methemoglobin, which causes dramatically shortened T1 times leading to a hyperintense appearance on T1-weighted imaging. The appearance on T2-weighted imaging remains hypointense, as intracellular methemoglobin has a strong paramagnetic effect.

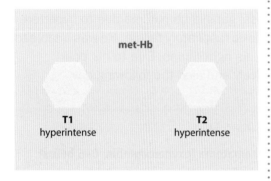

Late subacute hematoma (1 week – several months)

After the red cells lyse, methemoglobin becomes primarily extracellular, and remains hyperintense on T1-weighted imaging. On T2-weighted images, however, the extracellular methemoglobin is also hyperintense, thought to be due to decreased protein concentration.

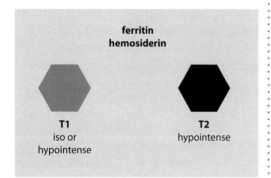

Chronic hematoma (several months and beyond)

Iron is permanently deposited as hemosiderin and ferritin, which remain trapped once the blood–brain barrier has been restored. The resultant strong susceptibility effects cause a very low signal on T2-weighted images. Chronic hematoma is isointense to slightly hypointense to brain on T1-weighted images. Chronic hematoma may also demonstrate peripheral enhancement.

Self-assessment

- *What is the differential diagnosis of multiple dark spots on gradient-echo MR?*

- Multiple foci of susceptibility effect on MR can be seen in hypertensive encephalopathy (with multiple microbleeds in the basal ganglia or cerebellum), cerebral amyloid angiopathy (with multiple cortical microbleeds), familial cavernomatosis, or diffuse axonal injury.

- *What is the most likely etiology of an intraparenchymal hemorrhage if post-contrast images demonstrate multiple enhancing lesions?*

- *What is the CTA "spot" sign?*

- The multiple enhancing lesions suggest metastatic disease, and hemorrhagic neoplasia would be a probable etiology for the intraparenchymal hemorrhage.

- The CTA "spot" sign describes a focus of enhancement within the periphery of a hematoma on angiographic-phase images of a CT angiogram. The "spot" sign is thought to be predictive of impending hematoma expansion and is a poor prognostic indicator.

Etiology of nontraumatic IPH

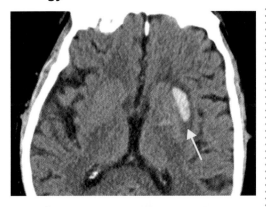

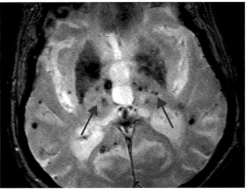

Hypertensive hemorrhage

Hypertensive hemorrhage is the most common cause of spontaneous intraparenchymal hemorrhage in older adults, as demonstrated in the index case. Hypertensive hemorrhage characteristically occurs in the basal ganglia, most commonly the putamen and external capsule, followed by the thalamus, pons, and cerebellum. A lobar distribution is less common. Hypertensive hemorrhages originating in the basal ganglia and brainstem have a propensity to extend into the nearby ventricular system, but subarachnoid extension is uncommon. MR imaging typically shows multiple foci of susceptibility (dark spots) in the basal ganglia on GRE, representing chronic microhemorrhages. Axial unenhanced CT (upper image) demonstrates a left putaminal hemorrhage (yellow arrow). GRE MR in a different patient (lower image) demonstrates multiple foci of susceptibility artifact scattered throughout the basal ganglia (red arrows) and subcortical regions.

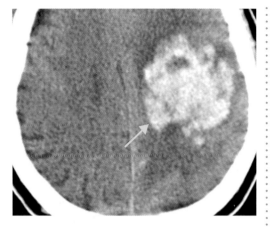

Cerebral amyloid angiopathy

Amyloid angiopathy is the result of vascular damage from amyloid deposition, and is the second most common cause of intraparenchymal hemorrhage in older adults. The hemorrhage tends to be lobar in location, as opposed to in the basal ganglia. GRE may also show numerous foci of susceptibility effect; however, these foci of micro-hemorrhage will typically also be within the cerebral hemispheres as opposed to the basal ganglia. Axial unenhanced CT demonstrates a large left frontoparietal lobar hemorrhage (arrow).

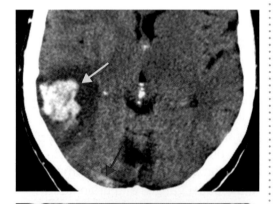

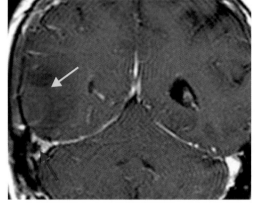

Venous thrombosis

Thrombosis of the deep venous sinuses is one of the most common causes of stroke in younger patients, especially females, since pregnancy and oral contraceptives are important risk factors. Parenchymal hemorrhage results from venous hypertension. There are three characteristic locations of the resultant hematoma: parasagittal high convexity due to superior sagittal sinus thrombosis, bilateral thalamic hematoma due to deep venous system thrombosis, and posterior temporal lobe hematoma due to transverse sinus thrombosis (as shown in this case). Two imaging signs of venous thrombosis are the "cord" sign, due to increased attenuation of the thrombosed sinus, and the "empty delta" sign, due to filling defect in the sinus seen on contrast-enhanced CT or MR. Axial unenhanced CT (upper image) demonstrates a right posterior temporal lobe hematoma (yellow arrow). There is high attenuation in the right transverse sinus (red arrow). Coronal T1-weighted post-contrast MR (lower image) demonstrates a filling defect in the right transverse sinus (red arrow). The hematoma (yellow arrow) is isointense to brain.

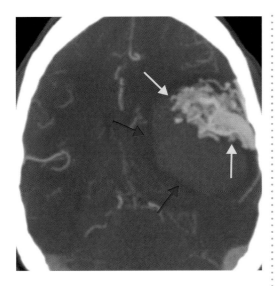

High-flow vascular malformation

Both AVM and dAVF are high-flow vascular malformations that may cause intraparenchymal hemorrhage. Although they may occur in any age group, younger people tend to be affected more commonly. An AVM is a developmental lesion characterized by abnormal connection between parenchymal arteries and veins, without intervening normal brain. dAVF is a diverse spectrum of disorders characterized by abnormal connection between a meningeal artery and a dural venous sinus or cortical vein. Coronal-oblique MIP from a CT angiogram demonstrates a large AVM (yellow arrows) with adjacent hematoma (red arrows).

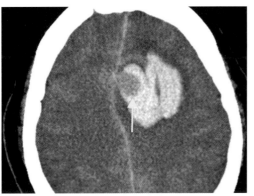

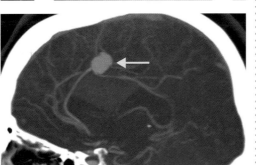

Aneurysmal hemorrhage

Although aneurysmal hemorrhage more commonly causes SAH, aneurysm rupture may also be associated with intraparenchymal hematoma. SAH is almost always present as well, and CTA (not MR) is the study of choice for the work-up of nontraumatic SAH. Aneurysmal hemorrhage can be seen at any age. Axial unenhanced CT demonstrates a left frontal hematoma with an adjacent rounded, relatively hypoattenuating structure (arrow), which was shown on sagittal MIP from a CT angiogram to represent a ruptured ACom aneurysm (arrow).

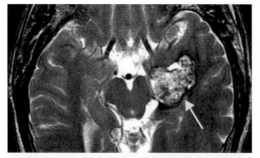

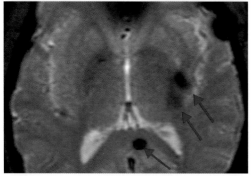

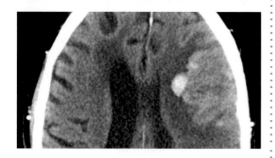

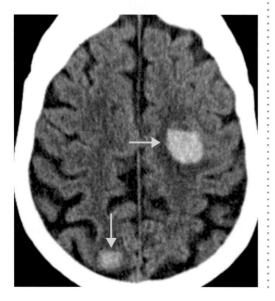

Cavernoma

A cavernoma is a low-flow vascular hamartoma that has a much lower risk of bleeding compared to high-flow vascular malformations. Cavernomas are often associated with developmental venous anomalies (DVA), which are abnormal veins draining normal brain. Although the appearance of a hemorrhage secondary to cavernoma is nonspecific, the presence of a nearby DVA may suggest the diagnosis. A familial form of multiple cavernomas is best seen on gradient-echo sequences as multiple dark spots due to micro-hemorrhages. Axial T2-weighted MR (upper image) demonstrates a left temporal lobe cavernoma (yellow arrow) with a typical lobulated shape and peripheral low signal intensity. Axial GRE in a different patient with multiple cavernomas (lower image) shows foci of susceptibility (red arrows) medial to the sylvian fissure and adjacent to the splenium of the corpus callosum.

Hemorrhagic transformation of embolic infarct

Symptomatic hemorrhage occurs in approximately 6–12% of patients receiving thrombolytic therapy for an ischemic infarct. Axial unenhanced CT in a patient who recently received intravenous thrombolytic therapy for treatment of an acute left MCA infarct demonstrates a left frontal hematoma in the MCA territory.

Hemorrhagic neoplasia

The most common primary brain tumor to cause hemorrhage is glioblastoma. Hemorrhagic metastatic tumors include lung and breast carcinoma, melanoma, renal cell carcinoma, thyroid carcinoma, and choriocarcinoma. Findings supporting neoplasia as the etiology of hemorrhage include vasogenic edema greater than expected relative to the size of the lesion, heterogeneous signal representing varying phases of breakdown of blood products, presence of multiple lesions, and regions of enhancement in a non-chronic hematoma. Axial unenhanced CT in a patient with melanoma demonstrates multifocal hemorrhages in the left frontal and right parietal lobes (arrows).

Further reading

Cordonnier, C., Klijn, C. J. M., van Beijnum, J., & Al-Shahi Salman, R. (2010). Radiological investigation of spontaneous intracerebral hemorrhage: systematic review and trinational survey. *Stroke: a journal of cerebral circulation*, 41(4), 685–690.

Delgado Almandoz, J. E., Schaefer, P. W., Forero, N. P., Falla, J. R., Gonzalez, R. G., & Romero, J. M. (2009). Diagnostic accuracy and yield of multidetector CT angiography in the evaluation of spontaneous intraparenchymal cerebral hemorrhage. *AJNR: American journal of neuroradiology*, 30(6), 1213–1221.

Fischbein, N. J., & Wijman, C. A. C. (2010). Nontraumatic intracranial hemorrhage. *Neuroimaging clinics of North America*, 20(4), 469–492.

Yousem, D. Y. (2011). Imaging of hemorrhage. *Neuroradiology – The Requisites*, ed. D. Y. Youssem, R. D. Zimmerman, R. I. Grossman. Maryland Heights, MO: Mosby. 3rd edn. (pp. 1–11).

Case 52   40-year-old man with a history of illicit drug use was found seizing and unconscious

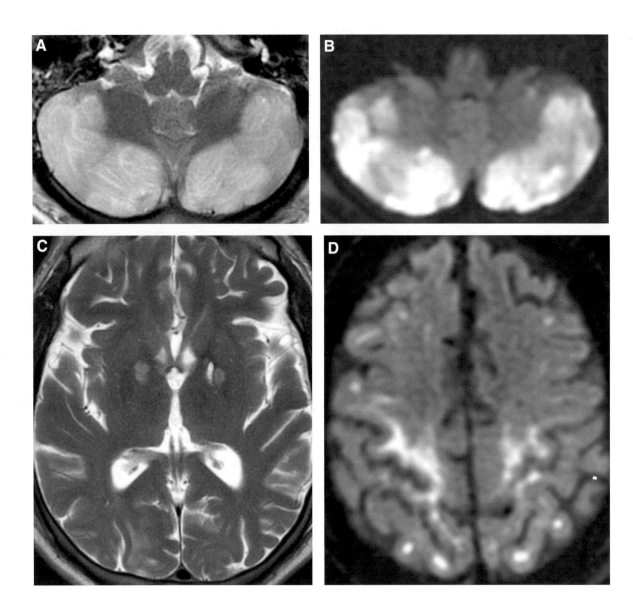

Diagnosis: **Cocaine-induced vasoconstriction syndrome**

Axial T2 (A) and DWI (B) MR images demonstrate T2 prolongation and reduced diffusion, consistent with acute bilateral cerebellar gray matter infarcts (yellow arrows). Axial T2-weighted image at the level of basal ganglia (C) reveals T2 prolongation in the globus pallidi bilaterally (red arrows). DWI at that level (not shown) did not demonstrate reduced diffusion, indicating chronic infarction. Axial DWI at the level of the cerebral convexities (D) shows reduced diffusion consistent with acute bilateral cortical and subcortical infarction (blue arrows). The presence of multiple acute supratentorial and infratentorial infarcts is highly suggestive of vasoconstriction syndrome, of which cocaine is a known cause.

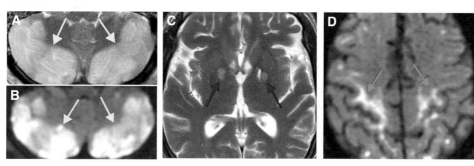

Discussion

Overview of street drug-induced neurological injury

- Cocaine use can result in significant neurological injury due to neurovascular complications, such as hemorrhage, stroke, and arteriopathy.
- Hemorrhage often results from transient blood pressure elevation due to the sympathomimetic action of the drug, and can occur in the brain parenchyma or subarachnoid space. Subarachnoid hemorrhage may be due to rupture of a pre-existing aneurysm or vascular malformation, or may result from extension of a parenchymal hemorrhagic infarct.
- Ischemic stroke may result from vasoconstriction or "moyamoya-like" arteriopathy. Cocaine may further predispose to ischemic stroke by causing hypercoagulability.
- Heroin inhalation injury, known as "chasing the dragon," produces cerebellar white matter injury without cortical infarction.

Imaging of reversible cerebral vasoconstriction syndrome

- Reversible cerebral vasoconstriction syndrome (RCVS) is characterized by hyperacute severe headache and multifocal vasospasm. The condition usually resolves by 3 months, but in severe cases may lead to permanent sequelae due to multiple infarcts. Together, vasoactive drugs and postpartum state account for more than half of cases. The distribution of abnormalities in RCVS is similar to that seen in posterior reversible encephalopathy syndrome (PRES), a syndrome thought to be due to loss of autoregulation of posterior circulation blood pressure. PRES is seen in diverse clinical scenarios, but most commonly in hypertension. On MRI, PRES typically features relatively symmetric hyperintensities on T2-weighted images, involving the cerebral convexities, cerebellum, and other territories. Acute infarcts, while still rare, are more common in RCVS.

- In RCVS, MRA and CTA show multiple vascular narrowings, more severe than in PRES.

Treatment of RCVS

- Anti-hypertensive agents, the mainstay of treatment in PRES, can worsen outcome in RCVS. RCVS is often treated with calcium channel blockers and steroids.

Clinical synopsis	This 40-year-old man with presumed cocaine-related fulminant vasoconstriction syndrome also presented with hepatic and renal failure, and extensive myocardial infarction. He died 5 days after admission.

Self-assessment

- *Name three types of cerebrovascular injury that can occur from cocaine use.*

  - Hypertensive hemorrhage, lacunar infarction, moyamoya-like arteriopathy, multifocal infarction due to vasoconstriction.

- *Compare and contrast the imaging appearances of PRES and RCVS, highlighting distinctions. What is the major treatment consideration for each?*

  - PRES and RCVS may both produce multiple areas of symmetric cortical and subcortical edema involving the cerebral convexities, cerebellum, and other territories, manifested as T2 prolongation on MRI. RCVS is distinguished from PRES by thunderclap headache accompanied by multiple areas of vasoconstriction on MRA or CTA. PRES is often treated with anti-hypertensive therapy, which may worsen RCVS. Treatment regimens for RCVS include calcium channel blockers and steroids.

- *True or false: heroin inhalation injury (from "chasing the dragon") causes cortical cerebellar infarction?*

  - False: Heroin inhalation causes cerebellar white matter injury.

Spectrum of cocaine abuse

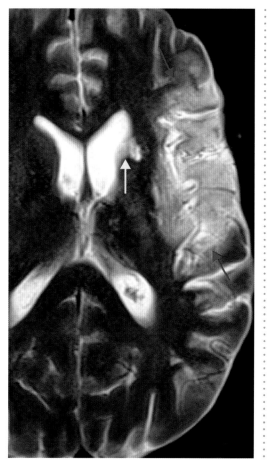

Acute and chronic infarction due to vasospasm

This 29-year-old man with a history of chronic cocaine abuse presented with acute aphasia. Axial T2-weighted image (left image) and DWI (middle image) show T2 prolongation and reduced diffusion in the left insula and anterior putamen and caudate head, consistent with acute infarction (yellow arrows). More laterally, T2 prolongation and subtle volume loss in the left temporal lobe (red arrows) without corresponding diffusion abnormality indicates prior infarction. Time-of-flight 3D MR angiogram of the circle of Willis (right image) shows multiple severe stenoses (blue arrows) throughout the middle cerebral and proximal anterior cerebral arteries.

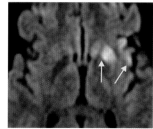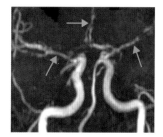

Chronic infarction

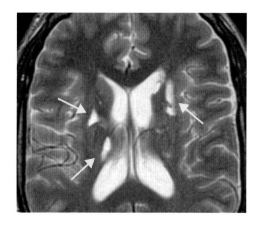

T2-weighted MR image in a 27-year-old male who was a habitual cocaine user shows multiple foci of T2 prolongation and volume loss in the basal ganglia (arrows), consistent with prior infarction.

Differential diagnosis of cocaine abuse

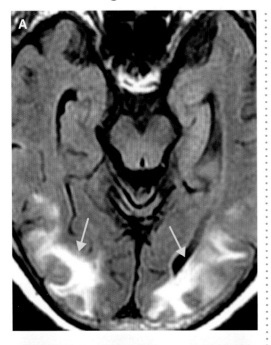

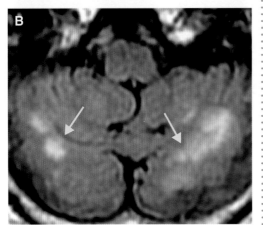

Posterior reversible encephalopathy syndrome

This 73-year-old hypertensive man presented with headache, visual loss, and change in mental status. Axial FLAIR MR images (A and B) show hyperintensity in the occipital and cerebellar sub-cortical white matter (yellow arrows). DWI (C) shows no evidence of acute infarction. Time-of-flight 3D MRA of the circle of Willis (D) shows no areas of vascular narrowing. Symptoms and findings resolved following treatment of hypertension, indicating PRES. PRES is distinguished from cocaine-related vasoconstriction by lack of history of cocaine use, the presence of hypertension, eclampsia, status epilepticus, or other risk factors, lack of infarction, and normal cerebrovascular imaging. Abnormalities in PRES are seen at typical watershed zones. "Companion lesions" may be seen in the deep white matter, basal ganglia, and brainstem.

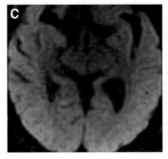

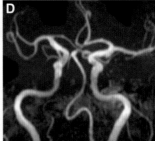

Further reading

Bartynski WS. Posterior Reversible Encephalopathy Syndrome, part 1: fundamental imaging and clinical features. *AJNR* 2008; 29: 1036–1042.

Geibpraset S, Gallucci M, Krings T. Addictive illegal drugs: structural neuroimaging. *AJNR* 2001; 31: 803–808.

Hagan IG, Burney K. Radiology of recreational drug abuse. *Radiographics* 2007; 27: 919–940.

Maloof NM, Harik SI. Clinical reasoning: a 33-year-old woman with severe post-partum occipital headache. *Neurology* 2012; 78: 366–369.

Miller TR, Shivashankar R, Mosse-Basha M, Gandhi D. Reversible cerebral vasoconstriction syndrome, part 1: Epidemiology, pathogenesis, and clinical course. *AJNR* 2015; 36: 1392–1399.

SECTION 5   MUSCULOSKELETAL

Case 53   42-year-old female presenting with fever and back pain

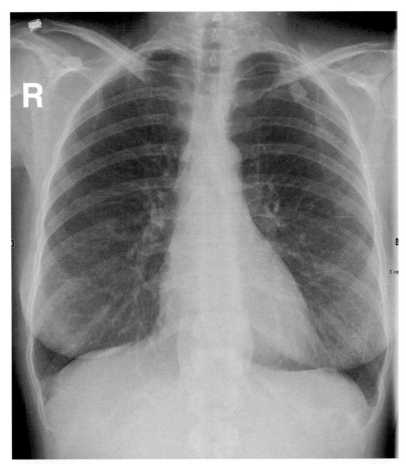

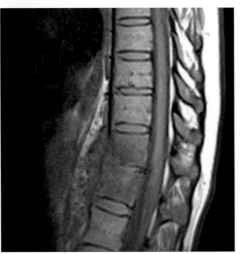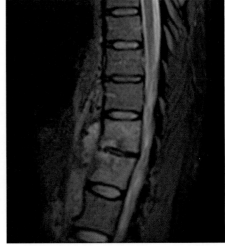

Diagnosis:
Spondylodiscitis
and paraspinal
abscess

PA chest radiograph (left image) demonstrates lateral displacement of the right and left paraspinal lines (yellow arrows). Sagittal T1-weighted (middle image) and STIR (right image) MR images show low T1 and high T2 signal intensity of two consecutive vertebral bodies (red arrows), with loss of definition of the vertebral endplates. In addition, there is a prevertebral fluid collection (blue arrows) consistent with an abscess.

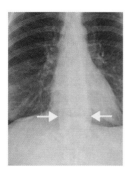 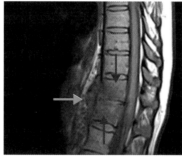 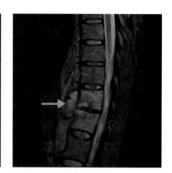

Discussion

Overview of spondylodiscitis

- Spondylodiscitis is septic inflammation of the spine involving the intervertebral disc and adjacent vertebral bodies, often with extension into the paravertebral soft tissues. The lumbar spine is the most common site.
- Spondylodiscitis has a bimodal age distribution, being more common in young (<20 years of age) and older (50–70 years of age) patients. Risk factors include diabetes, malignancy, compromised immunity, and intravenous drug use.
- The spinal column may become involved by infection via several routes of spread. Vascular spread of infection is thought to be due to Batson's paraspinal venous plexus. Contiguous spread of an adjacent infection can be seen in the setting of an infected aortic graft, mediastinal abscess, or retropharyngeal abscess. Direct contamination can be due to penetrating trauma or surgery.
- Clinical symptoms are nonspecific, which can delay the diagnosis. Back pain in the setting of fever is considered a "red flag" that should prompt imaging, especially in the presence of leukocytosis or elevated inflammatory markers (elevated C-reactive protein or erythrocyte sedimentation rate).
- Treatment is usually with antibiotics; however, if there is evidence of neurological compromise due to mass effect or large abscess, then surgery may be necessary.

Imaging of spondylodiscitis

- Chest radiograph has low sensitivity and specificity, but may show thickening of the paravertebral soft tissues, as in the index case. Later findings include decreased intervertebral disc space and endplate irregularity, although degenerative disc disease may appear identical.
- MRI is the preferred imaging modality when spondylodiscitis is suspected, due to its ability to identify paravertebral and epidural involvement, as well as involvement of the spinal cord itself. Findings consist of loss of definition of the affected vertebral endplates, with low signal intensity on T1-weighted images, and corresponding high signal intensity on T2/STIR images. Fluid-like signal may also be seen in the disc space and can help to differentiate infectious discitis from degenerative disc changes. In degenerative disease, the disc is typically dehydrated, demonstrating low T2 signal intensity (although this is variable). Post-contrast images may demonstrate a phlegmon or an abscess in the paravertebral soft tissues, the former demonstrating heterogeneous enhancement, and the latter, peripheral enhancement. In treated cases, follow-up MRI may show resolution of edema with fatty or sclerotic charges.
- Computed tomography can also be performed in the acute setting due to its ready availability. CT may demonstrate decreased intervertebral disc space and vertebral endplate irregularity and destruction, and can assess paravertebral soft tissue involvement, such as presence of phlegmon or abscess. CT is also a useful modality for pretreatment planning, such as percutaneous drainage of abscess or biopsy of the intervertebral disc. While degenerative disc disease may appear similar to spondylodiscitis on CT, it is important to note that the presence of gas in the intervertebral disc is considered pathognomonic for degenerative disc disease.

Clinical synopsis	The patient had a history of IV drug use. She was admitted, and after becoming afebrile, she was discharged with 6 weeks of IV antibiotic therapy (nafcillin). Post-treatment imaging of the spine demonstrated resolution of the paravertebral abscess.

Self-assessment

- *What is the most common pathogen that causes spondylodiscitis?*

  - Staphylococcus aureus.

- *Cite four risk factors for spondylodiscitis.*

  - Diabetes, IV drug use, spinal instrumentation, trauma.

- *What are the most common imaging findings of spondylodiscitis on MRI?*

- Loss of endplate definition with low T1 and high T2 signal intensity in the subchondral bone marrow, associated with high signal of the intervertebral disc on T2-weighted images.

Spectrum of spondylodiscitis

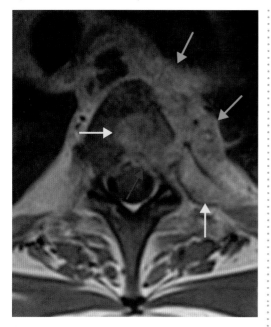

Bacterial spondylodiscitis complicated by epidural phlegmon

Infection of the spine may involve the adjacent soft tissues, including the paraspinal region (as in the index case) or the epidural space. Epidural spread may be a cause of spinal cord compression. Axial T1-weighted post-contrast MR of the thoracic spine demonstrates enhancement of the posterior aspect of the vertebral body and medial left rib (yellow arrows). There is posterior cortical break-through into the anterior spinal canal with lobulated, heterogeneously enhancing phlegmon extending to the epidural space (red arrow). An extensive left-sided prevertebral abscess (blue arrows) causes esophageal displacement to the right.

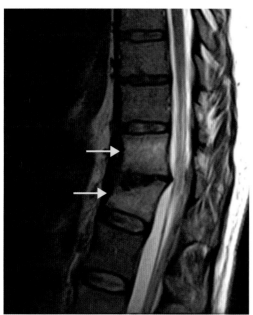

Pott's disease

Spondylodiscitis caused by *Mycobacterium tuberculosis,* known as Pott's disease, most often involves the thoracolumbar transition. It is most commonly seen in immunosuppressed (and HIV positive) patients. It usually starts in the anterior aspect of the vertebral body, leading to destruction, compression deformity, and focal kyphosis. Paraspinal abscess is frequently present and often demonstrates foci of calcification. Multilevel disease is common due to subligamentous spread; however, the intervertebral discs are characteristically spared. Sagittal T2-weighted MR demonstrates increased signal intensity of two adjacent vertebral bodies (arrows), with anterior wedging and focal kyphosis. There is endplate irregularity with loss of the T2 dark cortical line; however, the intervertebral disc is not increased in signal intensity.

Differential diagnosis of spondylodiscitis

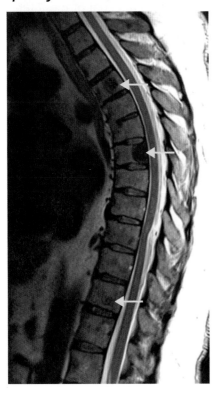

Metastatic disease

The vertebral column is a common site of bone metastasis. Metastatic disease to the spine rarely involves the disc space. Skip lesions are more common with metastatic disease, and rare with infection. The most common primary tumors causing vertebral metastases are breast, lung, and prostate. Sagittal T2-weighted MR image of the thoracic spine in a patient with prostate cancer shows multiple T2 hypointense lesions (arrows) in several vertebral bodies with intervening unaffected vertebral bodies. The intervertebral discs are preserved.

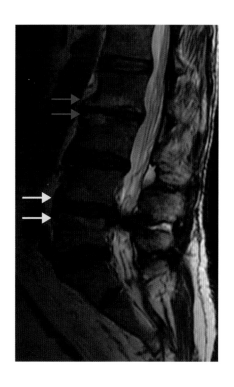

Modic endplate changes

Modic type 1 endplate changes (bone marrow edema pattern) may mimic infection. Further complicating differentiation, there may be increased T2 signal in a degenerated intervertebral disc. In contrast to infection, degenerative changes feature normal paraspinal tissues and inflammatory markers are normal. If radiographs or CT are available, the presence of vacuum phenomenon (air in an intervertebral disc) is considered pathognomonic of degenerative disc disease. Sagittal T2-weighted (upper left image), T1-weighted (lower left image), and STIR (right image) MR images demonstrate Modic type 1 changes at L4–L5 (yellow arrows), which are hyperintense on T2-weighted and STIR images and hypointense on T1-weighted images (following edema/fluid signal intensity). Note that Modic type 2 changes are present at L2–L3 (red arrows), which are hyperintense on both T1- and T2-weighted images, but hypointense on STIR (following fat signal intensity).

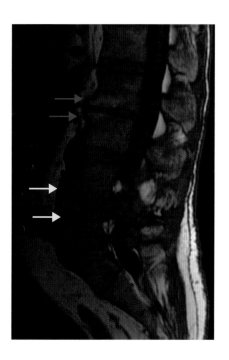

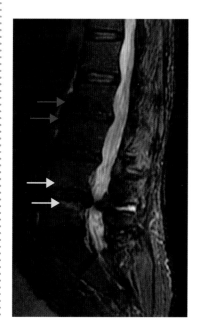

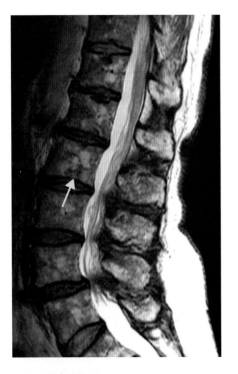

Acute Schmorl's node

A Schmorl's node is herniation of an intervertebral disc into a vertebral body endplate. An acute Schmorl's node may mimic infectious spondylo-discitis due to accompanying bone marrow edema at the vertebral endplate; however, the more focal nature of the process helps to make the distinction. Sagittal T2-weighted (upper left image), T1-weighted (lower left image), and STIR (right image) MR images demonstrate focal herniation of the L2–L3 intervertebral disc into the inferior end-plate of L2. The herniated disc is intermediate on T2, low signal intensity on T1, and slightly hyper-intense on STIR (arrows).

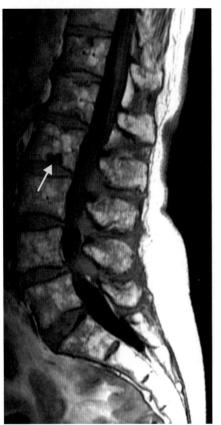

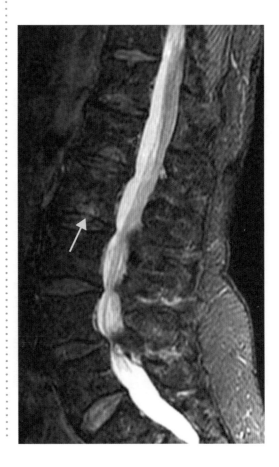

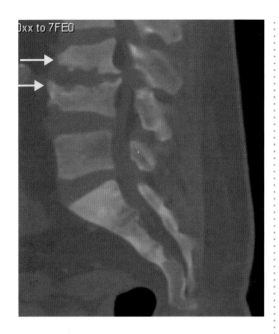

Oxx to 7FE0

Hemodialysis-induced destructive spondyloarthropathy

This condition is secondary to soft tissue and joint deposition of β2-microglobulin in patients who undergo dialysis for multiple years (mean of 8 years). The characteristic imaging features are discovertebral junction erosions with sclerosis, vertebral body compression, disc space narrowing, Schmorl's node formation, facet involvement with subluxation, and lack of osteophytes. The cervical and lumbar spines are most frequently affected, with multiple levels of involvement in more than 50% of patients. Although the radiological features may simulate an infectious process, clinical presentation and laboratory findings are inconsistent, and the multiple levels of involvement, lack of paravertebral soft tissue mass, and relatively mild bone marrow edema on T2-weighted images are atypical for osteomyelitis and discitis. Sagittal CT in a patient on chronic dialysis demonstrates narrowing of the L3–L4 disc space (arrows), associated with marked endplate irregularity and lack of paravertebral soft tissue stranding or mass. Patchy sclerosis of the sacrum is consistent with renal osteodystrophy.

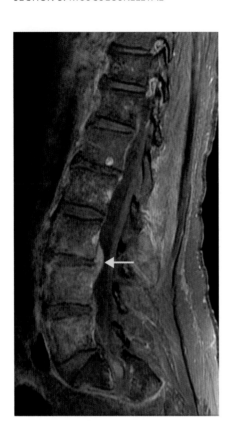

Enhancing extruded disc

Extrusion is a type of disc herniation where the neck of the herniation is smaller than the extruded fragment. A sequestered fragment is a type of extrusion where no continuity exists between the herniated disc material and the parent disc. Sagittal T1-weighted post-contrast MR image with fat suppression demonstrates an enhancing extruded disc (arrow) at the L3–L4 level, which could be mistaken for an epidural abscess. Note, however, the preserved hypointense endplate cortical lines, which would be unusual in discitis.

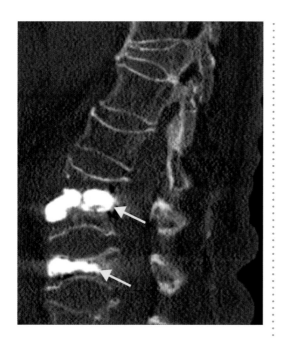

Epidural hematoma after vertebroplasty

One complication of interventional spinal procedures is hemorrhage. Sagittal CT (upper left image) demonstrates cement (yellow arrows) in two vertebral bodies after vertebroplasty, and multiple compression deformities. Sagittal T1-weighted MR images pre-contrast (lower left image) and post-contrast (right image) demonstrate a peripherally enhancing collection (red arrows) surrounding the superiormost augmented vertebra and extending in the epidural space posterior to the next superior vertebral body. Although this appearance may look similar to an epidural abscess, the intrinsic T1 shortening (increased signal on the T1-weighted image) and the lack of clinical and laboratory signs of infection are more suggestive of hematoma.

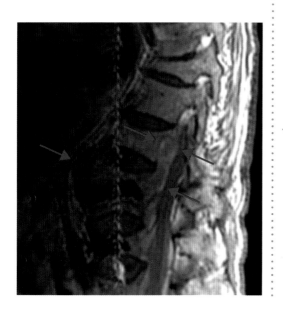

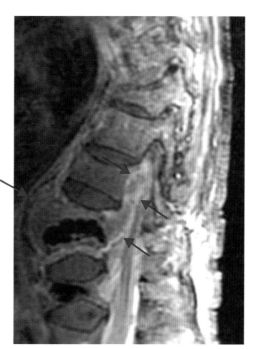

Neuropathic spine

Neuropathic spine is a destructive process that occurs in response to repeated trauma in the setting of diminished protective sensation, as can be seen in the setting of diabetes mellitus, syringomyelia, and rarely, syphilis. The thoracolumbar junction and lumbar spine are most often affected. Neuropathic spine may be difficult to differentiate from infection on imaging. Similar to neuropathic arthropathy involving other joints, however, debris, destruction, and disorganization can be seen in neuropathic spine. Facet involvement is also typical. If vacuum phenomenon is seen, then infection is considered extremely unlikely.

Further reading

Dziurzynska-Bialek E, Kruk-Bachonko J, Guz W, *et al.* Diagnostic Difficulties Resulting from Morphological Image Variation in Spondylodiscitis MR Imaging. *Pol J Radiol* 2012; 77(3):25–34.

Fardon DF, Milette PC. Nomenclature and Classification of Lumbar Disc Pathology: Recommendations of the Combined Task Forces of the North American Spine Society, American Society of Spine Radiology, and American Society of Neuroradiology. *Spine* 2001; 26:E93–E113.

Hong SH, Choi J, Lee JW, *et al.* Diagnostic MR Imaging Assessment of the Spine: Infection or an Imitation? *Radiographics* 2009; 29:599–612.

Meyer CA, Vagal AS, Seaman D. Put Your Back into It: Pathologic Conditions of the Spine at Chest CT. *Radiographics* 2011; 31:1425–1441.

Numaguchi Y, Rigamonti D, Rothman MI, *et al.* Spinal Epidural Abscess: Evaluation with Gadolinium-enhanced MR Imaging. *Radiographics* 1993; 13:545–559.

Case 54   59-year-old male with a history of metastatic colon cancer presented with left thigh pain

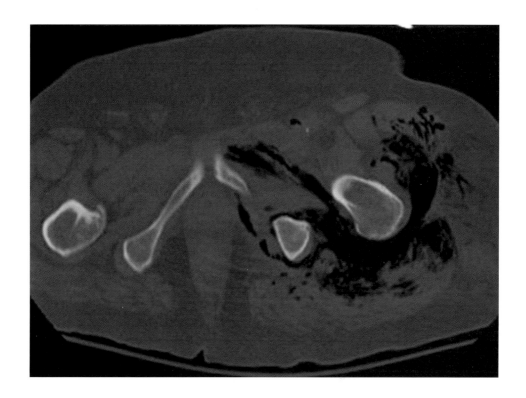

Diagnosis:
Necrotizing
fasciitis

Unenhanced axial CT of the pelvis demonstrates marked subcutaneous and deep fascial emphysema within the left thigh (yellow arrows) and in the left common femoral vein (red arrow).

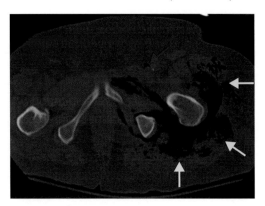

Discussion

Necrotizing fasciitis is a rapidly progressive infection that may involve any soft tissue layer.

- Immunocompromised and elderly patients are at increased risk. Predisposing factors include diabetes mellitus, superficial injury, cellulitis, surgery, and insect bites.
- Infection by a single organism occurs in about 15% of cases, with the remainder of cases caused by multiple aerobic and anaerobic organisms.
- Mortality rates range from 30–70%. Patients with severe, uncontrollable infection may die of septic shock with renal or multi-organ system failure.
- In addition to the risk of overwhelming systemic infection, affected patients are at risk for extensive soft tissue or limb loss.
- Given that necrotizing fasciitis tends to be rapidly progressive, time is of the essence in preventing morbidity and mortality.

Diagnosis may be challenging due to nonspecific and variable clinical presentation, most often with fever and vague pain. Therefore, it is important to have high clinical suspicion in susceptible patients.

- The classic clinical examination finding is dusky, "wooden" skin with mottled purple patches; however, this finding often does not develop until late in the course of disease.
- Presentations occur along a spectrum, and skin findings may even be normal.
- Early in the course of disease, pain may be absent or decreased relative to the extent of injury if there is damage to peripheral nerves. Common early clinical

findings include pain and tachycardia. Late findings include severe pain, skin discoloration, and multi-organ system failure.
- Although necrotizing fasciitis may affect any part of the body, the extremities, perineum (Fournier gangrene), and trunk are most commonly involved.

Necrotizing fasciitis may progress rapidly in a short period of time – initial radiographs may be normal or show only soft tissue swelling.
- The hallmark radiographic finding of soft tissue gas is seen only in a minority of cases.
- CT and MRI may be extremely helpful in diagnosis. Findings include edema, soft tissue gas, and fascial thickening and enhancement.
- Soft tissue gas can be difficult to detect on MR, but when present, can appear as focal susceptibility effect. Radiographs or CT may be helpful for confirmation.
- Ultrasound is more useful in the pediatric population. Findings include distorted fascial planes, subcutaneous edema, and fluid accumulation.

Aggressive and timely surgical debridement, IV antibiotic therapy, and supportive care are key in management.

Clinical synopsis   The patient underwent emergent surgical debridement and was treated with IV antibiotics.

Self-assessment

- *Name three typical CT findings in necrotizing fasciitis.*

- Soft tissue gas, ill- or well-defined fluid collections in the deep fascia, abscesses, fascial thickening and enhancement.

- *What is the appropriate next step when there is high clinical suspicion for necrotizing fasciitis?*

- If clinical suspicion is high, imaging should not delay emergent surgical intervention. Imaging is reserved for situations in which the patient is stable and further clarification is required for diagnosis.

Spectrum of necrotizing fasciitis

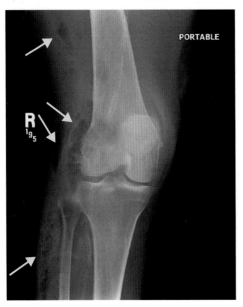

Radiographic diagnosis of necrotizing fasciitis

AP radiograph of the right knee in a 64-year-old woman with diabetes and chronic renal failure shows marked subcutaneous emphysema (arrows) and prominent vascular calcifications. The patient underwent emergent debridement and above-the-knee amputation.

Differential diagnosis of necrotizing fasciitis

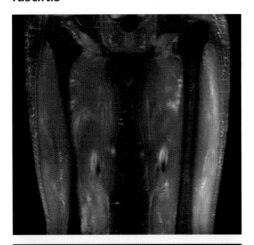

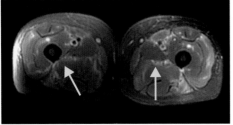

Myositis and fasciitis

Diffuse, bilateral, symmetrical inflammation is less typical of infection and more suggestive of an inflammatory process. Coronal and axial T2-weighted MR images of the thighs with fat suppression demonstrate patchy edema (T2 prolongation) involving the anterior, lateral, and posterior muscular compartments of both legs, consistent with myositis. There is some involvement of the fascial planes as well (arrows). This imaging appearance is nonspecific, and may be seen in a variety of inflammatory or idiopathic conditions including polymyositis, dermatomyositis, and myositis associated with connective tissue disorders.

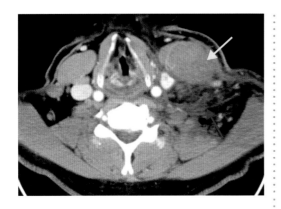

Focal idiopathic/infectious myositis

Axial contrast-enhanced CT of the lower neck in a patient who recently returned from a vacation in Fiji demonstrates asymmetric expansion of the left sternocleidomastoid muscle (yellow arrow), with adjacent fat stranding and fascial thickening (red arrow). The etiology was never well established, but was assumed to be infectious.

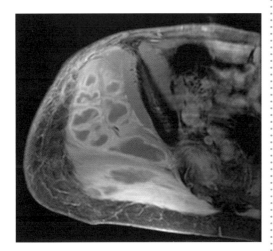

Pyomyositis

Pyomyositis is most common in HIV-positive and otherwise immunocompromised patients. Bacterial infection is typical, with *Staphylococcus aureus* being the most common pathogen; however, viruses (influenza, Coxsackie B), parasites (*Taenia solium*, *Toxoplasma*), and fungi (*Candida*, *Mucor*, *Aspergillus*) are sometimes involved. Axial T1-weighted post-gadolinium MRI with fat suppression in a 52-year-old male with MRSA pyomyositis demonstrates numerous ring-enhancing abscesses in the right gluteus medius and maximus muscles. The patient underwent emergent surgical debridement. Pyomyositis is defined as muscular infection with abscess formation.

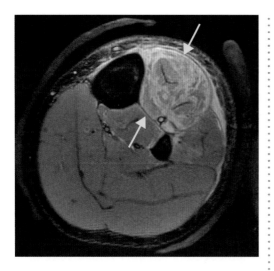

Compartment syndrome

Compartment syndrome occurs when high pressure within a fascial compartment restricts perfusion. Pain out of proportion to physical exam is typical. Emergent fasciotomy is the treatment of choice. In a young patient with thigh pain, axial STIR MR (upper image) shows expansion and edema of the anterior tibialis muscle (arrows) with overlying fascial and subcutaneous edema. T1 shortening within the anterior tibialis muscle on an unenhanced axial T1-weighted sequence (lower image) represents intramuscular hemorrhage.

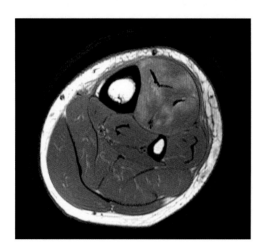

Further reading

Fugitt JB, Puckett ML, Quigley MM, Kerr SM. Necrotizing Fasciitis. *Radiographics* 2004; 24:1472–1476

Hasham S, Matteucci P, Stanley PR, Hart NB. Necrotising Fasciitis. *BMJ* 2005; 330:830–833 [Erratum in *BMJ* 2005; 330:1143]

Mulcahy H, Richardson ML. Imaging of Necrotizing Fasciitis: Self-Assessment Module. *AJR Integrative Imaging* 2010; 195:S66–69

Schulze M, Kotter I, Ernemann U, *et al.* MRI Findings in Inflammatory Muscle Diseases and their Noninflammatory Mimics. *AJR* 2009; 192(6):1708-1716

PART II Traumatic Conditions

Case 55   18-year-old male involved in head-on motor vehicle collision with closed head injury and admitting Glasgow coma scale score of 3

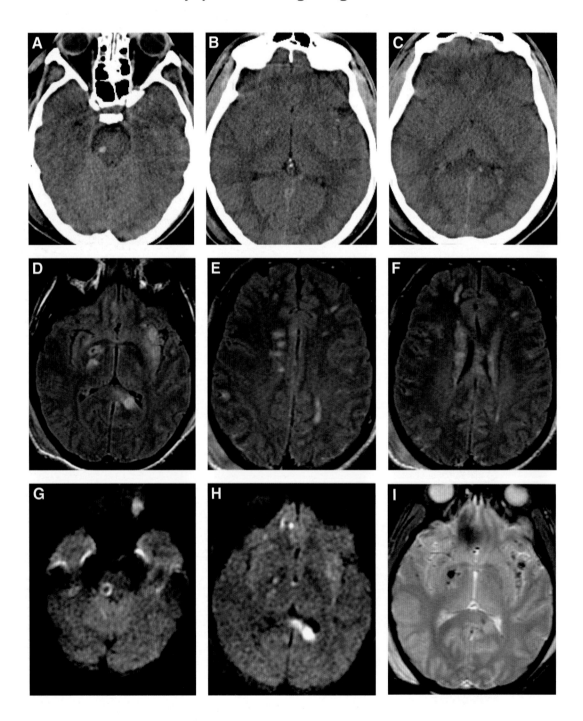

***Diagnosis:*
**Diffuse
axonal injury**

Unenhanced axial CT images (A–C) show multiple small foci of hemorrhage (arrows) in the right pons (A), right basal ganglia, left subinsular region (B) and left splenium of the corpus callosum (C).

Axial FLAIR MR images (D–F) demonstrate multiple corresponding signal abnormalities in the basal ganglia, subinsular region, splenium (D) and body of the corpus callosum (E) as well as gray–white junctions (E, F).

Axial diffusion-weighted imaging (DWI) (G, H) and gradient-recalled echo (GRE) (I) images show corresponding bright DWI and dark GRE foci in the right pons (G), left splenium (H), right basal ganglia, and left subinsular regions (I).

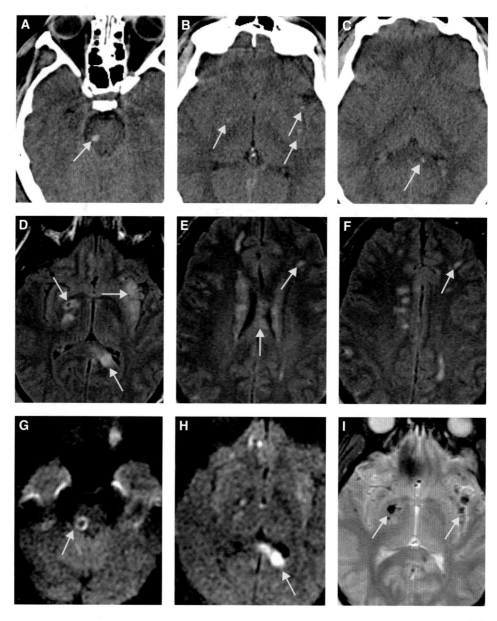

Discussion

Overview of diffuse axonal injury

- Diffuse axonal injury (DAI) is a common, potentially devastating traumatic brain injury resulting from acceleration–deceleration or rotational forces, such as those that occur in high-speed motor vehicle accidents, assaults (including child abuse), and falls.
- DAI is implicated in the majority of cases of unconsciousness and vegetative state after closed head injury. Most patients (90%) with severe DAI remain in a coma. Those who regain consciousness are often left with significant residual neurological deficits. Some experts consider concussion to be a mild manifestation of DAI.

Pathophysiology of DAI

- Microscopically, DAI reflects axonal disruption due to shear forces that stretch the axons as different density tissues slide across each other during injury. Axons that bridge the gray–white (corticomedullary) junction are therefore most commonly involved.
- Generally, it is not mechanical force itself that disrupts axons, but rather a precipitation of biological cascades that occurs over hours to days after the time of impact.
- Cytoskeletal and axonal cell membrane (axolemma) injury are key pathophysiological features. Stretching damages the cytoskeleton with disruption of sodium and calcium channels, leading to mitochondrial dysfunction and eventual cell death. Axonal transport is compromised at the site of cytoskeleton injury, resulting in accumulation of transported materials. The axon swells and ultimately tears, retracting toward the cell body and forming the so-called "retraction ball" that is a characteristic histological feature of DAI.
- Downstream from the initial injury, Wallerian degeneration begins within 1–2 days.

Imaging of DAI

- On imaging, DAI manifests as small lesions (1–15 mm) in the white matter, commonly at the corticomedullary junction, corona radiata, corpus callosum, brainstem, basal ganglia, and thalami.
- Initial CT is often normal (50–80%), with limited sensitivity due to the small size and the temporal evolution of DAI lesions. One should, therefore, always consider DAI when neurological deficits are disproportionate to imaging

findings after typical injury mechanisms such as high-speed motor vehicle accident (MVA).

- Compared to CT, diffusion-weighted MRI is much more sensitive for detecting punctate foci of cytotoxic edema, and GRE MRI is more sensitive for micro-hemorrhage (susceptibility effects).
- Ongoing research efforts focus on using magnetization transfer, diffusion tensor imaging (DTI), and perfusion imaging to gauge the degree of injury and, perhaps, to predict outcome.

Clinical synopsis	The patient's mental status improved during hospitalization with supportive treatment and he was transferred to a rehabilitation facility after 3 weeks. On discharge, the patient was able to respond non-verbally to simple commands.

Self-assessment

- *Define DAI, including mechanism of injury and a brief summary of the pathophysiology.*

  - DAI is injury to axons resulting from rotational or acceleration–deceleration forces such as those that occur in high-speed MVAs. There is direct and biochemically mediated injury to the axon that results in axonal separation, cell death, and downstream Wallerian degeneration.

- *What is the typical clinical scenario for DAI?*

  - Neurological deficits that are disproportionate to CT imaging findings after a typical high-speed injury.
  - Severe DAI may result in coma or other severe neurological syndrome with poor prognosis.

- *What are typical MR imaging features of DAI, including classic locations of injury?*

  - Small hyperintense lesions on FLAIR and DWI and susceptibility effect on GRE (microbleeds) in locations such as the corticomedullary junction, brainstem, corona radiata, and corpus callosum.

Spectrum of diffuse axonal injury

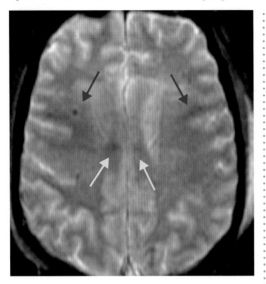

Subtle diffuse axonal injury

Imaging findings of less severe DAI can be subtle. Axial GRE image demonstrates faint curvilinear foci of susceptibility in the body of the corpus callosum (yellow arrows) and the corticomedullary junction bilaterally (red arrows). CT in this patient (not shown) was normal.

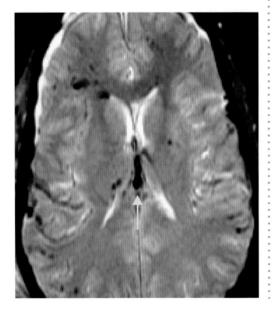

Diffuse axonal injury

Axial GRE image in a different patient shows numerous small microbleeds in the fornix (arrow) and corticomedullary junction, most prominent in the right frontal lobe.

Differential diagnosis of diffuse axonal injury

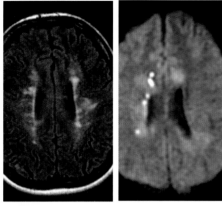

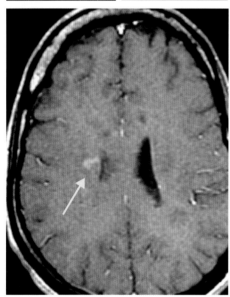

Multiple sclerosis

In a young patient with multiple sclerosis, there are multiple classic-appearing periventricular lesions on MR FLAIR imaging (upper left image) with several right-sided lesions demonstrating abnormal signal on DWI (upper right image). One presumably active lesion enhances on T1-weighted imaging (lower image) after the administration of intravenous gadolinium contrast (arrow).

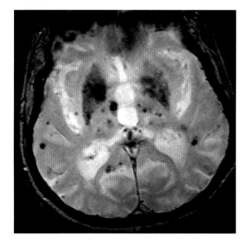

Chronic hypertension

Longstanding hypertension can lead to micro-hemorrhages in the cerebellum and deep gray matter, and is also often associated with confluent periventricular white matter changes from micro-vascular ischemia. Axial GRE MR imaging of a patient with long-standing hypertension shows multiple scattered foci of susceptibility representing microhemorrhages within deep gray matter structures including the basal ganglia and thalami.

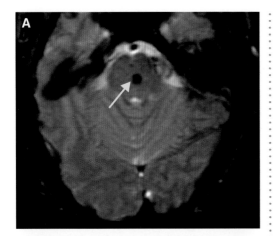

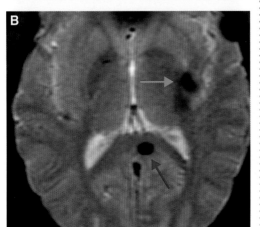

Multiple cavernomas

Serial axial MR GRE images in a patient with multiple cavernomas (A, B, and C) show multiple small round foci of susceptibility in the pons (yellow arrow), splenium (red arrow), left temporal lobe (green arrow), and subcortical white matter (blue arrows). Axial T2-weighted MR (D) demonstrates a large left medial temporal lobe cavernoma with characteristic heterogeneous central blood products (popcorn appearance) and a peripheral rim of hemosiderin (white arrow).

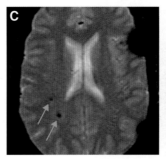

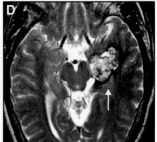

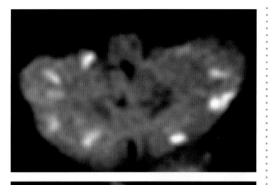

Embolic infarction

Multiple axial DWI images in a patient with atrial fibrillation show multiple scattered acute embolic infarcts. These are mostly peripheral in location, involving the cerebellum (top image) and supratentorial brain.

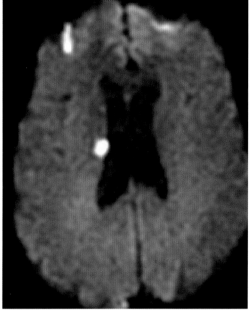

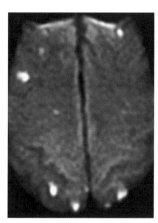

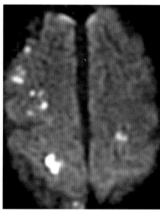

Further reading

Hardman JM, Manoukian A. Pathology of head trauma. *Neuroimaging Clinics of North America* 2002; 12(2):175-187

Iwata A *et al*. Traumatic axonal injury induces proteolytic cleavage of the voltage-gated sodium channels modulated by tetrodotoxin and protease inhibitors. *J of Neuroscience* 2004; 24(19):4605-4613

Kinoshita T *et al*. Conspicuity of diffuse axonal injury lesions on diffusion-weighted MR imaging. *Eur J Radiology* Oct. 2005; 56(1):5-11

Maas AI *et al*. Moderate and severe traumatic brain injury in adults. *Lancet Neurology* 2008; 7(8):728-741

Skandsen T *et al*. Prevalence and impact of diffuse axonal injury in patients with moderate and severe head injury: a cohort study of early MRI findings and 1-year outcome. *J Neurosurg* Oct. 23, 2009

Case 56   12-year-old male who presented with left-sided headache after motor vehicle accident

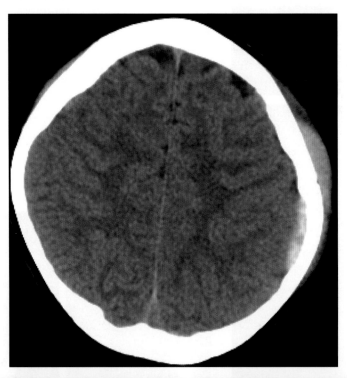

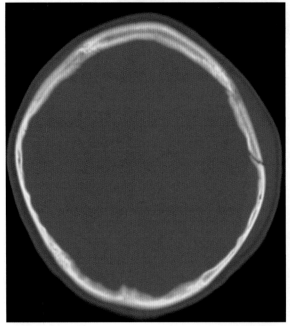

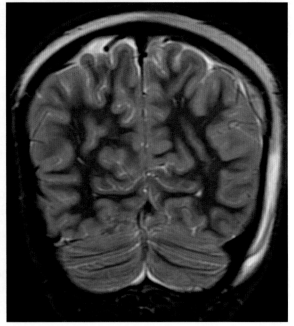

Diagnosis: Left parietal epidural hematoma with overlying fracture

Noncontrast axial CT in brain window (left image) demonstrates a hyperdense extra-axial collection over the left parietal convexity (yellow arrow). A small subgaleal hematoma is present superficially (red arrow). Bone windows (middle image) reveal an overlying non-displaced fracture (blue arrow). MRI was performed for clarification of which extra-axial space this hematoma occupied, as its small size made this difficult to discern on CT. T2-weighted coronal MRI (right image) shows that the hematoma (yellow arrow) is in the epidural compartment, superficial to the black line of the dura (green arrow).

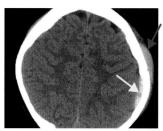 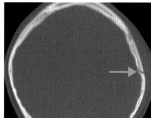 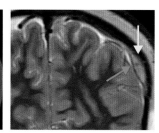

Discussion

Overview of epidural hematoma

- Epidural hematomas (EH) are intracranial extra-axial blood collections located between the periosteal layer of the inner calvarial table and the dura. 90% are due to arterial injury, while the remainder result from damage to a dural venous sinus near dural attachments. Trauma is the usual cause, with overlying skull fracture in greater than 85–95% of cases.

Arterial epidural hematoma

- The typical injury that results in epidural hematoma is a skull fracture with laceration of the middle meningeal artery (MMA). In children, traumatic MMA injury may result from stretching of the vessel without an overlying skull fracture. Given the location of the MMA, the majority of epidural hematomas are located along the temporal or temporo-parietal convexity.

Venous epidural hematoma

- Venous EH usually spans multiple cranial compartments and may cross the falx and tentorium. It is commonly seen in the posterior (transverse or sigmoid sinus injury) and middle cranial (sphenoparietal sinus injury) fossae and near the vertex (superior sagittal sinus injury). Posterior fossa EH are less common (5–10%) than supratentorial EH (90–95%). Because they result from slower venous bleeding, they tend to present in a delayed fashion, hence their worse prognosis. Venous EH are always located next to a dural sinus that has been transgressed by a fracture line. The involved sinus may be displaced by the collection but is usually not occluded.

Clinical presentation of epidural hematoma

- In 50% of cases, patients with EH present in a classical fashion: with an initial brief loss of consciousness followed by an asymptomatic period ("lucid interval"). After the lucid interval, precipitous decline in mental status develops rapidly. The overall mortality of unilateral EH is approximately 5%, rising to approximately 15–20% in cases where EH is bilateral. Prompt recognition and treatment of EH is essential to ensure good outcome. Epidural hematomas less than 1 cm in maximal thickness may not require surgical intervention. In some centers, a diagnostic angiogram may be performed to assess for active bleeding and possible therapeutic intervention such as embolization of the MMA.

Imaging of epidural hematoma

- On imaging, EH appear as lenticular or biconvex hyperdense extra-axial collections. They do not cross suture lines, as dural attachments act as barriers in the absence of suture injury. Rarely, EH can occur simultaneously with subdural hematomas. The combined biconvex and crescentic configuration of a mixed epidural–subdural hematoma has been named the "CT comma" sign.
- When it is small in size, it may be difficult to localize a hematoma to the epidural or subdural compartment by shape and confinement by dural structures. In these cases, MRI may be needed for clarification, as in the index case. On T2-weighted MRI, EH will be superficial to the thin hypointense dura, while subdural hematoma will be subjacent.
- Extra-axial hematomas, both subdural and epidural, produce variable mass effect on the underlying brain. Careful assessment for herniation, a potentially fatal complication, should be performed in all cases.
- Injuries associated with EH include contrecoup subdural hematomas and cerebral contusions. Air pockets within EH suggest paranasal sinus or mastoid fractures.
- In the acute setting, two-thirds of EH are hyperdense (50–80 HU). If there is active extravasation, a swirl of hypodense non-coagulated blood may be seen within the hyperdense collection ("swirl" sign). This sign may also be seen in anemic or coagulopathic patients. Over time, the EH will evolve into a mixed-density, and eventually, a hypodense collection.

Clinical synopsis	The patient experienced headache initially, followed by a several-hours-long lucid interval with subsequent recurrent headaches. Follow-up imaging showed unchanged size of the hematoma and he was treated conservatively.

Self-assessment

• *Name three features used to distinguish epidural from subdural hematomas.*

• EH are lentiform while subdural hematomas are crescent-shaped.
• EH are confined by sutural dural attachments, whereas subdural hematomas are confined by the falx and tentorium.
• EH classically present acutely in young, healthy individuals who have experienced overt trauma, while subdural hematomas are typically seen subacutely in elderly patients with brain atrophy, due to tearing of bridging subdural veins following minor or occult trauma. The lucid interval is another clinical characteristic that distinguishes EH.

• *How can other processes in the epidural space such as epidural abscess and dural-based neoplasm be distinguished from epidural hematoma?*

• Tissue characteristics and enhancement pattern on CT and MRI, effect on the underlying brain, clinical information, and presence or absence of associated traumatic injuries may help the radiologist differentiate among various entities.

Spectrum of epidural hematoma

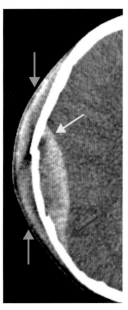
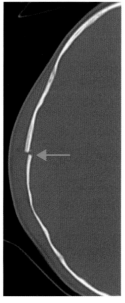

Mixed epidural–subdural hematoma with overlying skull fracture

In this patient with head trauma, axial and coronal unenhanced CT images show a large heterogeneous extra-axial collection at the right parieto-temporal convexity that does not cross dural suture attachments. As demonstrated on the axial image, the shape of the extra-axial collection is lenticular anteriorly (yellow arrow) and crescentic posteriorly (red arrow), illustrating the "CT comma" sign indicative of a mixed epidural–subdural hematoma. Heterogeneous hypoattenuation within the hematoma demonstrates the CT swirl sign – chronic liquefied clot is more homogeneous and focal. As in the index case, there is subgaleal hematoma (blue arrows) and a

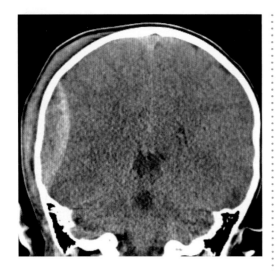

minimally displaced parieto-temporal bone fracture seen on bone windows (green arrow). In this location MMA injury is the likely culprit.

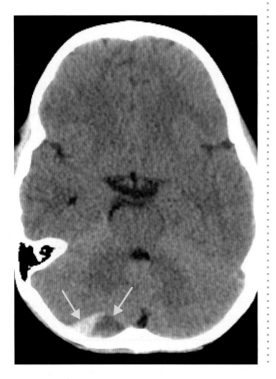

Posterior fossa epidural hematoma

Axial unenhanced CT shows a heterogeneous lentiform epidural hematoma in the right posterior fossa (arrows) that is confined by dural attachments. Epidural hematoma in the posterior fossa is especially dangerous due to limited space, with increased risk of herniation.

Differential diagnosis of epidural hematoma

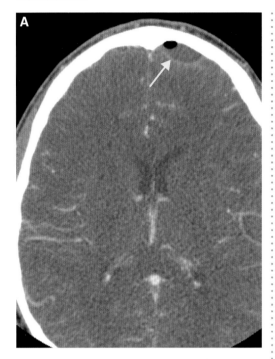

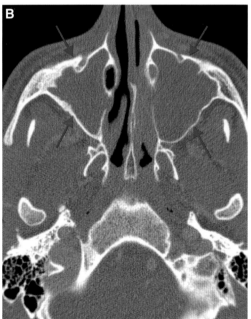

Epidural abscess

This patient presented with 2 weeks of progressive headache and facial pain. Axial enhanced CT (A and B) demonstrates an epidural abscess seen as a rim-enhancing, gas-containing, extra-axial collection along the left frontal convexity (yellow arrow). There is complete opacification of the maxillary sinuses (red arrows). Axial T2-weighted (C) and diffusion-weighted (D) MRI demonstrate fluid signal and reduced diffusion (yellow arrows). There is opacification of the frontal sinus (blue arrow in C). Axial fat-suppressed post-contrast T1-weighted image (E) shows avid enhancement of the thickened underlying dura (green arrows). Blood products in sterile extra-axial hematomas may produce heterogeneously reduced diffusion. This finding should be correlated with clinical signs of infection, as hematomas may become super-infected. Sterile chronic hematomas may exhibit peripheral enhancement.

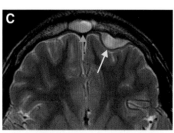

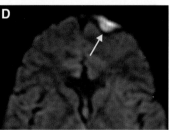

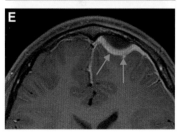

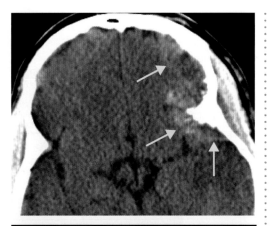

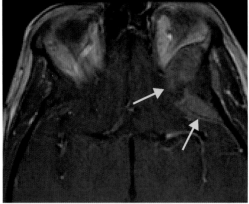

Epidural metastasis

Dural-based masses may mimic extra-axial hematomas on CT, particularly if they are hypercellular and, hence, hyperdense; however, masses are typically more irregularly shaped, may occur in unusual locations, and may result in adjacent bony changes such as erosion, hyperostosis, or periosteal reaction. Common primary solid tumors associated with dural metastasis include prostate and breast cancer in adults and neuroblastoma in children. In anemic patients, extramedullary hematopoiesis may explain multiple enhancing dural-based masses. In this patient with multiple dural-based metastases, axial unenhanced CT (upper image) shows heterogeneous attenuation of the brain (arrows) adjacent to the greater wing of the left sphenoid, with associated aggressive-appearing spiculated periosteal reaction. T1-weighted post-contrast MR (lower image) confirms that the extra-axial, dural-based mass demonstrates enhancement.

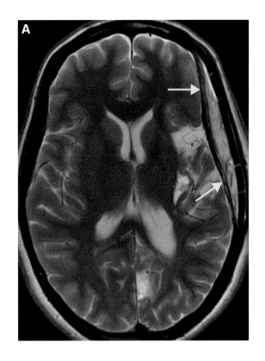

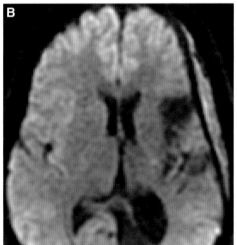

Epidural epidermoid

Like the previously described epidural abscess, epidermoid exhibits reduced diffusion. This is thought to be caused by material secreted by hypercellular keratinized squamous epithelium. Adjacent dural enhancement is similar to that seen in abscess. In contrast to abscess, however, clinical signs of infection are absent. In this patient who underwent previous left temporal lobe tumor resection, axial T2-weighted MR (A) demonstrates a heterogeneous, predominantly hyperintense extra-axial collection. The dura is a thickened hypointense line (yellow arrows) closely subjacent to the collection. The collection is slightly hyperintense on diffusion-weighted MRI (B). T1-weighted (C) and post-contrast T1-weighted (D) MRI show only enhancement of the thickened subjacent dura (arrows).

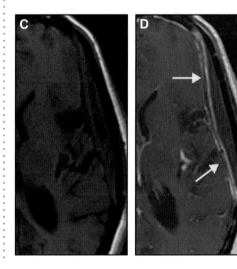

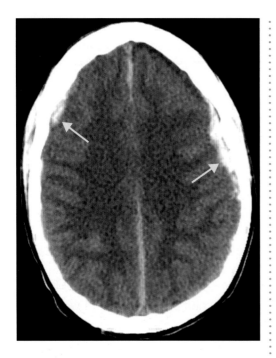

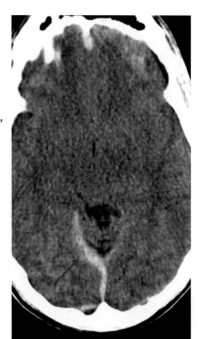

Subdural hematoma

Subdural hematomas are cresentic in shape and, unlike epidural collections, are not limited by insertion of the dura at the sutures. At times, they may be difficult to differentiate from leukemic or metastatic involvement of the dura extending into the subdural space. Density of the hematoma can be variable depending on chronicity. Axial CT demonstrates bilateral small high-attenuation acute subdural hematomas (yellow arrows) and hematoma tracking along the falx and tentorium (red arrow).

Further reading

Al-Nakshabandi NA. The swirl sign. *Radiology*. 2001;218 (2): 433.

Atlas SW. *Magnetic Resonance Imaging of the Brain and Spine*. New York, NY: Raven, 2008.

Güresir E, Beck J, Vatter H, Setzer M, Gerlach R, Seifert V, *et al*. Subarachnoid hemorrhage and intracerebral hematoma: incidence, prognostic factors, and outcome. *Neurosurgery*. Dec. 2008;63 (6): 1088-1093; discussion 1093-1094.

Sullivan TP, Jarvik JG, Cohen WA. Follow-up of conservatively managed epidural hematomas: implications for timing of repeat CT. *AJNR Am J Neuroradiol*. 1999;20 (1): 107-113.

Zimmerman R, Gibby A, Carmody R. *Neuroimaging, Clinical and Physical Principles*. New York, NY: Springer-Verlag, 2000.

Case 57   31-year-old jiu-jitsu player sustained neck trauma and presented with neck pain and dizziness

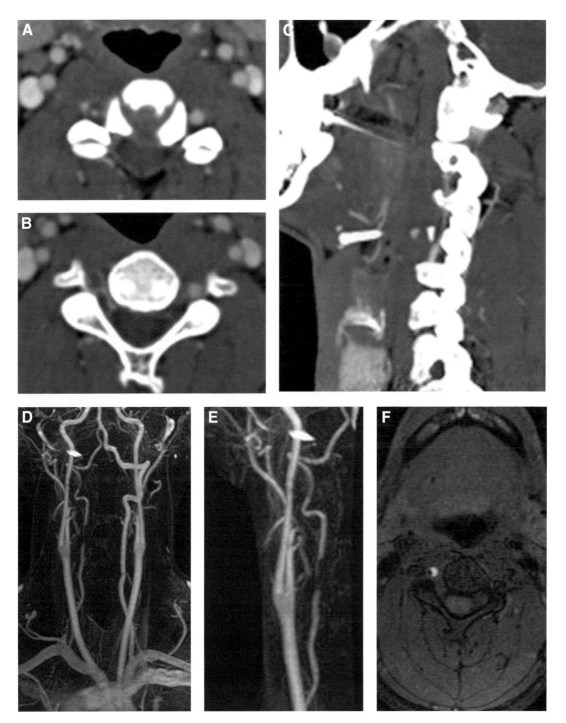

Diagnosis:
Vertebral artery dissection

Axial CTA with IV contrast (A, B) shows decreased caliber of the right vertebral artery (arrow) in comparison to the left, with soft tissue density encasing the patent lumen.

Sagittal CTA maximum intensity projection (MIP) of the right vertebral artery (C) shows eccentric stenosis of the mid right cervical vertebral artery (V2 segment), with soft tissue density along the stenotic segment (arrow).

Coronal (D) and sagittal (E) gadolinium-enhanced MRA MIP images show near-complete loss of normal flow signal at the same level (arrow).

Axial T1 fat saturation MRI (F) shows intramural hematoma as a crescent-shaped focus of high signal (arrow) that narrows the patent lumen (dark flow void).

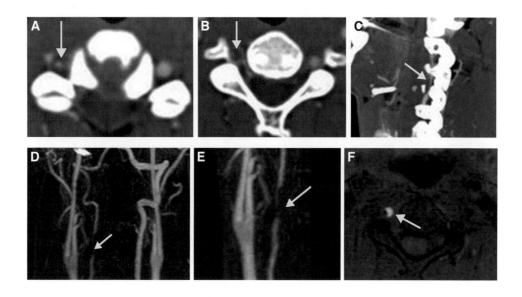

Discussion

Overview of vertebral artery dissection

- In vertebral artery dissection, blood enters the media from the true lumen via an intimal tear. This creates a false lumen with an intimomedial flap that may cause vascular stenosis or occlusion. In subadventitial dissection, rupture of the vasa vasorum results in accumulation of blood within the subadventitial media, which may produce pseudoaneurysms or frank adventitial rupture. Both patterns may occur simultaneously.
- Vertebral artery dissections may be spontaneous or result from major or minor trauma.
- Prompt diagnosis is essential to commence timely treatment and minimize complications such as embolic infarcts.

- Vertebral artery dissection is an important cause of stroke in younger patients. The incidence of spontaneous vertebral artery dissection is about 1 to 1.5 per 100,000 people per year, accounting for 0.4–2.5% of all ischemic strokes. In patients under 45 years of age, vertebral artery dissections cause up to 25% of strokes.
- Clinically, patients may present with occipital headache and neck pain (70%) or with signs and symptoms related to ischemia of the vertebrobasilar system (60%), including nystagmus, ataxia, vertigo, or nausea. Less common symptoms include paresthesias or weakness from cervical spinal cord ischemia or cervical nerve root impairment.
- The extracranial segments of the vertebral artery are thought to be more prone to dissection due to their increased mobility and proximity to bony structures. The horizontal V3 segment is particularly susceptible to traumatic dissection due to anchoring at the C2 foramen transversarium and the dura.

Imaging of vertebral artery dissection

- Unenhanced CT is often the first imaging study ordered in cases of vertebral artery dissection, especially when the presenting signs and symptoms are nonspecific. CT may be normal or show evidence of infarction or, rarely, subarachnoid hemorrhage in cases of adventitial rupture related to intradural (V4 segment) vertebral artery dissection.
- MRI/MRA and CTA are similar in sensitivity and specificity for vertebral artery dissection. Noninvasive imaging is generally preferred over conventional angiography except for rare situations in which endovascular intervention is being considered.
- CTA findings may include luminal irregularity, vascular stenosis, occlusion, intimal flap, and the "suboccipital rind" sign. Non-enhancing soft tissue density adjacent to the lumen suggests intramural hematoma (IMH). The "suboccipital rind" sign, a segment of non-enhancing soft tissue density adjacent to the vessel lumen, may be the only abnormality of the V3 segment where dissections may not significantly narrow the lumen. Mimics of the suboccipital rind sign include normal veins of the vertebral artery venous plexus and suboccipital venous sinus that may parallel the course of the vertebral artery; however, the suboccipital rind sign may be distinguished from these normal venous networks by absence of enhancement after administration of contrast.
- A normal anatomic variant that is occasionally mistaken for dissection is size discrepancy between the vertebral arteries. Congenitally small arteries may be distinguished from arteries with dissection by their uniform size from origin to terminus with a corresponding hypoplastic transverse foramen.
- MRI findings in vertebral artery dissection include IMH, intimal flap, and luminal irregularity, with or without associated stenosis or occlusion. IMH

appears as a crescent-shaped area of T1 shortening that surrounds or occludes the vertebral artery lumen. Axial T1-weighted imaging with fat suppression best depicts this finding by facilitating distinction of the fat that normally surrounds the blood vessel from the adjacent hematoma. While both fat and methemoglobin are inherently hyperintense on standard T1-weighted images, fat suppression accentuates the hyperintense hematoma, which is not saturated out. An important caveat is that acute or chronic intramural hematoma may be isointense to surrounding structures on T1 fat-suppressed imaging, as only subacute hemorrhage (containing methemoglobin) is hyperintense on T1-weighted images.

- Areas of acute infarction due to any ischemic cause, including dissection, will show abnormal signal on diffusion-weighted MRI.
- Angiographic imaging should be strongly considered in selected cases of cervical spine fracture, especially those that involve the transverse foramina. Connective tissue disorders such as fibromuscular dysplasia, Marfan syndrome, Ehlers–Danlos syndrome, and osteogenesis imperfecta type I all predispose to non-traumatic dissection.

Treatment of vertebral artery dissection

- Anticoagulation is the treatment of choice for extracranial vertebral dissection, given that the most common and serious complication is thromboembolism leading to cerebral infarction. In intracranial dissection, anticoagulation is more controversial. Subarachnoid hemorrhage due to adventitial rupture is a relative contraindication. Endovascular or surgical intervention may be employed in patients in whom anticoagulation is ineffective or contraindicated and in those with dissecting aneurysms.

Self-assessment

- *Briefly describe typical imaging characteristics of vertebral artery dissection on noncontrast CT, CTA, and MRI/MRA.*

- Unenhanced CT may be normal or show signs of infarction in the territory of the vertebral artery and its branches. Rarely, subarachnoid hemorrhage is seen in the context of intradural dissection with adventitial rupture. CTA findings may include the "suboccipital rind" sign, "string" sign of contrast in the narrowed arterial lumen, or luminal occlusion. On MRI/MRA, acute infarction may be seen on DWI. MRA findings associated with the dissected vessel are analogous to CTA findings. Detection of hyperintense methemoglobin-containing subacute thrombus may be improved by fat-saturated T1-weighted imaging.

- *Name a few conditions that may predispose to vertebral artery dissection.*

- Major or minor trauma, fibromuscular dyplasia, Marfan syndrome, Ehlers–Danlos syndrome, and osteogenesis imperfecta type I.

- *Describe two potential mimics of vertebral artery dissection that may be seen on CTA or MRI/MRA and how they may be distinguished from dissection.*

- Veins adjacent to the vertebral artery may be mistaken for the "suboccipital rind" sign but are generally less hyperintense on T1-weighted MRI than subacute thrombus. Unlike thrombus, veins show luminal enhancement after contrast administration. Small vertebral arteries, especially when asymmetric, can be mistaken for arteries that are narrowed by dissection. Arteries of small caliber from origin to terminus with corresponding small transverse foramina are likely to represent congenitally small arteries.

Spectrum of vertebral artery dissection

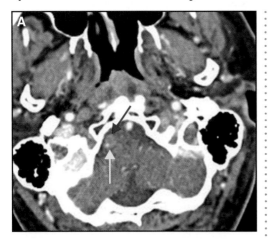

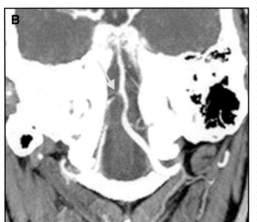

Spontaneous intradural vertebral artery dissection

This 39-year-old female presented with spontaneous headache, posterior auricular pain, and right eyelid droop. Axial (A) and coronal (B) CTA show severe stenosis of the intradural (V4) right vertebral artery (yellow arrows) with slightly hyperdense crescentic IMH adjacent to the stenotic segment (red arrow). AP (C) and lateral (D) conventional angiographic images performed after injection of contrast into the right vertebral artery show tapering of the intradural right vertebral artery (yellow arrows) just distal to the PICA origin.

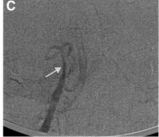
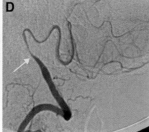

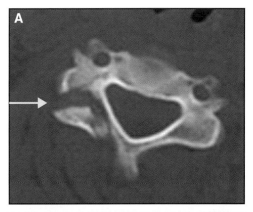

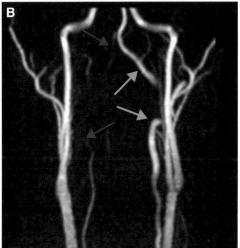

Traumatic vertebral artery dissection

In this 28-year-old male who was involved in a motor vehicle accident, axial noncontrast CT (A) shows a comminuted fracture of the right lateral mass of C3 (yellow arrow). Coronal MIP reformat from a post-gadolinium MRA (B) shows a long segment of loss of flow (red arrows). Note the normal left vertebral artery (blue arrows) for comparison. Axial T1-weighted MRI with fat suppression at the same level (C) and at the level of the intradural right vertebral artery (D) shows crescentic signal hyperintensity along the course of the artery, compatible with IMH (red arrows).

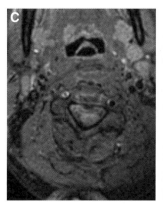 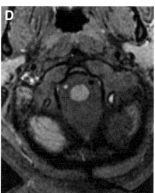

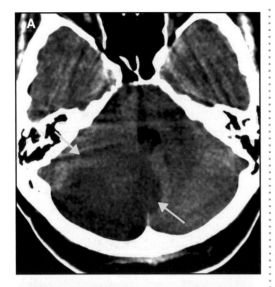

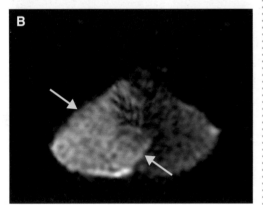

Right vertebral artery dissection with posterior inferior cerebellar artery territory infarct

This 51-year-old female developed hypertension after hysterectomy. Noncontrast CT (A) shows hypodensity of the posterior inferior cerebellar artery (PICA) territory with mass effect (yellow arrows). Axial DWI (B) reveals an acute infarct in the right PICA territory (yellow arrows). Coronal MIP reformat from a time-of-flight MRA of the circle of Willis (C) demonstrates attenuated flow-related enhancement throughout the intradural segment (V4) of the right vertebral artery (red arrow) and the right PICA. Axial T1-weighted image with fat suppression (D) shows T1 shortening along the course of the distal right cervical vertebral artery (red arrow), consistent with IMH.

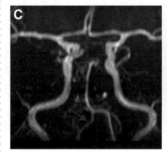

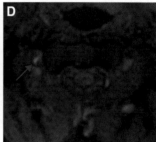

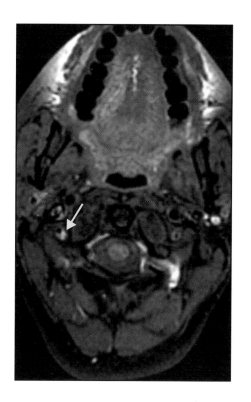

Right vertebral artery dissection with lateral medullary infarct

In this 39-year-old female with neck pain, axial T1-weighted MRI with fat saturation (left image) demonstrates IMH as crescentic signal hyperintensity at the right V2/V3 junction (yellow arrow). On FLAIR (middle image) and DWI (right image) sequences, there is a right lateral medullary infarct corresponding to the right PICA territory (red arrows).

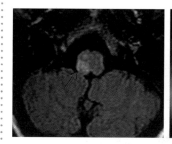 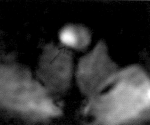

Further reading

Koh JS, Ryu CW, Lee SH, Bang JS, Kim GK. Bilateral vertebral-artery-dissecting aneurysm causing subarachnoid hemorrhage cured by staged endovascular reconstruction after occlusion. *Cerebrovasc Dis*. 2009;27(2):202–204. *Epub* Jan. 20, 2009.

Lum C, Chakraborty M, Schlossmacher M, Santos R, Mohan J, Sinclair, Sharma M. Vertebral artery dissection with a normal-appearing lumen at multisection CT angiography: the importance of identifying wall hematoma. *AJNR Am J Neuroradiol*. April 2009;30:787–792; originally published online Jan. 22, 2009, 10.3174/ajnr.A1455.

Provenzale JM, Sarikaya B. Comparison of test performance characteristics of MRI, MR angiography, and CT angiography in the diagnosis of carotid and vertebral artery dissection: a review of the medical literature. *AJR Am J Roentgenol*. Oct. 2009; 193(4):1167–1174.

Rodallec H *et al*. Craniocervical arterial dissection: spectrum of imaging findings and differential diagnosis. *Radiographics*. Oct. 2008;28:1711–1728.

Schievink WI, Roiter V. Epidemiology of cervical artery dissection. *Front Neurol Neurosci*. 2005;20:12–15.

SECTION 7 THORAX

Case 58   19-year-old motorcyclist presented with respiratory failure after a
            collision with a stationary truck

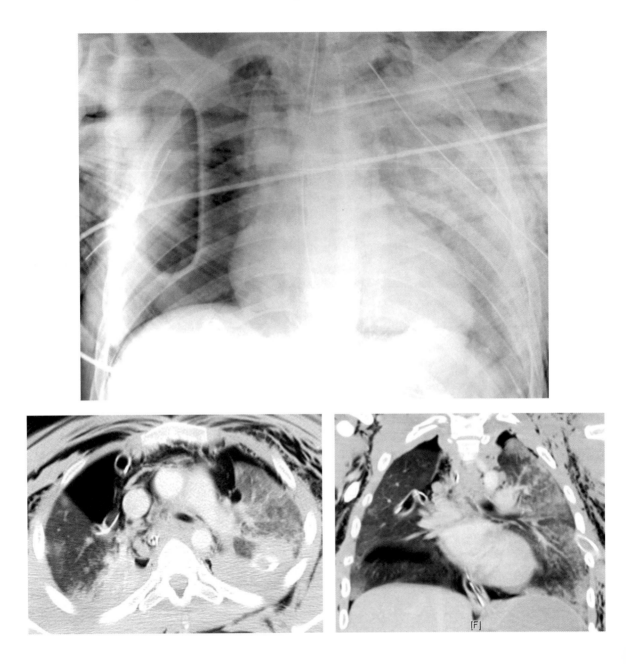

Diagnosis: Traumatic laceration of the right mainstem bronchus with pneumothorax and "fallen" lung

A portable chest radiograph shows extensive subcutaneous emphysema, the "visceral pleural line" sign of a right pneumothorax (yellow arrow), bilateral chest tubes, and a left upper lobe contusion (red arrow). Axial and coronal enhanced CT images also demonstrate extensive pneumomediastinum, bilateral pneumothoraces and pulmonary contusions, and narrowing and irregularity of the right mainstem bronchus (blue arrows); for comparison, note the normal contour and caliber of the left mainstem bronchus (green arrows). The right lung has fallen dependently towards the posterior chest wall despite placement of a chest tube.

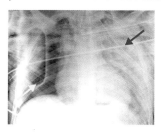 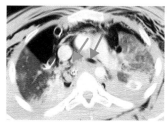 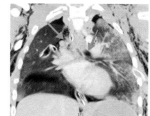

Discussion

Thoracic injuries are the third most common type of injury in trauma patients (after head and extremity injuries) and are implicated in approximately one-quarter of trauma-related deaths.

- Motor vehicle accidents are the mode of injury in more than two-thirds of cases of blunt thoracic trauma.
- Injuries to the heart and tracheobronchial tree carry the highest mortality of all injury types in blunt thoracic trauma.

In patients with suspected thoracic trauma, radiography is generally the modality of choice for initial evaluation; however, CT often reveals injuries even with normal radiographs.

- Radiographs facilitate identification of life-threatening injuries that require immediate attention, such as tension pneumothorax, hemothorax, mediastinal hemorrhage, and support line and tube misplacement. Superimposed objects (e.g., trauma boards and EKG leads) and suboptimal positioning of injured patients may complicate interpretation of portable radiographs.
- Chest CT images should be systematically interpreted in soft tissue windows (for evaluation of the heart, vasculature, esophagus, pleural collections, and the chest wall), lung windows (for evaluation of the lung parenchyma and tracheobronchial tree), and bone windows (for evaluation of the ribs and thoracic spine).
- IV contrast is recommended unless there is a known contraindication (such as allergy or known renal insufficiency). Water-soluble enteric contrast such as Gastrografin may be considered in cases with suspected esophageal injury.

- Multiplanar reformatted images are generally very useful in the evaluation of thoracic injury. 3D and MIP reconstructions are sometimes useful in the evaluation of complex cardiovascular and bone injuries, while minimum intensity projection (miniP) reconstructions are occasionally useful in the evaluation of airway injuries.
- Ultrasound may be used at the bedside for evaluation of the heart, pericardium, and pleural space. MRI currently does not play a role in the management of thoracic trauma.
- Common injuries in thoracic trauma include:

Lung	• Contusion • Aspiration • Laceration (hematocele, pneumatocele, hematopneumatocele)
Pleura	• Hemothorax • Pneumothorax (with or without tension physiology)
Heart and vessels	• Hemopericardium • Great vessel injury such as aortic transection • Cardiac rupture
Thoracic cage	• Rib fracture • Thoracic spine fracture • Thoracic spine ligamentous injuries • Sternal fracture
Other	• Diaphragmatic injury • Soft tissue injury

Clinical synopsis   Large air leak from the right chest tube, along with the imaging findings of a fallen right lung and massive subcutaneous emphysema, raised concern for a tracheobronchial laceration. The patient underwent bronchoscopy, which demonstrated a circumferential tear of the right mainstem bronchus below the carina. The patient recovered uneventfully after urgent right thoracotomy and repair of the right mainstem bronchus.

Self-assessment

- *Name three life-threatening thoracic injuries that may be identified on a portable chest radiograph in a patient with thoracic trauma.*

- Tension pneumothorax, large hemothorax, mediastinal hemorrhage, and misplacement of support lines and tubes.

- *When air-leak from a chest tube is identified in a patient with pneumothorax, what important complication should be suspected?*

- *Name three radiographic signs of pneumothorax.*

- Bronchopleural fistula.

- Absence of peripheral lung markings, "visceral pleural line" sign, hyperlucency at the bases and along the cardiac borders, "deep sulcus" sign, "double diaphragm" sign.

Spectrum of blunt chest trauma

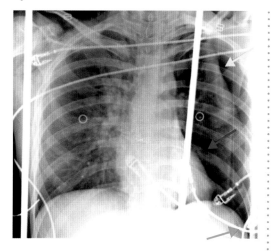

Pneumothorax

Extrapleural air tends to collect in the antero-medial thoracic base in supine patients. 10 to 50% of pneumothoraces are "occult" on plain radiographs, and identified only by CT. Small pneumothoraces may be radiographically subtle, and magnification should be used routinely in the assessment of trauma patients. Portable radiograph in a patient with a large left-sided pneumothorax illustrates absence of peripheral lung markings, the "visceral pleural line" sign (yellow arrow), hyperlucency in the base and along the left cardiac border (red arrow), and the "deep sulcus" sign (blue arrow).

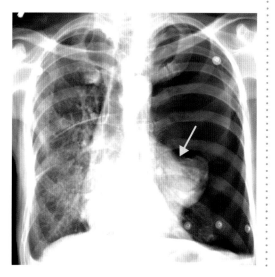

Tension pneumothorax

A frontal radiograph in a patient with a large tension pneumothorax demonstrates hyperlucency of the left hemithorax, with absence of vascular markings. The collapsed lung is seen medially (arrow). Tension physiology is manifested as flattening of the left hemidiaphragm, separation of the left-sided ribs, and tracheal and mediastinal shift. This diagnosis warrants immediate communication with the referring clinician given the risk for hemodynamic compromise related to diminished venous return.

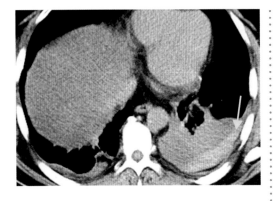

Hemothorax

An axial CT image of the lower chest demonstrates a hematocrit level in the left posterior hemithorax. The more dependent fluid (arrow) is similar in density to the intercostal muscles. In many cases, the finding is subtler than in the image presented in this case, or more difficult to differentiate from streak and other artifacts. The radiologist should, hence, maintain a high index of suspicion in cases of thoracic trauma (especially when rib or spinal fractures are present), and routinely interrogate pleural fluid with the region of interest (ROI) tool.

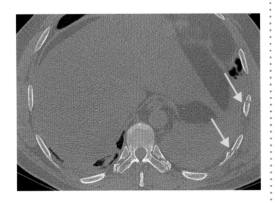

Rib fracture

Rib fractures are the most common injury in blunt chest trauma, occurring in about 50% of patients. When rib fractures are discovered, associated injuries should be sought: fractures of the upper ribs denote high-energy trauma and may be associated with injuries to the vessels and brachial plexus, while lower rib fractures are associated with injuries to the upper abdominal viscera. Conventional chest radiographs are less sensitive than dedicated rib series. CT is the most sensitive modality and allows for comprehensive assessment of associated injuries. Axial chest CT in bone windows shows non-displaced fractures of two adjacent left-sided ribs (arrows).

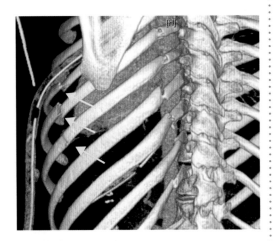

Multiple rib fractures

While isolated rib fractures cause limited morbidity, multiple or bilateral fractures may result in respiratory insufficiency due to paradoxical respiratory motion. "Flail chest" is defined as three or more contiguous ribs that are fractured in two or more places (segmental fractures). Fractures are most common in the middle to lower ribs, anteriorly and anterolaterally. More than half of patients with flail chest may have other serious injuries that require surgical management. A 3D volume-rendered posterior oblique CT image of the thorax demonstrates fractures of three contiguous left-sided ribs (arrows).

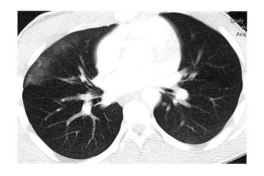

Contusion

Pulmonary contusion is the most common lung injury in blunt thoracic trauma. Non-segmentally distributed, ill-defined airspace opacities with 1–2 mm of subpleural sparing represent alveolar hemorrhage. Contusions are most common at the site of impact, but there may also be contrecoup injuries. Contusions are usually evident at the time of injury, and begin to clear at 24–48 hours. Axial CT in lung windows demonstrates pulmonary contusion as ill-defined airspace opacity with subpleural sparing in the anterior right middle lobe.

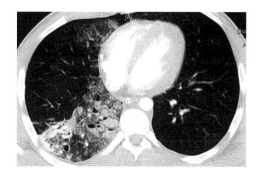

Hematopneumatocele (pulmonary laceration)

Pulmonary parenchymal lacerations manifest as cavities with thin or imperceptible walls due to recoil of inherently elastic lung tissue. They may contain air (pneumatocele), blood (hematocele), or both (hematopneumatocele). Shearing against the spine leads to paraspinal lacerations, while fractured ribs may produce peripheral lacerations. These injuries are more common in young patients with more flexible chest walls. Axial contrast-enhanced CT in lung windows demonstrates multiple pulmonary lacerations as small cavities with air–fluid levels in the paraspinal region of the right lower lobe. Ground glass opacity surrounding the lesions and in the anterior right middle lobe likely represents concurrent contusion.

Differential diagnosis of blunt thoracic trauma

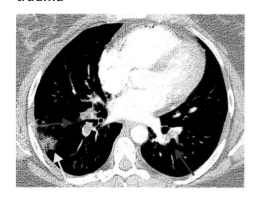

Pulmonary infarct

Pulmonary infarcts may occasionally simulate contusions. Unlike contusions, however, pulmonary infarcts are segmental and do not spare the subpleural region. Clinical history will differ between patients with contusions and patients with pulmonary infarcts. Axial image from a CT pulmonary angiogram demonstrates a pulmonary infarct as a peripheral, hypoenhancing, wedge-shaped opacity in the peripheral right lower lobe (yellow arrow). Filling defects representing pulmonary emboli are seen within multiple central pulmonary artery branches (red arrows).

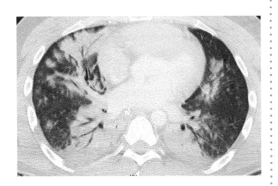

Pneumonia

Pneumonia has a variable imaging appearance and may resemble pulmonary contusion; however, clinical signs, symptoms, and history usually differ. Contrast-enhanced axial chest CT in lung windows demonstrates dense consolidation of the lower lobes with air bronchograms, as well as patchy nodular airspace opacities in the right middle lobe and the lingula. There are small bilateral pleural effusions layering dependently.

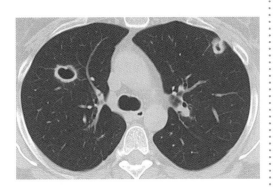

Inflammatory lung lesions (granulomatosis with polyangiitis)

In comparison to pulmonary lacerations, infectious and inflammatory cavitary lesions tend to have thicker walls. Clinical signs and symptoms also differ, and the lesions are not in a distribution typical for pulmonary lacerations. Axial CT demonstrates multiple cavitary lesions in both lungs in a patient with granulomatosis with polyangiitis (GPA, formerly known as Wegener's granulomatosis). There is no associated contusion, rib fracture, or other associated traumatic injury.

Further reading

Kaewlai R, Avery LL, Asrani AV, Novelline RA. Multidetector CT of blunt thoracic trauma. *RadioGraphics*. 2008. 28(6):1555–570.

Lomoschitz FM, Eisenhuber E, Linnau KF, Peloschek P, Schoder M, Bankier AA. Imaging of chest trauma: radiological patterns of injury and diagnostic algorithms. *Eur J Radiol*. Oct. 2003. 48(1):61–70.

Sangster GP, González-Beicos A, Carbo AI, Heldmann MG, Ibrahim H, Carrascosa P, Nazar M, D'Agostino HB. Blunt traumatic injuries of the lung parenchyma, pleura, thoracic wall, and intrathoracic airways: multidetector computer tomography imaging findings. *Emerg Radiol*. Oct. 2007. 14(5):297–310.

SECTION 8 ABDOMEN

Case 59   45-year-old male presenting with left upper quadrant pain and chronic
cough and multiple severe coughing spells

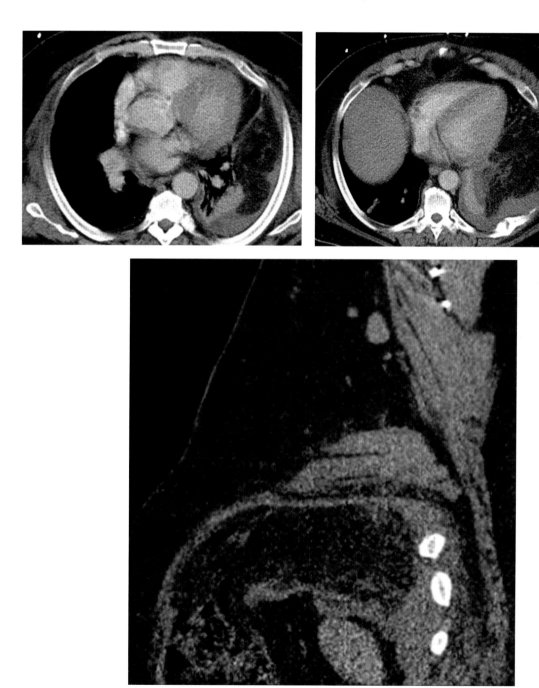

Diagnosis:
Diaphragmatic
hernia

Axial enhanced CT images (left and middle) demonstrate mixed solid and fat attenuation (yellow arrows) within the left thoracic cavity, associated with a small pleural effusion and enhancing compression atelectasis of the left lung base. There is herniation of the fat through the anterolateral chest wall (red arrows). Sagittal image from the same examination (right) shows a large defect in the anterolateral aspect of the diaphragm (blue arrow), with resultant thickening and folding of the shortened free edge of the diaphragm ("dangling diaphragm" sign). Mesenteric fat has herniated into the thorax (green arrow) through the diaphragmatic defect.

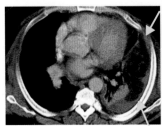 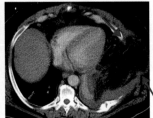 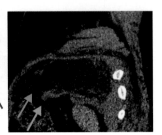

Discussion

Overview of diaphragmatic injury

- Diaphragmatic hernia is a disruption of the diaphragmatic muscular or tendinous fibers resulting in communication between the thoracic and abdominal cavities.
- Diaphragmatic hernia may result from penetrating injury (e.g., knife or gunshot wound) causing direct disruption of diaphragmatic fibers, or blunt trauma (e.g., motor vehicle accident) abruptly producing a pressure gradient between the thorax and abdomen. Secondary diaphragmatic injury may also occur due to diaphragmatic laceration from fractured ribs in trauma patients. A closed glottis at the time of trauma causes an elevated pressure gradient and further increases the risk of diaphragmatic injury. Chronic cough is a much less common cause of diaphragmatic rupture.
- Diaphragmatic injury is more readily diagnosed and more common on the left side, where herniation may include the stomach, colon, omentum, or spleen. Additionally, there is often congenital embryologic weakness in the left posterolateral aspect of the diaphragm, increasing susceptibility to injury. Conversely, the large size of the liver may offer protection against right diaphragmatic injury. Complications of diaphragmatic hernias include respiratory insufficiency, bowel obstruction, and incarceration with ischemia of the herniated viscera.

- Diagnosis of diaphragmatic injury may be delayed when caused by blunt trauma. In contrast to penetrating injuries, which are typically surgically explored, blunt diaphragmatic injury may initially present without herniation and may be diagnosed later when herniation of abdominal contents occurs. Careful evaluation of the sagittal and coronal CT reformations is especially helpful in detecting subtle diaphragmatic disruption.

Imaging of diaphragmatic injury

- Both direct and indirect signs of diaphragmatic injury can be detected by CT.
- A direct sign of diaphragmatic injury is a segmental diaphragmatic defect, which may be associated with muscle retraction (usually manifested as thickening) and hemorrhage. The "dangling diaphragm" sign is another direct sign of diaphragmatic injury and represents curling of the free edge of the ruptured diaphragm.
- Indirect signs of diaphragmatic injury include the "collar" sign and the "dependent viscera" sign. The first describes the waist-like constraint around herniated abdominal contents, and the latter, the apposition of herniated contents against the posterior thoracic wall due to loss of diaphragmatic support.
- Diaphragmatic scalloping (variation of costal insertion of fibers) may mimic injury due to indentation on underlying organs. Absence of a true diaphragmatic defect on sequential images helps to confirm this normal variant.

Clinical synopsis

The patient was diagnosed with diaphragmatic rupture caused by severe coughing spells due to pertussis respiratory infection. The patient was treated with intensive antibiotic and steroid courses. After symptomatic improvement, the patient underwent surgical repair of the diaphragm and chest wall.

Self-assessment

- *Why are diaphragmatic injuries more common on the left side?*

- There is often congenital weakness in the posterolateral aspect of the left hemidiaphragm, and left hemidiaphragmatic injury is easier to diagnose since abdominal contents herniate more easily on this side. Additionally, the liver likely affords some protective effect from injury to the right hemidiaphragm.

- *Why are blunt injuries to the diaphragm more often missed than direct penetrating injuries?*

- Penetrating injuries are often explored, although CT is increasingly being used to avoid surgical exploration in selected patients. Blunt trauma is often managed non-operatively, and diaphragmatic injury can be subtle if abdominal contents have not herniated into the thoracic cavity.

- *Cite two direct and two indirect signs of diaphragmatic rupture.*

- **Direct**: Segmental diaphragmatic defect and "dangling diaphragm" sign.
- **Indirect**: "Collar" sign and "dependent viscera" sign.

Spectrum of diaphragmatic rupture

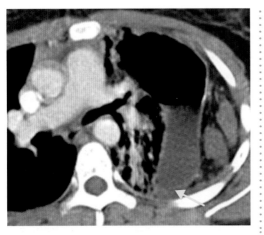

"Dependent viscera" sign

The "dependent viscera" sign is an indirect sign of diaphragmatic injury and is characterized by direct apposition of abdominal viscera against the posterior thoracic wall due to loss of diaphragmatic support. Axial enhanced CT demonstrates a left-sided diaphragmatic rupture, with the gastric fundus herniated into the thoracic cavity and in direct contact (arrow) with the posterior chest wall.

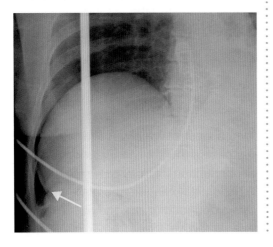

Pneumothorax

If a pneumothorax or displaced lower rib fractures are seen, diaphragmatic injury should be considered. While coronal and sagittal CT reconstructions are best, occasionally diaphragmatic injury is diagnosed by radiography. Supine chest radiography in a trauma patient demonstrates the "deep sulcus" sign, as well as indentation of the right hepatic lobe because of diaphragmatic constriction around the herniated liver (arrow).

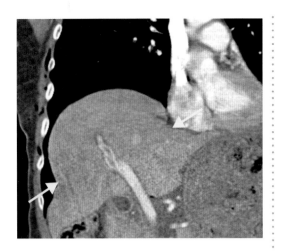

"Collar" sign

An indirect sign of diaphragmatic injury is herniation of abdominal contents through a defect, of which a variant is the "collar" sign, which describes a waist-like constriction around herniated viscera. Coronal contrast-enhanced CT in the same patient as the prior case demonstrates a mushroom-shaped hepatic hernia ("collar" sign; arrows) due to diaphragmatic rupture.

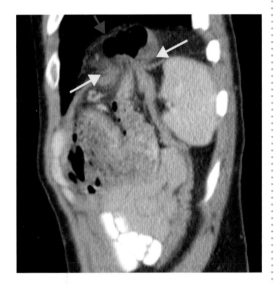

Remote, previously undiagnosed diaphragmatic injury complicated by bowel herniation

Sequela of diaphragmatic injury may manifest many years after the initial trauma. Although delayed diagnosis is more common in blunt than penetrating trauma, incarceration is more common with delayed diagnosis of penetrating trauma since penetrating defects are usually much smaller. Sagittal CT in a patient with a remote history of blunt trauma with symptoms of bowel obstruction demonstrates a diaphragmatic defect (yellow arrows) that was not diagnosed at the time of the prior trauma. There is herniation and incarceration of the splenic flexure of the colon (red arrow), which appears focally dilated above the diaphragm.

Differential diagnosis of diaphragmatic rupture

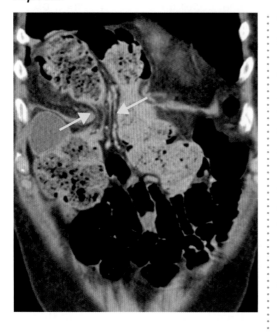

Congenital hernia

Congenital hernias are usually diagnosed in child-hood secondary to pulmonary symptoms. It is rare to encounter congenital hernias in adults. Boch-dalek hernia occurs posterolaterally, typically on the left, with approximately 150 reported cases in the adult literature. Morgagni hernia is even rarer, comprising 2% of congenital hernias, with 12 reported symptomatic adult cases in the lit-erature. Morgagni hernia is related to a congenital defect in the anteromedial diaphragm, usually on the right. Coronal CT demonstrates a Morgagni hernia (arrows) anteriorly and to the right of mid-line, through which a portion of the colon herni-ates. The patient had no history of trauma.

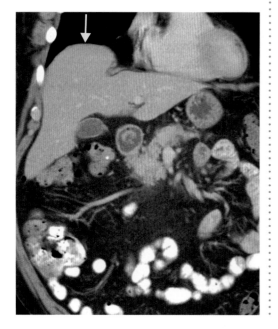

Diaphragmatic eventration

Diaphragmatic eventration is a congenital focal area of replacement of diaphragmatic muscle by fibroelastic tissue, causing elevation of the affected portion of the diaphragm. It is more common on the left. In contrast to congenital dia-phragmatic hernia, the diaphragm remains intact. Coronal CT demonstrates a focal area of thinning of the diaphragm over the liver (arrow). Careful evaluation of contiguous CT slices confirmed that the diaphragm was intact.

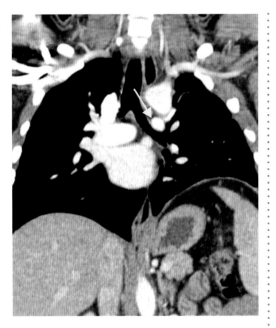

Pulmonary hypoplasia

Pulmonary hypoplasia is incomplete development of a portion of the lungs, resulting in an abnormally low number or size of bronchopulmonary segments or alveoli. It most often occurs secondary to other fetal abnormalities that interfere with normal development of the lungs, such as congenital diaphragmatic hernia and congenital pulmonary airway malformation. Coronal enhanced CT image demonstrates an intact diaphragmatic contour, with small left lung and small left pulmonary artery (arrow), consistent with pulmonary hypoplasia.

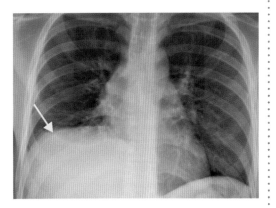

Diaphragmatic paralysis

Unilateral elevation of one hemidiaphragm may be due to phrenic nerve injury. Frontal chest radiograph demonstrates elevation of the right hemidiaphragm (yellow arrow). Coronal enhanced CT demonstrates a large anterior mediastinal mass (red arrow), causing right phrenic nerve paralysis and subsequent right diaphragmatic elevation. The most reliable method to confirm diaphragmatic paralysis is the fluoroscopic sniff test.

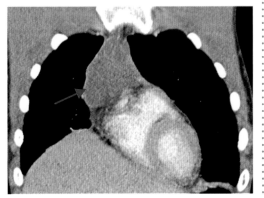

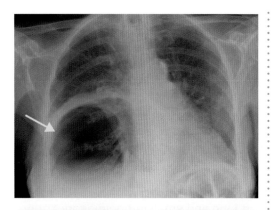

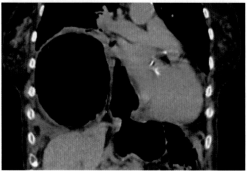

Hiatal hernia

Hiatal hernia consists of herniation of variable portions of the stomach into the chest, through the esophageal hiatus. Hiatal hernia can be classified as a sliding hernia, when the gastroesophageal (GE) junction is superiorly displaced, or a para-esophageal hernia, when the gastric fundus herniates adjacent to the normally located GE junction. A paraesophageal hernia has an increased risk of incarceration in comparison to the sliding type. Frontal chest radiograph shows a large lucent structure (arrow) projecting over the base of the right hemithorax, which could be mistaken for diaphragmatic rupture. Coronal CT image reveals an atypical hiatal hernia, with the gastric fundus located in the right hemithorax.

Further reading

Bodanapally UK, Shanmuganathan K, *et al.* MDCT Diagnosis of Penetrating Diaphragm Injury. *EurRadiol* 2009; 19:1875–1881.

Cadichon B. Pulmonary hypoplasia, in Kumar, P., Burton, B. K., *Congenital Malformations: Evidence-based Evaluation and Management*. 2007, ch. 22.

Desir A, Ghaye B. CT of Blunt Diaphragmatic Rupture. *Radiographics* 2012; 32:477–498.

Iochum S, Ludig T, Walter F, *et al.* Imaging of Diaphragmatic Injury: A Diagnostic Challenge? *Radiographics* 2002; 22:S103–118.

Nason LK, Walker CM, McNeeley MF, *et al.* Imaging of the Diaphragm: Anatomy and Function. *Radiographics* 2012; 32:E51–E70.

Rodríguez MR, de Vega VM, Alonso RC, *et al.* MR Imaging of Thoracic Abnormalities in the Fetus. *Radiographics* 2012; 32:E305–321.

34-year-old male with abdominal and pelvic injuries after a motor vehicle collision

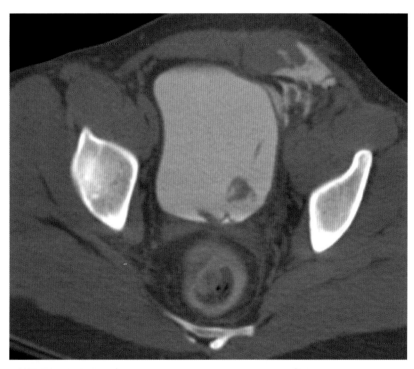

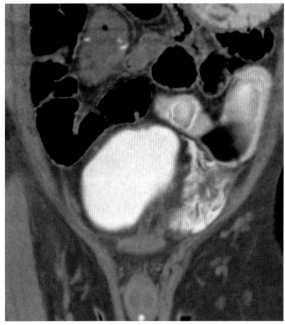

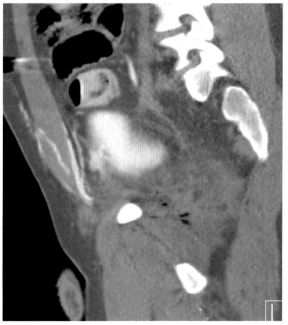

Diagnosis:
Extraperitoneal
bladder
rupture

Axial (left image), coronal (middle image), and sagittal (right image) CT cystogram (with some enteric contrast from a previous examination) demonstrates contrast extravasation from the distended bladder into the extraperitoneal space (yellow arrows) and superficial soft tissues, consistent with a complex extraperitoneal bladder rupture. Filling defects (red arrows) within the bladder likely represent blood clots.

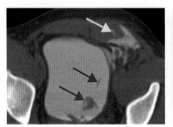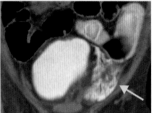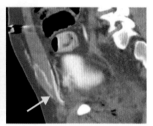

Discussion

Imaging and classification of bladder injuries

- Evaluation of bladder injuries may be accomplished by CT cystogram or conventional cystography, which require retrograde filling of the bladder with 300–400 mL of diluted contrast material by gravity. The bladder must be adequately distended to reliably detect wall disruption. Identifying the site of contrast extravasation is important in localizing the site of rupture. In many trauma centers, CT cystography has supplanted conventional cystography as the preferred modality.
- Accurate classification of bladder injuries is essential in guiding management in the trauma setting. Bladder injuries can be classified into five types based on cystography findings:
  - **Type 1:** Bladder contusion resulting from an incomplete tear in the bladder mucosa. Imaging findings may be normal or simply show mild focal wall thickening.
  - **Type 2:** Intraperitoneal rupture, most commonly occurring at the bladder dome as a result of blunt trauma to a distended bladder. There is increased risk for chemical peritonitis. Conventional and CT cystography findings include contrast extravasation into the peritoneal cavity. Contrast is often most visible in the paracolic gutters and between loops of small bowel.
  - **Type 3:** Interstitial injury resulting from a tear of the serosal surface. This is rare, and imaging findings include a mural defect without contrast extravasation. There may be intravasation of contrast within the bladder wall.

- **Type 4:** Extraperitoneal rupture often occurs anterolaterally near the base of the bladder and is usually associated with pelvic fractures. Conventional and CT cystography findings of extravasation into the extraperitoneal space of Retzius are classified as simple, or Type 4A. With extension into the scrotum, perineum, and thigh, extraperitoneal rupture is classified as complex, or Type 4B.
- **Type 5:** Combined intraperitoneal and extraperitoneal bladder rupture.

Treatment of bladder injuries

- Bladder contusions (Type 1) and interstitial injuries (Type 3) are treated conservatively, with urinary diversion by Foley catheter placement.
- Intraperitoneal ruptures (Type 2) and combined intra- and extraperitoneal ruptures (Type 5) are treated with surgical repair.
- Extraperitoneal ruptures (Type 4) may be treated conservatively with urinary diversion unless the bladder neck is injured, in which case surgical intervention may be required.

Clinical synopsis   The patient was treated conservatively with Foley catheter placement until the urine cleared of blood. Surgical intervention was not required in this case.

Self-assessment

- *What are the imaging findings associated with intraperitoneal rupture, and what is the usual management?*

- The typical imaging appearance is free fluid in the peritoneal cavity on CT performed without cystography. CT cystography shows extravasation from the dome of the distended bladder into the peritoneal cavity. Surgical repair is usually required.

- *What are the imaging findings associated with extraperitoneal bladder rupture, and what is the usual management?*

- Extraperitoneal rupture due to injury to the bladder base is typically identified by contrast extravasation into the prevesical space of Retzius (simple or Type 4A). This may produce the "molar tooth" sign. With extension of contrast into the perineum, thigh, or scrotum, extraperitoneal rupture is classified as complex, or Type 4B. Free fluid in the space of Retzius may indicate the diagnosis on CT without cystography. Concomitant pelvic fractures should be suspected in Type 4 injury. Foley catheter placement is the treatment of choice unless there is injury to the bladder neck, which may require surgical intervention.

• *What is the imaging modality of choice to identify bladder injuries?*

• CT cystography or (less commonly) conventional cystography. In order to achieve high sensitivity, both imaging studies require retrograde filling of the bladder to ensure adequate distention.

Spectrum of bladder injuries

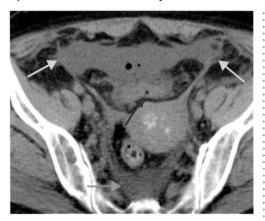

Extraperitoneal bladder rupture

Axial noncontrast CT of the pelvis demonstrates fluid in the space of Retzius (yellow arrows) containing small locules of gas. There is a tiny focus of gas (red arrow) in the neck of the decompressed bladder. The space of Retzius is an extraperitoneal space anterior to the bladder, and is a common location for fluid to accumulate in extraperitoneal rupture. Additional findings include presacral fluid (blue arrow). A calcified uterine fibroid is seen incidentally.

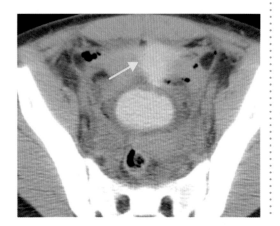

Postsurgical extraperitoneal bladder injury

Axial CT cystogram demonstrates extravasation of contrast from the distended bladder anteriorly into the space of Retzius (arrow) after appendectomy. Several locules of extraluminal gas are noted in the anterior peritoneal cavity, consistent with immediate postoperative state.

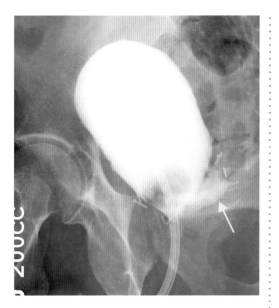

Conventional cystography: extraperitoneal bladder injury as a complication of prostatectomy

Frontal image from a conventional cystogram demonstrates extravasation of contrast (arrow) from the base of the bladder due to injury to the bladder during surgery. Clips are present within the adjacent surgical bed.

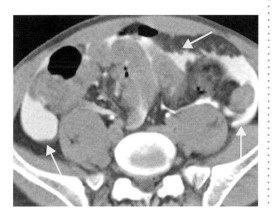

Intraperitoneal bladder rupture

Intraperitoneal bladder rupture (Type 2 injury) is often caused by blunt trauma in the setting of a distended bladder and typically requires surgical repair. Axial image from a CT cystogram demonstrates extravasated contrast (arrows) surrounding small bowel loops and in the paracolic gutters. *Case courtesy Cheryl Sadow, MD.*

Differential diagnosis of bladder injury

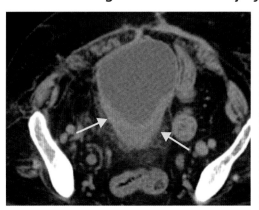

Cystitis

Cystitis is inflammation of the bladder wall due to infection or noninfectious etiologies such as mechanical irritation, drugs (e.g., cyclophosphamide), or radiation. CT findings include bladder wall thickening, perivesical inflammatory fat stranding, and low-density bladder wall edema. Complications of cystitis include abscess formation and, in chronic cases, malignancy. Noncontrast CT shows thickening of the posterior bladder wall (arrows) with perivesical fat stranding.

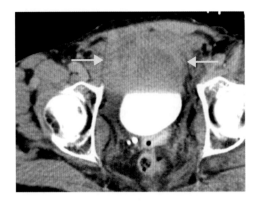

Pelvic hemorrhage in space of Retzius

Enhanced axial CT of the pelvis demonstrates partial filling of the bladder with contrast and a moderate amount of high attenuation material (arrows) in the prevesical space of Retzius representing hemorrhage. The presence of hemorrhagic fluid within this space raises clinical suspicion for bladder injury, but CT cystogram needs to be performed for accurate diagnosis. In this case, no contrast extravasation from the bladder was identified.

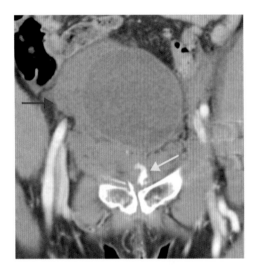

Active hemorrhage due to pelvic fractures

Pelvic fractures can cause vascular injury, which may simulate extravasation of contrast from the bladder, especially if there is any contrast within the urinary system at time of imaging. Coronal enhanced CT shows active extravasation of contrast above the pubic symphysis (yellow arrow). In this case, however, enhancement is in the arterial phase and the free contrast is similar in attenuation to the enhanced iliac vessels. No contrast material is seen in the bladder. There is a moderate amount of hemorrhage surrounding the right bladder wall (red arrow). Multiple pelvic fractures were present but are not pictured. In the context of pelvic fractures and hematoma, CT cystogram is indicated to assess for bladder injury.

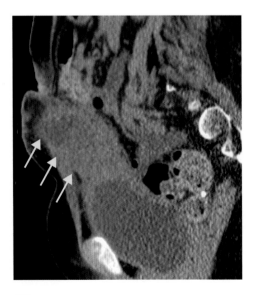

Urachal remnant

A urachal remnant is the result of incomplete obliteration of the allantoic duct, the embryonic connection between the umbilicus and dome of the urinary bladder. The spectrum ranges from a patent urachus providing communication between the bladder dome and umbilicus to a urachal cyst that does not communicate with either the umbilicus or the bladder. Urachal remnants may be mistaken for pelvic hematoma or extravasation, particularly if there is communication with the bladder on cystography. Sagittal unenhanced CT (upper image) demonstrates a patent urachus communicating between the bladder dome and the

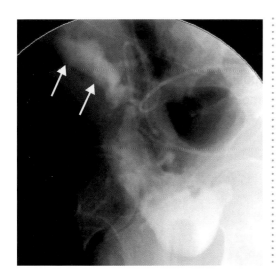

umbilicus (arrows). Sagittal view from a conventional cystogram (lower image) demonstrates contrast communicating between the umbilicus and the bladder (arrows), but no contrast collects within the peritoneal cavity or extraperitoneal space, distinguishing urachal remnant from bladder injury.

Further reading

Morgan DE *et al.*: CT cystography: radiographic and clinical predictors of bladder rupture. *AJR Am J Roentgenol.* 174(1):89–95, 2000

Myers DL: Interstitial cystitis. *Med Health R I.* 92(1):22–26, 2009

Sandler CM: Bladder trauma. In: Pollack HW, ed. *Clinical Urology*. Vol. II. Philadelphia, Pa: Saunders, 1990; 1505–1521.

Vaccaro JP *et al.*: CT cystography in the evaluation of major bladder trauma. *Radiographics.* 20(5):1373–1381, 2000

Grade		
I	Subcapsular hematoma	<10% of surface area
	Laceration	<1 cm in depth
II	Subcapsular hematoma	10–50% of surface area
	Intraparenchymal hematoma	<10 cm diameter
	Laceration	1–3 cm in depth
III	Subcapsular hematoma	>50% of surface area (or expanding in size) or actively bleeding
	Intraparenchymal hematoma	>10 cm diameter or expanding or actively bleeding
	Laceration	>3 cm in depth
IV	Intraparenchymal hematoma	ruptured with active bleeding
	Laceration	parenchymal disruption involving 25–75% of the hepatic lobes or 1–3 Couinaud segments within one lobe
V	Laceration	parenchymal disruption involving >75% of the hepatic lobes or >3 Couinaud segments within one lobe
	Vascular	venous injuries involving the IVC or major hepatic veins
VI	Vascular	hepatic avulsion

- In hemodynamically stable patients, contrast-enhanced CT of the abdomen and pelvis is the imaging modality of choice. CT allows rapid assessment of extent and severity of hepatic injury, particularly active extravasation and vascular injury, as in the index case, in addition to injuries involving other organs. Unstable patients usually undergo emergent exploratory laparotomy without imaging.

Clinical synopsis	The patient was diagnosed with severe hepatic injury, including active extravasation into the peritoneum. Due to hemodynamic instability, interventional radiologists performed angiography and arterial embolization. The patient was then transferred to the ICU.

Self-assessment

- *What is the most common cause of hepatic injury?*

- *What additional injuries should be sought with the finding of left hepatic lobe injury?*

- Blunt trauma. Additional causes are penetrating and iatrogenic trauma.

- Left hepatic lobe injuries may be associated with concurrent bowel and pancreatic injuries.

Spectrum of hepatic trauma

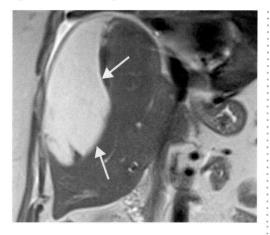

Subcapsular hematoma

Subcapsular hematomas most often occur at the anterolateral aspect of the right hepatic lobe, and can be associated with an overlying rib fracture. They are lenticular in shape and can flatten the adjacent liver parenchyma. Coronal T2-weighted MRI demonstrates a large, hyperintense subcapsular fluid collection (arrows) in this patient on warfarin with a history of minor trauma.

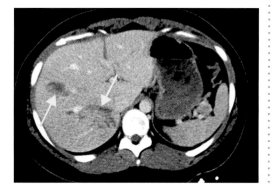

Grade III hepatic laceration

A grade III hepatic laceration is >3 cm in depth. Axial contrast-enhanced CT demonstrates multiple linear, low-attenuation defects (arrows) involving the right lobe of the liver, with the largest >3 cm in length.

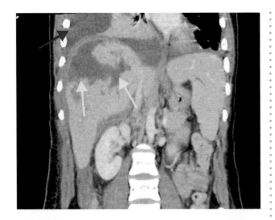

Grade III/IV hepatic laceration

Enhanced coronal CT demonstrates an irregular region of low attenuation >3 cm in diameter (yellow arrows) extending from the liver capsule into the hepatic parenchyma. A grade III injury is >3 cm in diameter, which this clearly is; however, there is probable disruption of at least 25% of the parenchyma, which would make this a grade IV injury. Note the presence of a large adjacent hemothorax (red arrow).

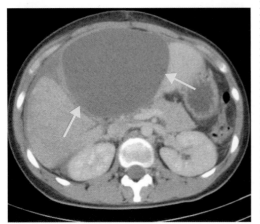

Post-traumatic biloma

A biloma is the result of a sequestered bile leak. They are typically slow-growing and may take weeks to months to develop due to the slow rate of bile leakage. Axial enhanced CT in a patient who suffered hepatic trauma requiring angiographic embolization 3 weeks earlier demonstrates a large, well-defined low-attenuation collection (arrows) splaying the hepatic parenchyma. This collection was subsequently drained and was proven to be a biloma.

Differential diagnosis of liver trauma

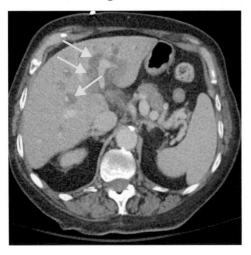

Cholangitis

Acute cholangitis is infection (usually bacterial) of the biliary system and is potentially life-threatening. It may be caused by obstruction of the biliary tree. CT findings may be nonspecific, and correlation with clinical presentation is essential. On imaging, it is important to attempt to assess for the cause and degree of biliary obstruction. Trauma is not a feature of the clinical history. This 67-year-old male presented with jaundice, abdominal pain, and fever. Axial enhanced CT demonstrates biliary ductal dilatation as tubular areas of decreased attenuation (arrows) adjacent to the portal veins throughout the liver. A common bile duct stone was found on ERCP (not shown).

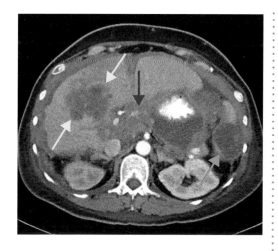

Hepatic metastasis

Liver metastasis is the most common malignant liver lesion. Metastasis may be isolated or multiple. Hypervascular liver metastases include neuroendocrine, thyroid, and renal cancers, as well as melanoma and sarcoma. Hypovascular liver metastases include lung, gastrointestinal, pancreas, bladder, and uterine cancers. Lymphoma may also present as a low-attenuation hepatic mass. Enhanced axial CT in a patient with metastatic colon cancer demonstrates an ill-defined, low-attenuation mass in the right lobe of the liver (yellow arrows). There is also low-attenuation retroperitoneal lymphadenopathy (red arrow), a low-attenuation splenic mass (blue arrow), and trace ascites.

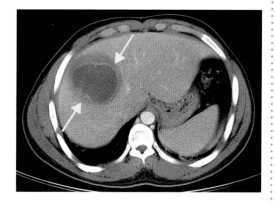

Pyogenic hepatic abscess

The most common pyogenic organisms to cause hepatic abscesses are *Klebsiella pneumoniae* in adults and *Staphylococcus aureus* in children. Abscess and metastasis may appear similar on CT; however, the clinical history is useful for differentiating between the two entities. Treatment consists of IV antibiotics and percutaneous drainage. Axial enhanced CT demonstrates a well-defined, low-attenuation, rim-enhancing lesion (arrows) in the right lobe of the liver in this patient who presented with fevers and abdominal pain.

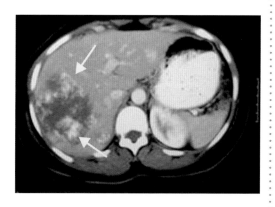

Hepatic hemangioma

A hemangioma is the most common benign tumor in the liver. It is composed of a network of vascular elements that are irregular in size and shape. Axial enhanced CT demonstrates a large hypoattenuating right hepatic lobe lesion (arrows) with the typical enhancement pattern of a hemangioma with peripheral, discontinuous, nodular enhancement. Delayed imaging (not shown) of hemangioma would show progressive centripetal filling in from periphery to center of the lesion.

Further reading

Horton, K. *et al*. CT and MR Imaging of Benign Hepatic and Biliary Tumors. *Radiographics*. March 1999; 19: 431–451

Malaki, M., Mangat, K. Hepatic and Splenic Trauma. *Trauma*. July 2011; 13(3): 233–244

Shanmuganathan, K., Jen-Dar, C., Mirvis, S. E. Imaging Blunt Hepatic Trauma. *Applied Radiology*. April 2000; 29(4)

Yoon, W. *et al*. CT in Blunt Liver Trauma. *Radiographics*. January 2005; 25: 87–104

Zealley, I. A., Chakraverty, S. The Role of Interventional Radiology in Trauma. *BMJ*. February 8 , 2010; 340: C497.

Case 62   38-year-old male complaining of diffuse abdominal pain after a motor vehicle collision

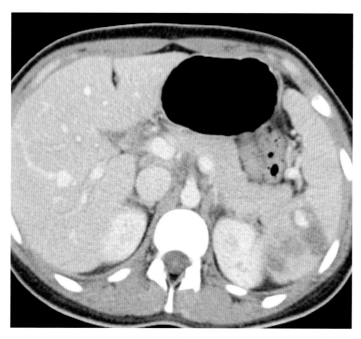

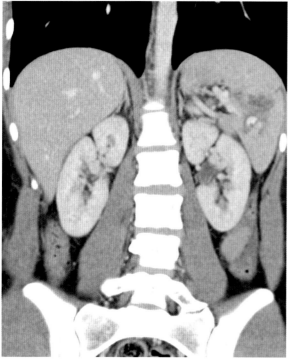

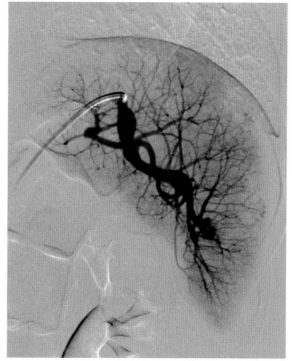

Diagnosis:
Grade 3 splenic laceration with splenic artery pseudo-aneurysms

Axial (left image) and coronal (middle image) enhanced CT demonstrate an irregular, low-attenuation defect (yellow arrows) in the spleen greater than 3 cm in length, consistent with a grade 3 laceration. There is a round focus of increased attenuation adjacent to the laceration (red arrows) that is similar in attenuation to the arterial tree, consistent with a vascular injury (active extravasation or pseudoaneurysm). Subsequent digital subtraction angiogram (right image) of the splenic artery confirms the presence of two adjacent pseudoaneurysms in the lower pole of the spleen (blue arrow).

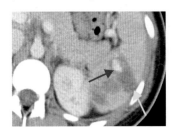 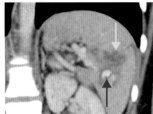 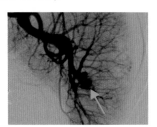

Discussion

Overview of splenic trauma

- The spleen is the abdominal organ that is most often injured in trauma. The majority of splenic injuries are caused by blunt abdominal trauma. Associated injuries frequently involve the left hemithorax, pancreatic tail, and left hepatic lobe.

Imaging of splenic trauma

- Contrast-enhanced CT is the imaging modality of choice in suspected splenic trauma. Splenic laceration appears as a low-attenuation, irregular, linear, or wedge-shaped hypodense defect extending from the splenic margin. It may be associated with hemoperitoneum, active extravasation, pseudoaneurysm, or subcapsular hematoma.
- High-grade injuries may result in vascular disruption, which can be seen as active extravasation or a traumatic pseudoaneurysm, as in the index case. Contrast extravasation or "blush" on CT suggests active hemorrhage.

Grading of splenic trauma

- The most commonly used grading system is published by the AAST:

Grade	
I	Laceration <1 cm depth; or subcapsular hematoma involving <10% of splenic surface area.
II	Laceration 1–3 cm depth; or subcapsular hematoma involving 10–50% of splenic surface area; or intraparenchymal hematoma <5 cm in diameter.
III	Laceration >3 cm depth; or subcapsular hematoma involving >50% of splenic surface area or expanding with active hemorrhage; or intraparenchymal hemorrhage >5 cm diameter.
IV	Laceration extending to the splenic hilum; or ruptured intraparenchymal hematoma with active bleeding.
V	Shattered spleen.

Treatment of splenic trauma

- Treatment of traumatic splenic injury varies by institution.
- Imaging findings are critical to the multidisciplinary management of the patient, as the natural course may vary from spontaneous hemostasis to hemodynamic instability. While the former is often managed with watchful waiting or serial imaging, the latter requires emergent transcatheter embolization or splenectomy.
- Due to the deleterious effects of splenectomy on immune function, the trend is for conservative treatment except in unstable or potentially unstable patients.

Clinical synopsis The patient underwent successful angiographic coil embolization of the splenic artery.

Self-assessment

- *Name three types of injuries that typically occur with splenic trauma.*

- Subcapsular hematoma, laceration, fracture, pseudoaneurysm, and active extravasation.

- *What is the imaging modality of choice for evaluation of splenic trauma?*

- Contrast-enhanced CT is the imaging modality of choice because it is readily available at most institutions and provides a fast and accurate assessment of the extent of injury and associated complications.

- *Name three other sites that should be carefully inspected for injury when splenic injury is diagnosed.*

- Left lobe of the liver, pancreatic tail, and left hemithorax.

Spectrum of splenic trauma

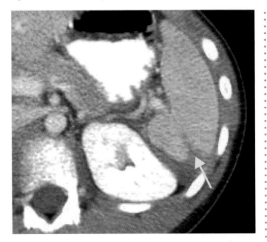

Laceration (grade II)

Enhanced axial CT image demonstrates a hypodense, wedge-shaped defect (arrow) extending from the splenic surface. The laceration is between 1 and 3 cm in depth, consistent with a grade II injury. Splenic lacerations may be irregular, linear, or wedge-shaped and may be associated with extravasation, pseudoaneurysm formation, hemoperitoneum, or subcapsular hematoma.

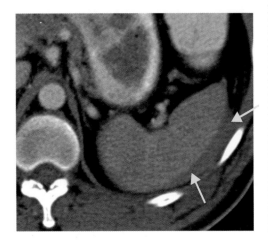

Subcapsular hematoma (grade III)

Contrast-enhanced axial CT demonstrates a crescentic, low-attenuation collection (arrows) along the lateral margin of the spleen, with flattening of its normal contour, consistent with a subcapsular hematoma. Hematomas can be intraparenchymal or subcapsular in location. Intrasplenic hematomas may be hypo- or hyperdense on noncontrast CT, with poor enhancement on postcontrast images. This case is a grade II splenic injury as the subcapsular hematoma involves between 10 and 50% of the splenic surface area.

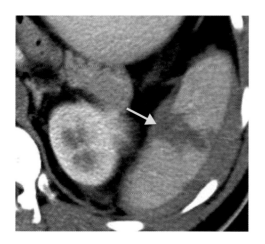

Splenic fracture (grade IV)

Axial contrast-enhanced CT shows an irregular, transverse, low density band (arrow) coursing through the splenic midpole with separation of the ventral and dorsal fragments. Splenic fracture is defined as a laceration extending from the outer cortex to the hilum with complete separation of fragments. Multiple fractures result in a shattered spleen.

Differential diagnosis of splenic trauma

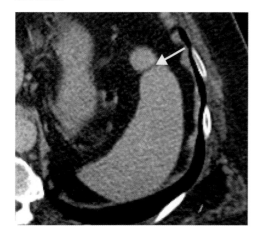

Splenic cleft

Grooves that normally separate the splenic lobules may appear as notches or clefts. Notches and clefts are usually seen along the inferior margin of the spleen and can be as deep as 2–3 cm. A cleft should not be mistaken for a laceration in a trauma patient. Axial enhanced CT demonstrates a splenic cleft as a thin, regular, hypoattenuating line (arrow) in the anterior aspect of the spleen. At the edges of the cleft, there are subtle indentations in the splenic contour.

Splenic abscess

Splenic abscesses are usually a complication of infarction, trauma, septic embolism, or direct extension of infection. Diagnosis is critical for appropriate management, as splenic abscesses are associated with high mortality if unrecognized. The typical appearance of splenic abscess is a low-density intrasplenic fluid collection with internal gas or fluid–fluid levels. There may be perilesional enhancement. Axial contrast-enhanced CT demonstrates a large intrasplenic collection with a gas–fluid level (arrow) and several locules of gas medially. The collection extends into the splenic hilum.

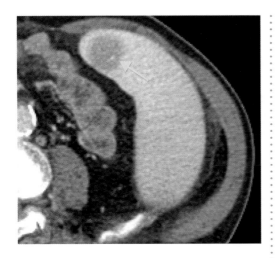

Splenic metastasis

Splenic metastases are rare. They may present as single or multiple masses. Colorectal and endometrial cancer are the most common primary malignancies associated with solitary splenic metastasis. Breast, lung, colorectal, and ovarian carcinomas, and melanoma, are the most common primary malignancies that present with disseminated splenic metastases. Axial contrast-enhanced CT shows an ill-defined, round, hypodense mass in the anterior aspect of the spleen (arrow) in this patient with metastatic lung cancer.

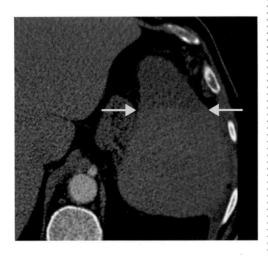

Splenic infarct

Splenic infarction occurs when the splenic artery or one of its branches is occluded. Splenic infarcts are most commonly caused by cardiac thromboembolism, such as from atrial fibrillation. Other etiologies of thrombosis include pancreatitis, infection, myelofibrosis, sickle cell disease, malignancy, and vasculitis. On CT, splenic infarction is most commonly seen as a poorly enhancing region of decreased density, which classically is peripheral and wedge-shaped. Axial unenhanced CT demonstrates a triangular-shaped region of decreased attenuation in the anterior spleen (arrows).

Further reading

G Agrawal, P Johnson, E Fishman. Splenic artery aneurysms and pseudoaneurysms: clinical distinctions and CT appearances. *AJR* 2007; 188:992–999.

S Anderson, J Varghese, B Lucey, et al. Blunt splenic trauma: delayed phase CT for differentiation of active hemorrhage from contained vascular injury in patients. *Radiology* April 2007; 243:88–95.

CD Becker et al. The trauma concept: the role of MDCT in the diagnosis and management of visceral injuries. *Eur Radiol* 2005; 15 Suppl. 4:105–109.

N Dalrymple, J Leyendecker, M Oliphant. (2009) *Problem Solving in Abdominal Imaging*. Philadelphia, PA: Elsevier.

AM de Schepper, F Vanhoenacker. (2000) *Medical Imaging of the Spleen*. Berlin: Springer-Verlag.

F Ferrozzi, D Bova, F Draghi, *et al*. CT findings in primary vascular tumors of the spleen. *AJR* 1996; 166:1097–1101.

G Gayer, R Zissin, S Apter, *et al*. CT findings in congenital anomalies of the spleen. *Br J Radiol* 2001; 74:767–772.

LS Rabushka, A Kawashima, EK Fishman. Imaging of the spleen: CT with supplemental MR examination. *Radiographics* March 1994; 14:307–332.

35-year-old male who lost control of his bicycle and fell onto his right side presented with right flank pain

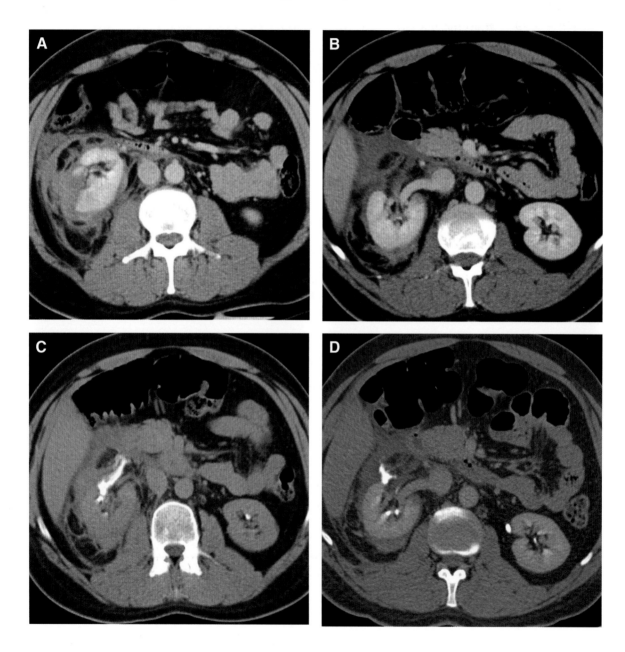

**Diagnosis:
Renal
laceration
extending into
the collecting
system
(Grade IV
traumatic
renal injury)**

Contrast-enhanced axial CT (A,B) demonstrates a deep right renal laceration (yellow arrows) with hyperdense, hemorrhagic perinephric fluid. A small hypoenhancing parenchymal contusion is also seen medially (red arrow). Delayed, excretory phase axial images (C,D) show excreted contrast leakage from the injured collecting system (blue arrows).

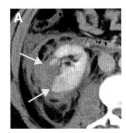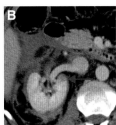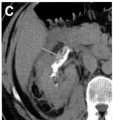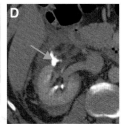

Discussion

Overview of renal trauma

- The kidneys are the most commonly traumatically injured organ in children and the third most commonly injured organ (after the spleen and liver) in adults. Blunt trauma accounts for 90% of renal injuries.

Imaging of suspected renal injury

- Imaging is not essential in every case of suspected renal injury. Established indications for imaging differ for adults and pediatric patients, and also depend on the mechanism of injury (blunt versus penetrating injury).
- Blunt abdominal trauma in adults: patients with gross hematuria OR microscopic hematuria with shock (systolic blood pressure <90 mmHg) should be imaged. Microscopic hematuria in the absence of shock is not an indication for imaging.
- Blunt abdominal trauma in children: patients with microscopic or gross hematuria should be imaged, irrespective of blood pressure.
- Penetrating trauma: all patients, irrespective of age or whether hematuria is present, should be imaged.
- Contrast-enhanced CT is the primary modality for assessing renal injury. Imaging during multiple phases of enhancement is often required for adequate evaluation of the renal parenchyma, vasculature, and collecting system. Routine images are obtained in the portal venous phase. Delayed phase images, if necessary, are typically obtained 3–5 minutes after the initial injection of contrast material. Ideally, a radiologist is present at the CT scanner at the time of imaging to decide whether delayed phase images are needed.

- If a renal laceration is detected during the portal venous phase, or if there is unexplained perinephric fluid, a delayed scan should generally be performed to assess for extension of injury into the collecting system. Extravasation of opacified urine from the collecting system confirms this injury.
- If a contrast blush is detected on the portal venous phase, delayed imaging (in a hemodynamically stable patient) can help differentiate a contained traumatic pseudoaneurysm or arteriovenous fistula from active intraparenchymal bleeding: free contrast extravasation persists on delayed phase imaging, while the contained vascular injuries will wash out. Stable patients with active bleeding (persistent and/or enlarging contrast blush) are often referred for emergent angiographic embolization.

Classification of traumatic renal injuries

- Various classification systems exist. The most commonly referenced grading system is the organ injury scale (OIS) from the AAST.

Grade	Injury description	
I	Contusion	Microscopic or gross hematuria
	Hematoma	Subcapsular, nonexpanding hematoma without laceration
II	Hematoma	Nonexpanding perirenal hematoma confined to renal retroperitoneum
	Laceration	<1 cm parenchymal depth of renal cortex without urinary extravasation
III	Laceration	>1 cm parenchymal depth of renal cortex without urinary extravasation or collecting system rupture
IV	Laceration	Parenchymal laceration extending through the renal cortex, medulla, and collecting system
	Vascular	Traumatic thrombosis of a segmental renal artery branch or injury to the main renal artery without complete renal devascularization
V	Laceration	Completely shattered kidney
	Vascular	Avulsion of the renal hilum with complete renal devascularization, or traumatic main renal artery thrombosis

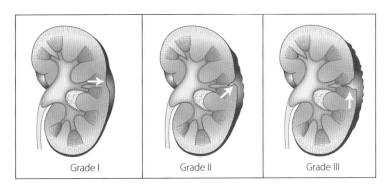

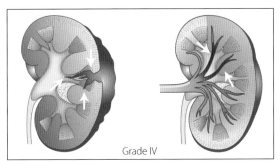

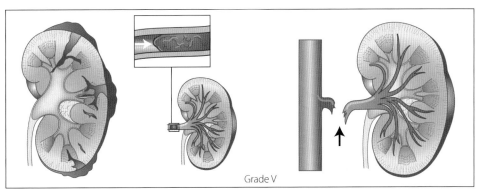

Renal trauma grading scale

Clinical synopsis

The patient was managed without surgical intervention and discharged from the Emergency Department. Following discharge, he developed hematuria and a repeat emergent CT was performed to reassess the injury and evaluate for complications. There was no change in the renal laceration and the urinary leak had resolved. The patient recovered uneventfully without further treatment.

Self-assessment

- *Is imaging required in all trauma patients with hematuria?*

- No. Imaging is not required in adult blunt trauma patients with microscopic hematuria.

- *What pre-existing renal abnormalities predispose patients to traumatic renal injury?*

- Congenital anomalies (e.g., horseshoe kidney, renal ectopia, polycystic kidney disease, congenital ureteropelvic junction obstruction).
- Chronic hydronephrosis.
- Cysts.
- Tumors.

- *What are some of the complications that can be seen with traumatic renal injury?*

- Urinoma (if there is collecting system injury).
- Delayed bleeding.
- Pseudoaneurysm.
- Abscess.
- Hypertension.

Spectrum of traumatic renal injury

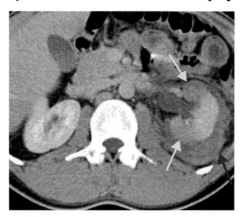

Contusion

Axial contrast-enhanced CT in the parenchymal phase shows ill-defined areas of decreased parenchymal enhancement (yellow arrows). There is a mixed density perinephric hematoma (red arrow). Contusions are typically round or oval-shaped and are categorized as grade I injuries. They may look similar to renal infarcts; however, contusions enhance and retain contrast on delayed phase images, whereas infarcts do not enhance. This is an OIS grade I injury (contusion with perinephric hematoma).

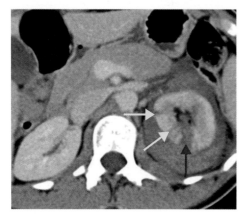

Laceration

Axial contrast-enhanced CT in the parenchymal phase shows linear, non-enhancing parenchymal defects representing superficial (yellow arrows) and deep (red arrow) lacerations. As in this case, renal lacerations are often seen in conjunction with perinephric hematoma, which indicates capsular rupture. The depth of the laceration (greater than or less than 1 cm) and the presence or absence of collecting system injury are key factors for accurate grading. This is at least an OIS grade III injury. Delayed images would be necessary to distinguish between grade III and grade IV injury involving the collecting system.

Subcapsular hematoma

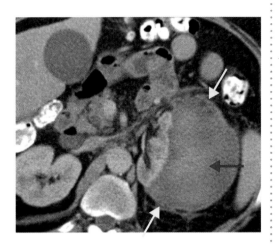

Axial contrast-enhanced CT in the parenchymal phase shows a large crescent-shaped hematoma contained by the renal capsule (yellow arrows) and exerting significant mass effect on the left kidney. Amorphous increased attenuation within the hematoma reflects clotted blood (red arrow). If hematoma persists, impairment of blood flow into the kidney due to compression may result in hypertension, as occurred in this patient. New onset hypertension due to a subcapsular collection is referred to as "Page kidney" (named after Irvine Page, who discovered the condition in 1939 by wrapping cellophane around dogs' kidneys).

Active hemorrhage due to vascular injury

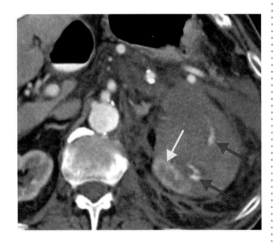

Axial contrast-enhanced parenchymal phase CT shows a large hematoma in the left upper quadrant with surrounding fat stranding. There is posteromedial mass effect on the left kidney (yellow arrow). Ectopic areas of intense contrast blush (red arrows; similar in intensity to the aorta) indicate vascular injury. These are usually located within a laceration or hematoma. The appearance is nonspecific, and delayed images can help differentiate active arterial extravasation (in which enhancement persists on delayed images) from a post-traumatic pseudoaneurysm or AV fistula (which wash out on delayed images).

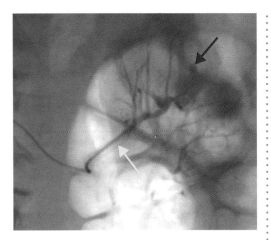

Pseudoaneurysm

Selective conventional arteriogram of the left renal artery (yellow arrow) shows a small pseudoaneurysm (red arrow) in the upper pole of the left kidney. It is critical to identify pseudoaneurysms (contained foci of extravasation), as rupture can result in catastrophic blood loss. Penetrating trauma is a common cause. Pseudoaneurysms may be identified in either the acute or subacute setting. Increasing or new hematuria should prompt repeat imaging to unmask a pseudoaneurysm that was initially filled with acute thrombus.

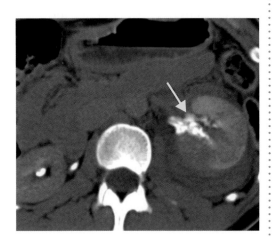

Urinary extravasation due to collecting system injury

Extravasation of contrast from the urinary collecting system (arrow) in this axial delayed phase contrast-enhanced CT image indicates at least a grade IV injury. Most urinary leaks resolve spontaneously without surgical intervention. Urinomas (urine collections lined with fibrous tissue) are a common complication, and these may become secondarily infected. Follow up CT is used to monitor urinary leaks and guide percutaneous drainage of collections.

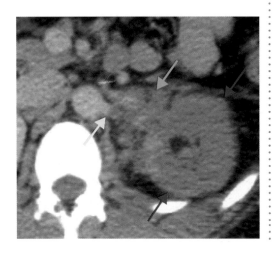

Traumatic renal artery thrombosis

Axial parenchymal-phase contrast-enhanced CT shows abrupt cut-off of the left main renal artery (yellow arrow), hypoenhancement of the left kidney (red arrows), and hematoma surrounding the renal artery and hilum (blue arrow) in this patient with grade V traumatic renal injury. It is imperative to detect and treat global renal ischemia urgently, since permanent loss of renal function occurs after about 4 hours.

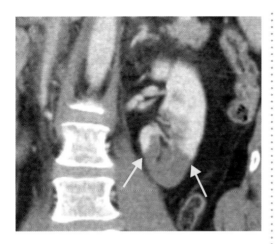

Post-traumatic segmental infarct

As demonstrated by this coronal parenchymal-phase contrast-enhanced CT image in a patient with grade IV traumatic renal injury, segmental infarcts are typically well-demarcated, wedge-shaped areas of parenchymal nonenhancement (arrows). A rapid deceleration mechanism causes arterial intimal dissection, which leads to thrombosis and infarction in the distribution of the affected artery.

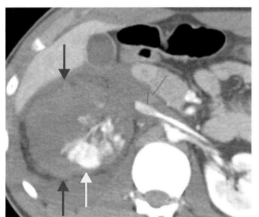

Shattered kidney

This grade V injury is characterized by gross disruption of the renal parenchyma due to a combination of lacerations and subsegmental infarcts. This axial contrast-enhanced portal venous phase CT shows a shattered and partially devascularized right kidney (yellow arrow) surrounded by a large hematoma (red arrows). The IVC (blue arrow) is flattened due to hypovolemic shock.

Differential diagnosis of traumatic renal injury

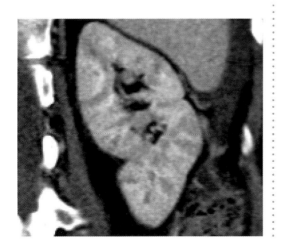

The absence of a history of trauma and pertinent positive findings in the clinical history are key in differentiating renal trauma from these mimics.

Striated nephrogram due to pyelonephritis

There are numerous hypoenhancing wedge-shaped areas that give the kidneys a striated appearance on this coronal nephrographic phase contrast-enhanced CT in a patient with bilateral pyelonephritis. The linear areas of decreased enhancement can mimic lacerations or traumatic subsegmental infarcts. This appearance may also be seen in renal vein thrombosis, acute tubular necrosis, and acute hydronephrosis.

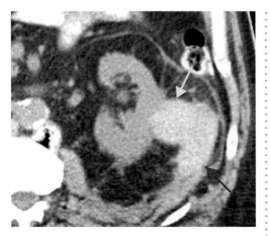

Ruptured hemorrhagic renal cyst

If the amount of bleeding is out of proportion to the severity of trauma, a pre-existing renal abnormality should be considered. Thus, short-interval follow-up MRI or CT should be performed after resolution of acute hematoma. Axial enhanced CT demonstrates a hyperdense left renal cyst (yellow arrow) with rupture into the perinephric space (red arrow). The presence of a cyst or tumor increases the risk of traumatic hemorrhage, and vascular masses such as renal cell carcinoma and angiomyolipoma (AML) commonly rupture and bleed.

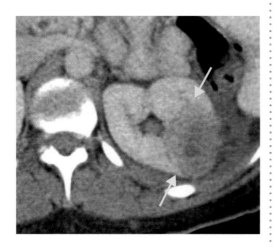

Pyelonephritis with renal abscess

Pyelonephritis affecting a focal area of the renal parenchyma can mimic contusion or infarct. This region of ill-defined hypoperfusion (arrows) on an axial contrast-enhanced CT image in the parenchymal phase was due to a developing abscess. Focal pyelonephritis and abscess tend to have ill-defined margins and are less geographic in distribution. Affected patients may be septic and will lack a history of trauma.

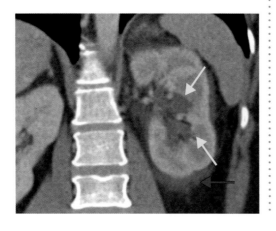

Forniceal rupture due to hydronephrosis

In severe or acute hydronephrosis, backflow pressure into the calyces can cause rupture of a fornix, which allows water-attenuation urine to leak out of the collecting system and into the perinephric space, surrounding the kidney and mimicking perinephric urine from traumatic collecting system injury. Coronal enhanced CT demonstrates fullness of the collecting system with calyceal blunting (yellow arrows) and water-attenuation perinephric fluid (red arrow).

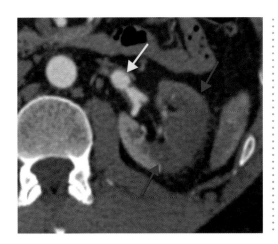

Renal infarction

Infarction may be due to trauma, embolism, or arterial thrombosis. Infarcts are typically wedge-shaped, cortically based, hypoenhancing areas of parenchyma. This axial contrast-enhanced CT image in the nephrographic phase demonstrates a pseudoaneurysm (yellow arrow) of the renal artery and subsegmental infarction of the left kidney (red arrows), due to distal embolism.

Further reading

Page, I. H. (1939). The production of persistent arterial hypertension by cellophane perinephritis. *JAMA* 113(23), 2046–2048

Park, S. J., Kim, J. K., Kim, K. W., & Cho, K.-S. (2006). MDCT findings of renal trauma. *AJR. American journal of roentgenology* 187(2), 541–547.

Ramchandani, P., & Buckler, P. M. (2009). Imaging of genitourinary trauma. *AJR. American journal of roentgenology* 192(6), 1514–1523.

Srinivasa, R. N., Akbar, S. A., Jafri, S. Z., & Howells, G. A. (2009). Genitourinary trauma: a pictorial essay. *Emergency radiology* 16(1), 21–33.

Torreggiani, W. C., & Marchinkow, L. O. (2001). CT Findings in Blunt Renal Trauma 1 OBJECTIVES, 201–214.

West, O. C., Tamm, E. P., Fishman, E. K., & Goldman, S. M. (2001). Imaging of Renal Trauma: A Comprehensive Review 1 OBJECTIVES, 55905, 557–574.

Case 64   37-year-old female with worsening right lower quadrant pain and fever
after laparoscopic appendectomy

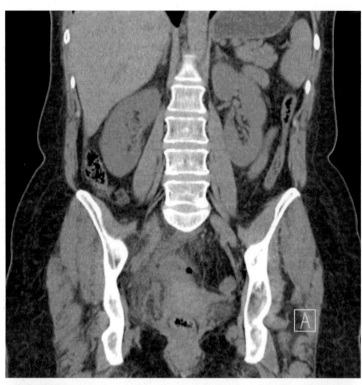

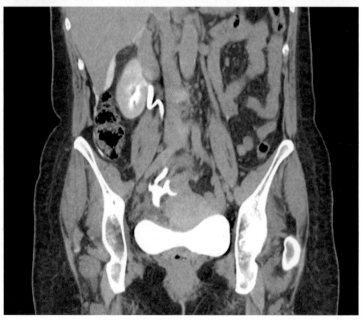

Diagnosis:
Distal right
ureteral
injury

Unenhanced coronal CT of the abdomen and pelvis (left image) demonstrates fat stranding and fluid in the right hemipelvis, in the vicinity of the right distal ureter (yellow arrows). Delayed coronal CT (right image) obtained 15 minutes after administration of IV contrast demonstrates opacification of the right renal collecting system and ureter, with an irregular collection of extraluminal contrast denoting injury of the distal right ureter (red arrow).

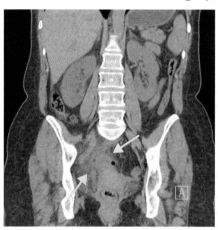 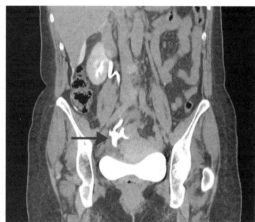

Discussion

- Ureteral injury may result from blunt, penetrating, or iatrogenic trauma. The most common cause of ureteral injury is iatrogenic trauma (80–90%) incurred with gynecologic, urinary tract, retroperitoneal, and pelvic surgeries.
- Delayed diagnosis is common due to the nonspecific clinical presentation.
- Penetrating injury may result in direct transection of the ureter and is usually accompanied by other intra-abdominal injuries. Blunt trauma from deceleration mechanisms may cause avulsion at the ureteropelvic junction.
- The AAST classification of ureteral injury is as follows:
  - Grade I – Hematoma; contusion or hematoma without devascularization
  - Grade II – Laceration; <50% transection
  - Grade III – Laceration; >/= 50% transection
  - Grade IV – Laceration; complete transection with <2 cm devascularization
  - Grade V – Laceration; avulsion with >2 cm devascularization
  - *Advance one grade for bilateral injury, grades I–III.
- Contrast-enhanced CT of the abdomen and pelvis must include a delayed phase (10–20 minutes after contrast administration) to adequately assess the renal collecting systems and ureters. A less frequently used alternative is fluoroscopic retrograde pyelography. Scintigraphy may be used in patients who are unable to receive iodinated contrast (e.g., due to renal failure or contrast allergy).

- Treatment varies based on severity. A ureteral stent may be left in place for 4–8 weeks to promote uroepithelial healing. Associated urinomas may be drained percutaneously. Early identification leads to improved clinical outcomes. When diagnosis is delayed, ureteral strictures may form, necessitating balloon dilatation. Surgery is typically reserved for cases of complete ureteral transection or strictures that do not improve with balloon dilatation.

Clinical synopsis   The patient was admitted to the hospital for a short period of time, and a ureteral stent was left in place for approximately 8 weeks. Upon removal of the ureteral stent, repeat imaging showed no extraluminal contrast or urinary obstruction, indicating complete ureteral healing.

Self-assessment

- *What is the most common cause of ureteral injury?*

- Iatrogenic trauma.

- *Which imaging phase of a contrast-enhanced CT is optimal for diagnosis of ureteral injuries, 30 seconds, 70 seconds, or 10–20 minutes after IV contrast?*

- The delayed/excretory phase (10–20 minutes after administration of IV contrast) is necessary for opacification of the ureters and identification of extraluminal contrast collections.

Spectrum of ureteral injury

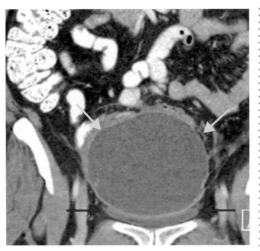

Iatrogenic ureteral injury (3 different patients)

Portal venous phase enhanced coronal CT (upper image) of the pelvis demonstrates a large, round, midline fluid collection (yellow arrows) compressing the bladder (red arrows). The differential diagnosis included abscess and urinoma. Delayed phase axial CT (lower image) obtained 20 minutes later demonstrates opacification of the irregular collection, which indicated contiguity with the collecting system and confirmed the diagnosis of urinoma.

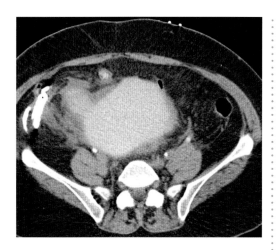

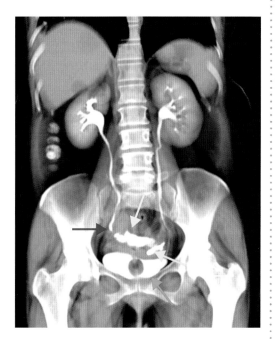

In a different patient, a MIP coronal CT image obtained in the delayed phase demonstrates an irregular collection of extraluminal contrast (yellow arrows) near the distal right ureter, which has an acute cut-off (red arrow). The intact left ureter fills the bladder (blue arrow), which contains a Foley catheter balloon.

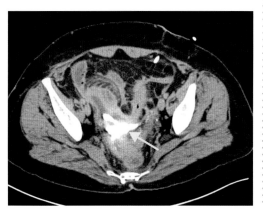

In a different patient, delayed axial enhanced CT of the pelvis demonstrates extraluminal pooling of contrast in the right hemipelvis (arrow), in the region of the right distal ureter. There is surrounding reactive inflammatory stranding and free fluid, consistent with extravasation of urine.

Differential of ureteral injury

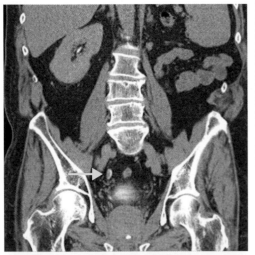

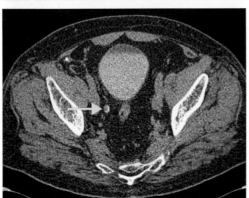

Transitional cell carcinoma (TCC)

TCC accounts for approximately 10% of upper urinary tract neoplasms; 25% are ureteral. Hematuria is typical. Ureteral TCC is often multicentric, necessitating imaging of the entire urinary tract in staging and follow-up. Coronal and axial delayed phase enhanced CT images demonstrate a soft tissue density filling defect in the distal right ureter (arrows).

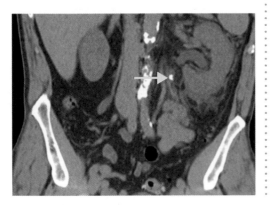

Ureteral calculus

CT imaging findings of calculi include the "soft tissue rim" sign caused by the edematous surrounding ureter, which may differentiate a ureteral calculus from a phlebolith. Most stones <5 mm in size pass spontaneously. Unenhanced coronal CT demonstrates an obstructing radiopaque stone (arrow) in the proximal left ureter, with left hydronephrosis and perinephric stranding.

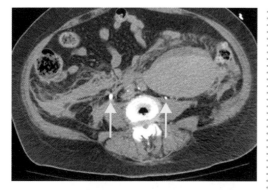

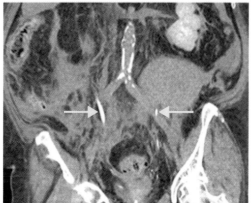

Retroperitoneal hematoma (RPH)

RPH may occur in the setting of trauma or invasive procedures, or due to hemorrhage of vascular lesions such as angiomyolipomas. Patients with coagulopathy are particularly susceptible. Delayed contrast-enhanced axial and coronal CT images of a patient who experienced trauma demonstrate free right retroperitoneal hemorrhage and stranding in addition to a large, left RPH with a hematocrit level. The ureters (arrows) are opacified and are separate from these injuries, without extraluminal contrast to indicate ureteral injury.

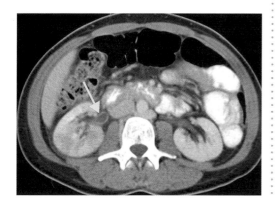

Ureteral infection

In this patient with fever, flank pain, and pyuria, contrast-enhanced axial CT demonstrates thickening and abnormal enhancement of the right proximal ureteral uroepithelium (arrow). The right kidney is enlarged and edematous, with heterogeneous perfusion and mild perinephric stranding, indicating pyelonephritis. If the patient lacked septic presentation, urothelial malignancy could also be considered.

Further reading

Browne R et al. Transitional cell carcinoma of the upper urinary tract: spectrum of imaging findings. *Radiographics*. 25: 1609–1627, November 2005.

Ortega SJ et al. CT scanning for diagnosing blunt ureteral and ureteropelvic junction injuries. *BMC Urol*. 8(3): 2008.

Parpala-Spårman T et al. Increasing numbers of ureteric injuries after the introduction of laparoscopic surgery. *Scand J Urol Nephrol*. 42(5):422–427, 2008.

Ramachandani P, Buckler PM. Imaging of genitourinary trauma. *AJR*. 192(6): 1514–1523, June 2009.

Case 65   28-year-old female with diffuse lower abdominal pain referred from an outpatient clinic for clinical suspicion of uterine perforation during a therapeutic abortion

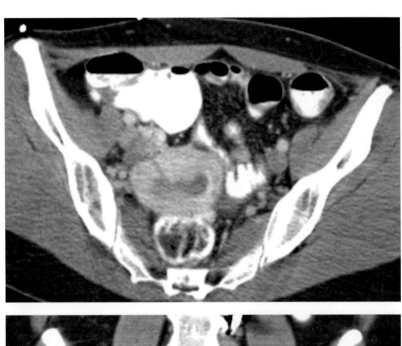

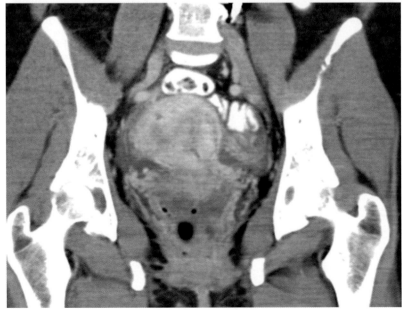

Diagnosis:
Uterine perforation as a complication of therapeutic abortion

Axial and coronal contrast-enhanced CT of the pelvis show a linear low-attenuation defect (arrows) through the right anterior, inferior wall of the uterus and a small amount of free fluid, consistent with focal uterine perforation secondary to instrumentation.

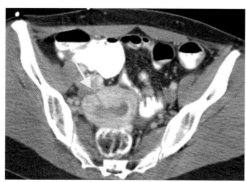 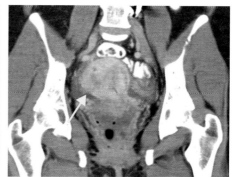

Discussion

The majority of patients with uterine rupture have a history of prior cesarean section.

- Uterine rupture most commonly occurs in women of childbearing age during pregnancy, labor, or the postpartum period. Uterine perforation may also occur due to instrumentation or trauma. Any site of prior uterine incision is predisposed to perforation.
- Classic vertical cesarean section scars are more likely to rupture before labor, while transverse lower uterine segment scars more frequently rupture during or after labor.
- Overall, the most common site of rupture is the anterior lower uterine segment, which is the thinnest portion of the myometrium in pregnant patients and the most common site of scarring from prior low transverse cesarean section.
- Less commonly, rupture of the uterine body occurs during pregnancy.

Ultrasound, MRI, or CT can be used to evaluate suspected uterine rupture.

- All modalities may demonstrate an extrauterine hematoma, ascites, or hemoperitoneum.
- Ultrasound may show discontinuity in the myometrium with protrusion of the amniotic sac in a pregnant patient.
- MRI may be most useful when anatomy is difficult to delineate by ultrasound, for instance in the presence of multiple fibroids or congenital fetal anomalies. MRI findings include a linear defect with high signal on both T1- and T2-weighted images that is clearly distinct from the normal incision site. CT is readily available in the acute setting and may demonstrate analogous findings.
- If the patient is pregnant with a viable fetus, radiation dose should be considered in the risk–benefit analysis.

Treatment of uterine perforation

- Treatment of partial perforation in non-pregnant patients may be conservative, with antibiotic administration.
- Uterine rupture during pregnancy is a surgical emergency.

Clinical synopsis The patient was admitted to the hospital. Since the myometrial defect was small, the patient was treated with antibiotics.

Self-assessment

- *Where does uterine rupture most commonly occur and why?*

- The anterior lower uterine segment is the most common site of rupture. The low transverse cesarean section is performed inferiorly and the lower uterine segment is thinnest portion of the myometrium in pregnant patients.

- *In non-pregnant patients, what are two causes of uterine rupture?*

- Uterine instrumentation and trauma are the leading causes of perforation in non-pregnant patients.

Spectrum of uterine rupture

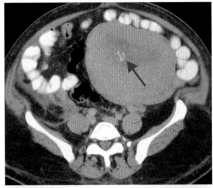
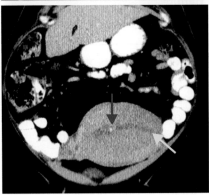

Postpartum uterine rupture (CT)

Postpartum uterine rupture presents with persistent bleeding that does not respond to oxytocin or uterine massage. Axial and coronal contrast-enhanced CT in a 28-year-old postpartum female demonstrates a linear defect extending through the left lateral myometrium (yellow arrow on the coronal image). The uterus is enlarged and globular, with fluid distending the endometrium. Foci of increased attenuation in the endometrium represent active bleeding (red arrows).

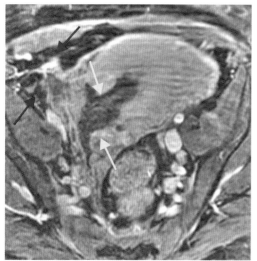

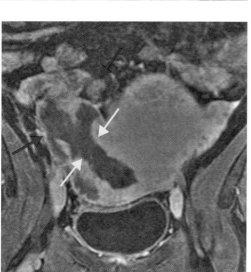

Postpartum uterine rupture (MR)

In a different case, axial and coronal post-contrast T1-weighted MR images with fat suppression in a recently postpartum female demonstrate a full thickness defect (yellow arrows) in the right lower uterine wall with an adjacent hematoma (red arrows). MRI is useful to distinguish uterine rupture from bladder flap hematoma and normal cesarean section scar.

Differential diagnosis of uterine rupture

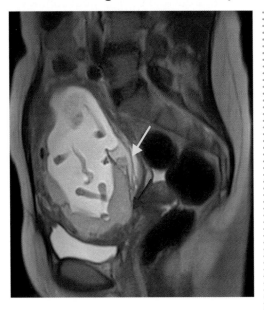

Placental abruption

Placental abruption, a common cause of third tri-mester bleeding, is defined as abnormal separation of the placenta from the uterus between 20 weeks gestation and birth. Ultrasound is typically the modality of choice, with MRI used in selected cases. Imaging findings include areas of hemorrhage that vary in appearance based on the location, size, and timing. Small abruptions may resolve without ther-apy. Early delivery may be required if there are signs of placental insufficiency. Sagittal T2-weighted MRI demonstrates separation of the posterior placenta from the myometrium (yellow arrow), with an inter-posed heterogeneous collection representing hem-orrhage. There is placenta previa, with the placenta covering the cervical os (red arrow).

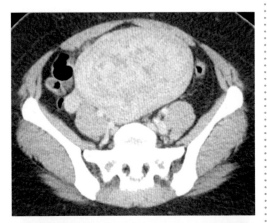

Degenerating fibroid

Uterine fibroids (also known as leiomyomas) are benign, smooth muscle proliferations in the myo-metrium. They can be submucosal, mural, or sub-serosal in location, and can grow very large. Typical clinical presentations include pain and bleeding, although fibroids are a common incidental finding in asymptomatic patients as well. Treatment options include uterine artery embolization, hormonal ther-apy, myomectomy, and hysterectomy. Axial and coronal contrast-enhanced CT images show a large uterine mass with heterogeneous cystic areas.

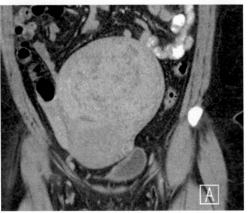

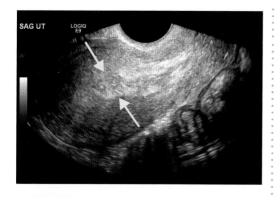

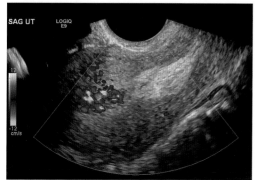

Retained products of conception

Retained placental tissue may be present after delivery, miscarriage, or termination of pregnancy. Importantly, absence of internal flow does not exclude the diagnosis. Management may be supportive (allowing the tissue to pass spontaneously). Dilatation and curettage may be performed when the amount of retained tissue is greater than 1 cm in maximum dimension. Sagittal grayscale transvaginal ultrasound images of the uterus without and with color Doppler demonstrate heterogeneous, echogenic material (arrows) eccentrically located within the endometrium (calipers) with internal blood flow towards the fundus.

Further reading

Catanzarite VA, Mehalek KE, Wachtel T, Westbrook C. Sonographic diagnosis of traumatic and later recurrent uterine rupture. *Am J Perinatol.* Apr. 1996;13(3): 177–180.

Dash N, Lupetin AR. Uterine rupture secondary to trauma: CT findings. *J Comput Assist Tomogr.* 1991; 15(2):329–331.

Hamrick-Turner JE, Cranston PE, Lanstrip BS. Gravid uterine dehiscence: MR findings. *Abdom Imaging.* 1995;20:486–488.

Lydon-Rochelle M, Holt V, Easterling T, Martin D. Risk of uterine rupture during labor among women with a prior cesarean delivery. *N Engl J Med.* July 2001;345:3.

Shrout AB, Kopelman JN. Ultrasonographic diagnosis of uterine dehiscence during pregnancy. *J Ultrasound Med.* May 1995;14(5):399–402.

Section 9.1 Axial Skeleton Trauma

Case 66   21-year-old male with quadriplegia after diving into a shallow pond. The patient struck his head against an embankment, with his head flexed, chin against chest

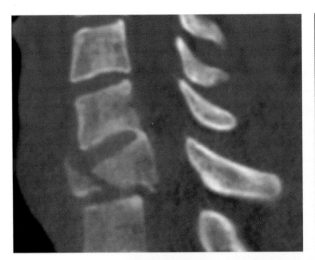
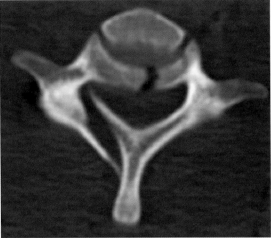

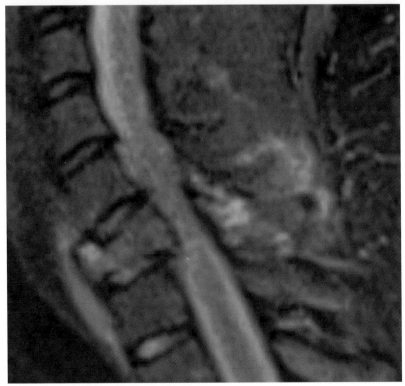

Diagnosis:
Flexion
teardrop
fracture at C7

Sagittal and axial CT images (left and middle images) demonstrate a small anterior teardrop fragment (yellow arrow) and retropulsion of the C7 vertebral body into the spinal canal. There is also posterior column injury, depicted by widening of the interspinous distance (red arrows) and displaced fracture of the lamina (blue arrow). The prevertebral soft tissues are thickened.

Sagittal STIR MRI (right image) demonstrates compression of the spinal cord at C7 with disruption of the ligamentum flavum (green arrow), and interspinous ligaments (white arrow). History of traumatic hyperflexion along with these findings supports the diagnosis of flexion teardrop fracture.

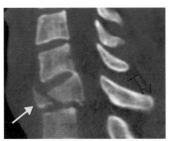 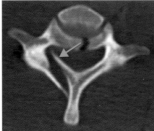 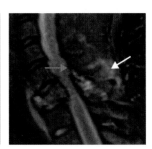

Discussion

Approximately 3–4% of trauma patients suffer cervical spine injury, with spinal cord injury in approximately 12,000 patients per year in the US.

- Traumatic cervical cord injury is fatal in about half of cases.
- Classification systems for cervical spinal cord injuries take into account the complex anatomy of the vertebrae and ligamentous stabilizers.
- The Subaxial Cervical Spine Injury Classification (SLIC) system is based on fracture morphology, status of the discoligamentous complex, and neurological status. The SLIC is similar to, but slightly different from, the Thoracolumbar Injury Classification and Severity Score (TLICS) scoring system discussed in Case 67 (e.g., a distraction morphology is 3 points for SLIC and 4 points for TLICS). Operative management is recommended for patients with SLIC scores of five or greater.

Subaxial Cervical Spine Injury Classification (SLIC)

Fracture morphology	Score
None	0
Compression	1
Burst	2
Distraction	3
Rotation/Translation	4
Disco-Ligamentous Complex	
None	0
Indeterminate	2
Disrupted	3
Neurologic Function	
Intact	0
Root injury	1
Complete cord injury	2
Incomplete cord injury	3
Ongoing compression with deficits	+1
Total *	

* Total score $\leq$ 3, nonoperative treatment is recommended; score = 4, either surgery or nonoperative treatment is indicated; and scores $\geq$ 5, surgery is recommended.

A helpful schema when considering spinal fractures is the three-column concept, which is used by spine surgeons to categorize the injured structures.

- The distinguishing feature of SLIC is emphasis on morphology rather than mechanism of injury.

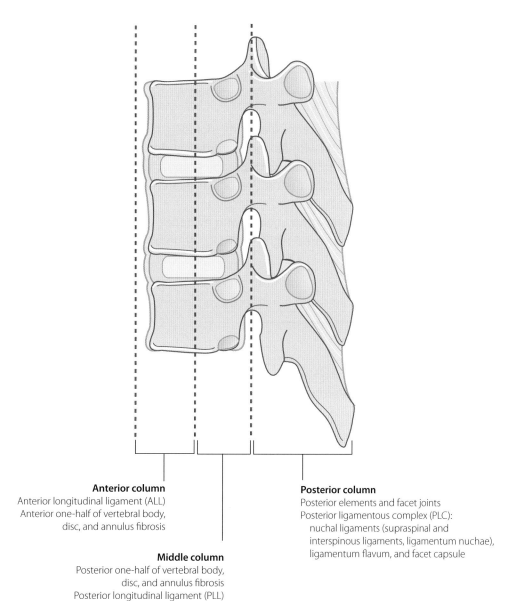

Anterior column
Anterior longitudinal ligament (ALL)
Anterior one-half of vertebral body,
disc, and annulus fibrosis

Posterior column
Posterior elements and facet joints
Posterior ligamentous complex (PLC):
 nuchal ligaments (supraspinal and
 interspinous ligaments, ligamentum nuchae),
 ligamentum flavum, and facet capsule

Middle column
Posterior one-half of vertebral body,
disc, and annulus fibrosis
Posterior longitudinal ligament (PLL)

Three column schema for diagnosis of spinal fractures

- Flexion teardrop fracture results from compression forces applied downwardly and posteriorly on the anterior column (e.g., from diving or sports-related activities).
- Downward posterior forces are concentrated within the anterior, inferior corner of the vertebral body, which leads to the classic "teardrop" fragment that usually becomes displaced anteriorly.
- There is usually disruption of posterior column ligaments secondary to distraction forces with posterior displacement of the vertebral body.

In flexion teardrop injury, there is posterior displacement of the intact-appearing posterior vertebral body into the central canal, which results in spinal cord injury.

- This posterior displacement of the intact-appearing vertebral body is distinct from "burst" fracture, in which axial loading causes fracture of the posterior aspect of the vertebral body and retropulsion (posterior displacement) of a fracture fragment.
- Injury to posterior elements including the posterior ligamentous complex (PLC) is common with flexion teardrop injuries. Although the ligamentous complex is not directly visualized on radiographs, radiographic signs suggestive of PLC injury include distraction of the posterior column, interspinous widening, and facet fractures and dislocations.
- Anterior column injuries with evidence of PLC injuries are considered unstable and are scored highly on SLIC, generally requiring surgical intervention.

| *Clinical synopsis* | The patient underwent anterior corpectomy of C7 for decompression of the spinal cord and nerve roots and anterior interbody fusion at C6–C7 and C7–T1. |

Self-assessment

- *Describe the causal mechanism and appearance of flexion teardrop fracture.*

- Flexion teardrop fracture occurs secondary to compression forces applied downwardly and posteriorly, with the forces concentrated within the anteroinferior corner of the vertebral body, or "teardrop," which is fractured and displaced anteriorly. There is typically posterior displacement of the vertebral body into the central canal, resulting in neurological injury.

- *What is the difference between flexion teardrop fracture and a burst fracture?*

- In flexion/axial loading injuries (flexion teardrop fracture), there is posterior displacement of the vertebral body. Importantly, the posterior cortex remains intact. Burst fractures, on the other hand, are distinguished by posterior cortical disruption with posterior displacement of a fracture fragment.

- *Name the structures in the anterior, middle, and posterior columns of the cervical spine.*

- Anterior: ALL, anterior one-half of vertebral body, disc, and annulus fibrosis.
- Middle: Posterior one-half of vertebral body, disc, and annulus fibrosis, PLL.
- Posterior: Posterior elements and facet joints, and the posterior ligamentous complex (PLC), which includes the nuchal ligaments (supraspinal and interspinous ligaments, ligamentum nuchae), ligamentum flavum, and facet capsule.

Spectrum of flexion teardrop injury

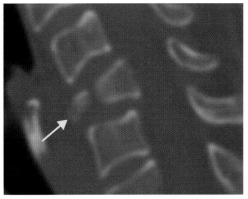

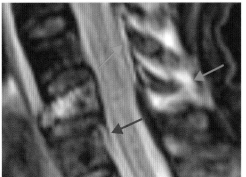

C5 flexion teardrop fracture

A 48-year-old male presented after a forward fall due to syncope. Sagittal CT demonstrates a C5 teardrop fragment (yellow arrow) and retropulsion of the vertebral body. The posterior cortex is intact. STIR MRI illustrates disruption of the PLL (red arrow) and ligamentum flavum (blue arrow), with edema of the interspinous ligament (green arrow).

Differential diagnosis of flexion teardrop injury

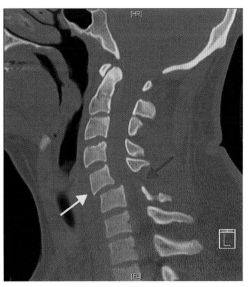

Flexion with translation injury

A 22-year-old male presented after a head-on motorcycle collision with a wall. Sagittal CT demonstrates anterior subluxation of C5 on C6 (yellow arrow) and interspinous widening (red arrow) with a jumped facet at C5–C6 (blue arrow). A small facet fracture fragment is seen posterior to the superior aspect of the C6 facet. Sagittal STIR MRI demonstrates hyperintense acute epidural hematoma ventrally, abutting the spinal cord (green arrows), as well as high signal (edema) within the cord at C5–C6 (white arrow). This pattern of injury is consistent with flexion and translation injury.

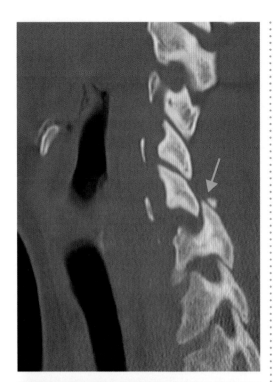

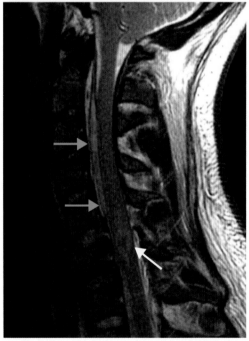

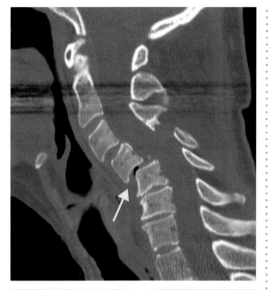

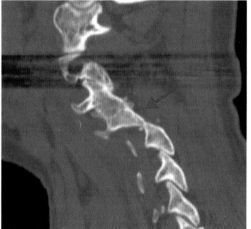

Flexion with rotation injury

Flexion rotation injuries may cause unilateral or bilateral facet dislocations. A 76-year-old female presented after a mechanical fall, with neck pain and no neurological deficits. Sagittal midline (upper) and left parasagittal (middle) CT images of the cervical spine demonstrate anterior subluxation of C4 on C5 (yellow arrow) and jumped left-sided facet at C4–C5 (red arrow). Axial CT image (lower) shows displaced fractures of the C4 laminae (blue arrows). This pattern of injury can be seen in forceful head rotation with flexion. Facet fractures are common with this injury pattern, and interspinous widening signifies injury to the PLC. These fractures require surgical stabilization. This patient underwent C3–C6 laminectomy and spinal fusion.

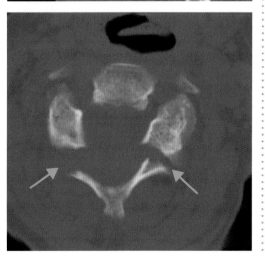

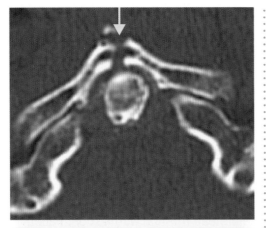

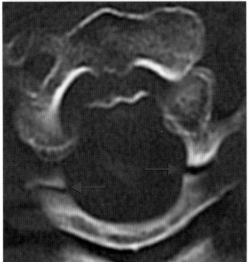

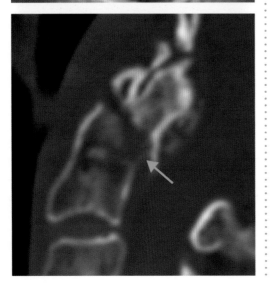

Axial loading injury (compression): Jefferson fracture with type II dens fracture

A Jefferson fracture is a burst fracture of C1 caused by an axial loading injury, and is often associated with other cervical spine fractures, such as flexion teardrop fractures of C2, lateral mass fractures, and dens fractures, as in this case. Axial CT images (upper and middle images) of an 83-year-old female who presented after a mechanical fall demonstrate a minimally displaced fracture of the anterior arch of C1 (yellow arrow) and bilateral posterior arch of C1 fractures (red arrows), consistent with Jefferson fracture. A sagittal CT image (lower image) also demonstrates a displaced fracture through the base of the odontoid process (blue arrow), representing a type II dens fracture (a type I dens fracture involves the superior-most portion of the odontoid process and a type III dens fracture involves the lateral masses of C2).

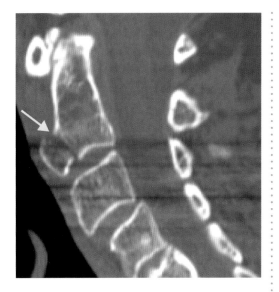

Forced extension injury: extension teardrop fracture

Sagittal CT image through the cervical spine demonstrates an anteroinferior corner fracture of C2 (arrow), consistent with extension teardrop fracture. The typical mechanism is forced extension of the neck. These fractures result from avulsion of the anterior aspect of the inferior vertebral body endplate by the ALL. In older patients, these injuries tend to occur at C2 due to degenerative anterior fusion of lower cervical vertebral bodies that alters spinal dynamics. The resultant hyperextension teardrop fracture fragment is usually larger in craniocaudad extent than it is in its anteroposterior dimension. This is unlike flexion teardrop fracture, where the fragment is typically wider than it is tall. Additionally, the extension teardrop fracture is more common in the upper cervical spine, whereas the flexion teardrop injury typically occurs in the lower cervical levels.

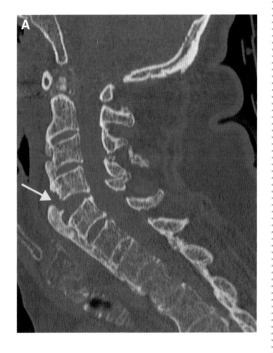

Hyperextension injury with cord compression and vertebral artery dissection in a patient with diffuse idiopathic skeletal hyperostosis (DISH)

Patients with DISH and other conditions that fuse the spine, such as ankylosing spondylitis, are at increased risk for serious fractures with even apparently minor trauma. This elderly male with DISH presented after a fall. Sagittal CT (A) demonstrates acute fracture of the anterior/inferior corner of C4 with fracture of the anterior bridging osteophytes (yellow arrow) and widened C4–C5 disc space anteriorly. Sagittal T2-weighted MR (B) shows cord compression at C4 without cord signal change. There is disruption of the anterior longitudinal ligament (red arrow) and a hyperintense prevertebral hematoma (blue arrows). Axial CT (C) also shows a fracture of the right transverse foramen (green arrow). Sagittal MIP image from a CT angiogram (D) demonstrates segmental dissection of the right vertebral artery (white arrow) seen on the (D) demonstrates.

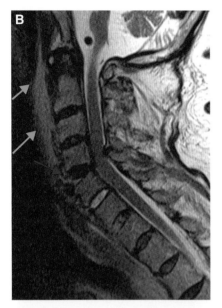

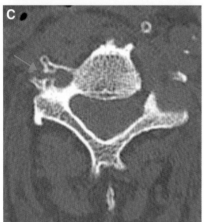

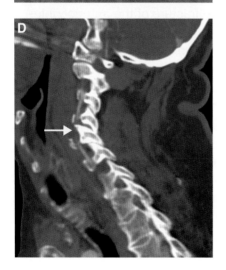

Further reading

Herkowitz, H. N., Rothman, R. H., Simeone, F. A. *Rothman–Simeone, The Spine*. Philadelphia: Saunders Elsevier, 2006.

Patel, A. A. *et al.* Subaxial cervical spine trauma classification: the Subaxial Injury Classification system and case examples. *Neurosurg Focus* 25, E8 (2008).

Pimentel, L. & Diegelmann, L. Evaluation and management of acute cervical spine trauma. *Emerg. Med. Clin. North Am.* 28, 719–738 (2010).

Radcliff, K. & Thomasson, B. G. Flexion–distraction injuries of the subaxial cervical spine. *Seminars in Spine Surgery* 25, 45–56 (2013).

Vaccaro, A. R. *et al.* The subaxial cervical spine injury classification system: a novel approach to recognize the importance of morphology, neurology, and integrity of the disco-ligamentous complex. *Spine* 32, 2365–2374 (2007).

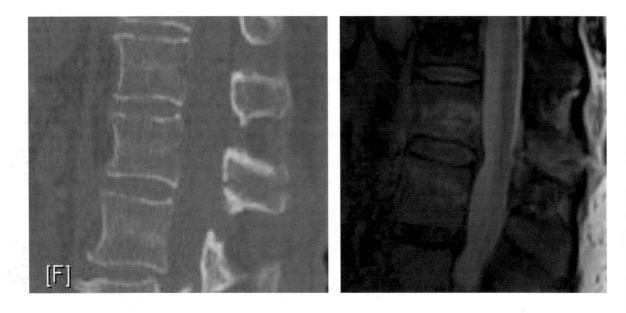

Diagnosis:
Flexion distraction injury at L1

Sagittal CT of the thoracolumbar spine demonstrates a transversely oriented fracture through the spinous process of L1 (yellow arrow). No other fractures are evident. Mechanism of injury (restrained motor vehicle accident) and fracture pattern raised concern for flexion distraction injury; thus, MRI was performed. Sagittal STIR MRI of the lumbar spine demonstrates disruption of the supraspinous ligament at the spinous process of L1 (red arrow), edema within the interspinous ligaments (blue arrows), and fracture of the L1 vertebral body (green arrow).

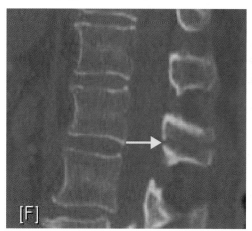 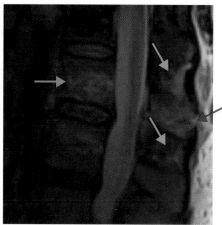

Discussion

In thoracic and lumbar trauma, the thoracolumbar junction is the most common site of injury – more than 50% of injuries occur between T11 and L1.

- In the upright position, the center of gravity of the human body is immediately anterior to the thoracolumbar spine. At rest, there are compressive forces on the vertebral bodies and distractive forces on the posterior ligamentous structures.
- The posterior ligamentous complex (PLC), consisting of the supraspinous ligament, interspinous ligaments, articular facet capsules, and ligamentum flavum, plays a key role in maintaining spinal stability when there is injury to the vertebral bodies.
- Injury to the PLC usually requires surgical correction to prevent kyphotic progression with vertebral body collapse.

Thoracolumbar injuries can be scored and classified according to the thoracolumbar injury classification and severity score (TLICS), which was developed by the Spine Trauma Study Group.

- Scoring requires assessment of three parameters: injury morphology, integrity of the PLC, and neurological status. This classification system assesses biomechanical and neurological spinal stability, and influences management decisions.
- A useful framework for understanding spinal injury divides the spine into anterior, middle, and posterior compartments (see "Flexion teardrop fracture" case for further explanation).

TLICS scoring system

Injury category	Point value
Injury morphology	
Compression	1
Burst	2
Translation or rotation	3
Distraction	4
PLC status	
Intact	0
Injury suspected	2
Injured	3
Neurologic status	
Intact	0
Nerve root involvement	2
Spinal cord or conus injury, complete	2
Spinal cord or conus injury, incomplete	3
Cauda equina syndrome	3

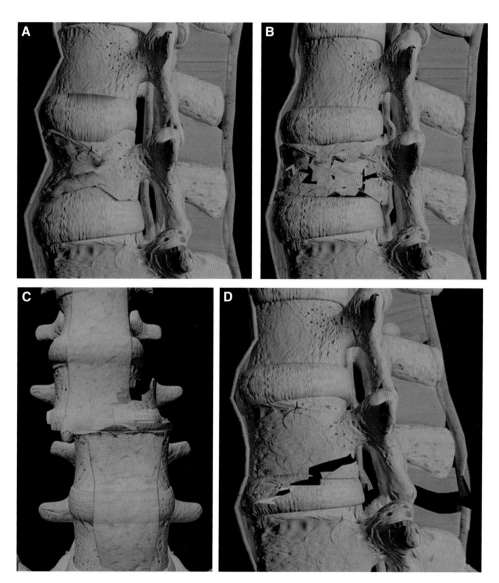

Computer-generated graphic of thoracolumbar fracture injury morphology with TLICS scoring:
A: Compression (1 point). B: Compression with burst fracture (2 points). C: Translation or rotation
(3 points). D: Distraction (4 points).
Copyright: *Radiographics*, used with permission: Khurana, B., Sheehan, S. E., Sodickson, A.,
Bono, C. M. & Harris, M. B. Traumatic thoracolumbar spine injuries: what the spine surgeon
wants to know. *Radiographics* 33, 2031–2046 (2013).

Fracture pattern is predictable for a given mechanism of injury.

- Compression fracture is distinguished by decreased vertebral body height or
  disruption of the endplate. While minor compression injuries from axial loading
  most commonly occur at the anterior portion of the vertebral body, stronger
  forces can cause a burst fracture, characterized by disruption of the posterior
  cortex and retropulsion of fracture fragments.

- Translational injuries occur with torsional and shear forces, which produce rotation and/or displacement of one vertebral body relative to the adjacent one.

Flexion distraction injury results from distractive forces on the PLC rather than axial loading.

- This injury pattern is rare, accounting for less than 10% of all thoracolumbar fractures. Severe disruption of the ALL and PLC results in unstable injury. Injury to the PLC usually does not heal adequately without surgical correction.
- Flexion distraction injuries usually occur in the setting of lap-belt restraints and are commonly associated with significant intra-abdominal injuries.
- There are often associated injuries to the vertebral body or the disc. If the fulcrum of force is anterior to the vertebral column, the vertebral body may not be injured and injury may be confined to the PLC; however, if the fulcrum of the force is within the anterior column, compression or burst fracture may occur. Particular attention should be paid to the PLC to avoid satisfaction of search in the context of a compression or burst fracture.

Imaging and clinical features of PLC injury.

- Characteristics of PLC injury on radiographs and CT include splaying of spinous processes, widening of facet joints, horizontal split fracture of the lamina or spinous process (as in the index case), empty facet joints, and vertebral body translation.
- Neurological deficits occur in only 10 to 15% of cases of flexion distraction injury.

Clinical synopsis Surgical stabilization was not performed in this case due to concomitant aortic injury. The patient was managed with bracing and physical therapy.

Self-assessment

- *How does the mechanism of flexion distraction injury differ from that of compression fracture?*

  - Flexion distraction injury occurs secondary to distractive forces on the PLC rather than axial loading that causes compression fracture.

- *What is a typical clinical scenario in which flexion distraction injury occurs and what associated injuries should be sought?*

  - Flexion distraction injury with damage to the PLC may occur in motor vehicle accidents with restrained passengers or drivers wearing lap belts. Injury to the vertebral bodies, discs, and intra-abdominal structures should be assessed for.

- *Name three components of the PLC.*

  - Supraspinous ligament, interspinous ligament, articular facet capsule, and ligamentum flavum.

Spectrum of flexion distraction injuries

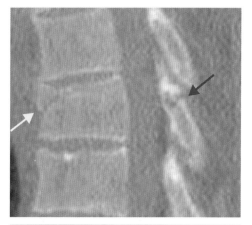

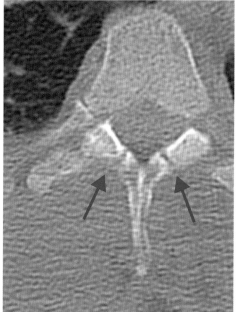

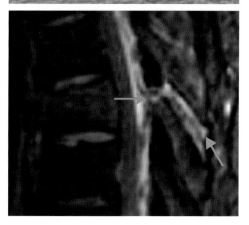

Superior end plate compression fracture with flexion distraction injury

Sagittal CT demonstrates an anterior flexion deformity of T7 with less than 25% height loss (yellow arrow). Fractures of the laminae are evident on both the sagittal (upper image) and axial (middle image) reconstructions (red arrows). There is no posterior cortical disruption or retropulsion of fragments into the spinal canal. Sagittal STIR MRI also demonstrates edema of the interspinous ligaments (blue arrow) and disruption of the ligamentum flavum (green arrow), consistent with PLC injury. The overall pattern is typical for flexion distraction injury.

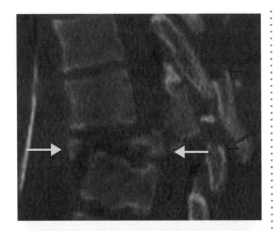

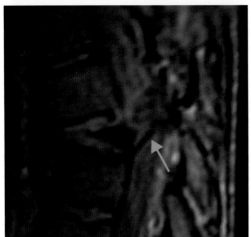

Severe flexion distraction injury with translation

Sagittal CT of the thoracic spine in a patient involved in a high-speed motor vehicle accident demonstrates marked compression of the T8 vertebral body (yellow arrows) with retropulsion into the spinal canal and anterolisthesis of T7 on T8. Concurrent fractures of the posterior elements (red arrows) with disruption of the PLC indicate severe flexion distraction injury. Sagittal STIR MR better demonstrates the retropulsed vertebral body fragments (blue arrow) that contribute to severe cord injury.

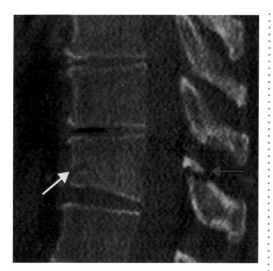

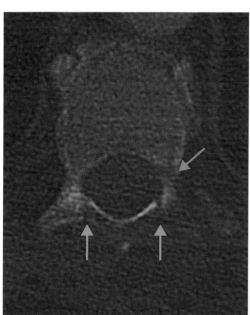

Anterior compression fracture with flexion distraction

This patient presented with a flexion distraction injury after a 30-foot backward fall from a ladder. Sagittal CT shows an anterior compression fracture of the T11 vertebral body with mild height loss (yellow arrow). The spinous process is fractured (red arrow). Axial CT shows bilateral laminar (blue arrows) and left pedicle (green arrow) fractures.

Differential diagnosis of flexion distraction injury

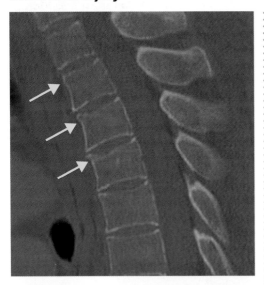

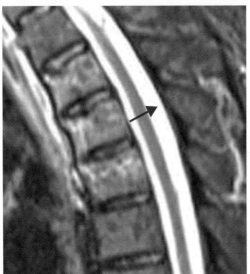

Compression injuries

Compression fractures occur in the anterior column due to axial loading, whereas flexion distraction causes injury to the posterior column by creating tension on the posterior elements and PLC. This patient presented with back pain after a minor motor vehicle accident. Sagittal CT and STIR MRI demonstrate subtle compression deformities of T3, T4, and T5 (note endplate depression, yellow arrows) with correlating vertebral body edema on STIR MRI. There is no fracture within the posterior column. The ligamentum flavum is intact (red arrow), and there is no edema within the interspinous ligaments.

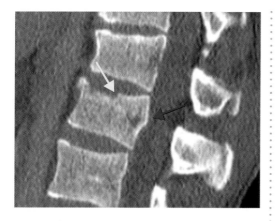

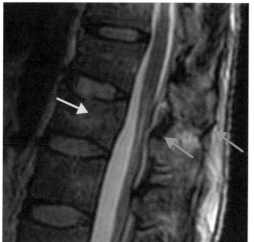

Burst fracture with intact PLC

Burst fractures are caused by more severe axial loading, leading to fracture of the posterior aspect of the vertebral body. It is important to assess the integrity of the PLC if a burst fracture is identified. Sagittal CT demonstrate superior endplate compression of the L1 vertebral body (yellow arrow) with disruption of the posterior cortex and minimal retropulsion (red arrow), consistent with a burst fracture. Sagittal T2-weighted MR demonstrates edema within the L1 vertebral body (yellow arrow). This burst fracture is distinguished from flexion distraction injury by the intact ligamentum flavum and supraspinous ligament (PLC, blue arrows). Like compression fractures, burst fractures are caused by axial loading injury; however, middle and posterior column injuries are more common with burst fractures.

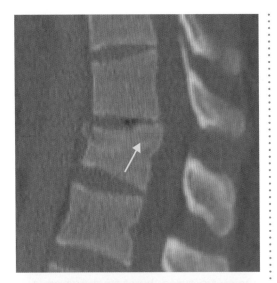

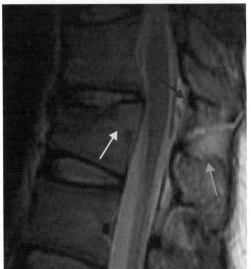

Burst fracture with PLC injury

Neurological deficits, degree of retropulsion into the spinal canal, and injury to PLC are factors that guide management of burst fractures. In a different patient with burst fracture, sagittal CT and T2-weighted MR demonstrates compression deformity of a thoracic vertebral body with the fracture line extending into the posterior aspect of the vertebral body (yellow arrows). There is minimal retropulsion of the posterior segment. T2-weighted MRI shows associated marrow edema. Unlike in the previous case, there is PLC injury, indicated by disruption of the ligamentum flavum (red arrow) and tear of the interspinous ligaments (blue arrow).

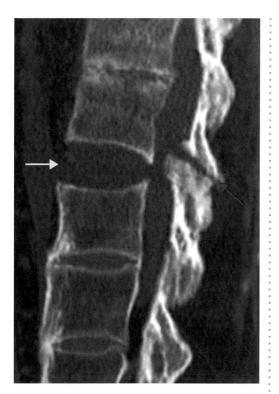

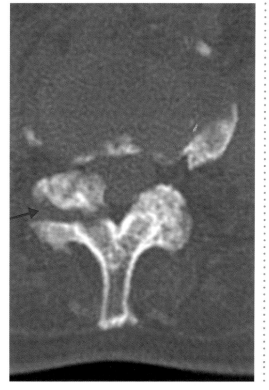

Intervertebral disc and facet fracture

Sagittal CT shows widening of the L1–L2 disc space (disc fracture, yellow arrow) and fracture of a fused facet joint (red arrow) in a patient with history of ankylosing spondylitis who experienced a minor fall. Axial CT confirms fracture of the right L1–L2 facet (red arrow). Anterior and posterior fusion of the vertebral bodies and facet joints, as seen in this case, is typical for ankylosing spondylitis. Clinicians must have a high index of suspicion for injury in patients with ankylosing spondylitis, DISH, and other conditions that fuse the spine, even with relatively minor trauma. These patients may experience "carrot stick fractures," where the inflexible spine cannot bend in response to injury, but rather fractures like a snapped carrot stick.

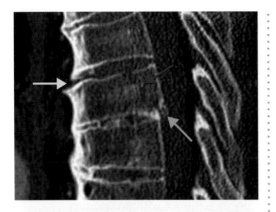

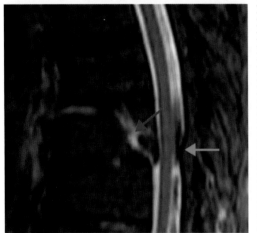

Hyperextension injury

This 85-year-old man with DISH was a restrained driver whose vehicle was rear-ended. He experienced spinal hyperextension and presented with back pain. Sagittal CT and STIR MRI through the thoracic spine reveal discontinuity of an anterior osteophyte mass at T6–T7 (yellow arrow) and a fracture line traversing the T7 vertebral body (red arrows), with minimal retropulsion (blue arrow). These findings are typical for hyperextension injury. The PLC, including the ligamentum flavum (green arrow), appears intact, and there is no edema within the spinal cord.

Further reading

Bagley, L. J. Imaging of spinal trauma. *Radiol. Clin. North Am.* 44, 1–12, vii (2006).

Dundamadappa, S. K. & Cauley, K. A. MR imaging of acute cervical spinal ligamentous and soft tissue trauma. *Emerg Radiol.* 19, 277–286 (2012).

Herkowitz H. N., Rothman R. H., & Simeone F. A. *Rothman–Simeone, The Spine.* Philadelphia: Saunders Elsevier, 2006.

Khurana, B., Sheehan, S. E., Sodickson, A., Bono, C. M. & Harris, M. B. Traumatic thoracolumbar spine injuries: what the spine surgeon wants to know. *Radiographics* 33, 2031–2046 (2013).

Looby, S. & Flanders, A. Spine trauma. *Radiol. Clin. North Am.* 49, 129–163 (2011).

Case 68   50-year-old male presented with hemodynamic instability after
a head-on motor vehicle collision at 40 miles per hour

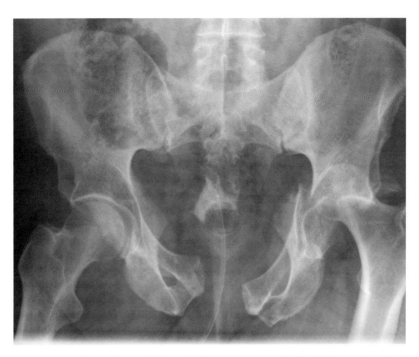

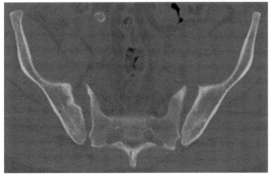

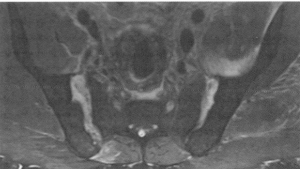

Diagnosis:
Anterior
posterior
compression
(APC) type 2
pelvic ring
injury

AP radiograph of the pelvis (left image) demonstrates a displaced fracture through the roof of the left acetabulum (yellow arrow) with posterior dislocation of the hip. There is marked pubic symphyseal diastasis (red arrow) of greater than 2.5 cm, with apparent broadening of the right iliac wing. Axial CT (middle image) demonstrates widening of the anterior aspects of the right greater than left anterior sacroiliac (SI) joints (blue arrows). Axial proton density MRI with fat suppression (right image) shows disruption of both anterior SI ligaments (green arrows) and confirms widening of the anterior SI joint spaces. Thickening and edema of the right posterior SI ligament (white arrow) suggests sprain or partial tear, in contrast to the normal left posterior SI ligament. This is an anterior posterior compression (APC) type 2 injury given the pubic symphysis diastasis of > 2.5 cm and widening of the anterior sacroiliac joints.

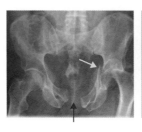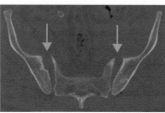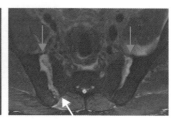

Discussion

The pelvis is a ring structure composed of the sacrum and paired innominate bones, which are joined anteriorly at the pubic symphysis (anterior arch) and posteriorly at the sacrum via the SI joints (posterior arch).

- The pubic symphysis, which is the weakest portion of the pelvic ring, is stabilized by the superior and inferior pubic ligaments.
- The posterior arch is stabilized by the anterior and posterior interosseous SI ligaments. The anterior SI ligaments resist internal rotation, while the stronger posterior SI ligaments resist external rotation and vertical displacement.

Pelvic ring injuries usually occur in high-impact trauma due to transfer of a large amount of kinetic energy: motor vehicle accidents, falls from height, and crush injuries are the most common etiologies.

- Associated injuries may be caused by primary impact, osseous fragments, or secondary to shear forces, and include vascular disruption, hemorrhage, urogenital injury, lumbosacral plexus disruption, and long bone fracture.
- As in other complex fracture scenarios, understanding the mechanism of injury can refine the search for additional injuries. Analogous to injury of other ring structures such as the mandible, fracture in one portion of the pelvic ring should prompt a search for fracture or ligamentous injury in a second location.

In the setting of trauma, the pelvic ring can be radiographically evaluated using a standard AP view, pelvic inlet and outlet (Ferguson) views, and in some cases, with CT or MRI.

- The inlet view is useful for characterizing anterior–posterior fracture displacement, while the outlet view is useful for identifying vertical displacement.
- CT or CT cystography is useful for evaluation of the pelvic organs in severe trauma, and for further evaluation of pelvic fractures identified by radiography.
- In the emergency setting, pelvic MRI image can be abbreviated to coronal STIR and coronal T1-weighted imaging. These limited sequences have high sensitivity for fracture, avascular necrosis of femoral head, and soft tissue injury. MRI should be considered when radiographically occult or insufficiency-type fractures are suspected.

The Young and Burgess classification, based on the force vector, classifies pelvic ring injuries as lateral compression (50–70%), APC (20–30%), vertical shear (14%), or combined mechanism injuries.

- APC injury results from head-on motor vehicle collisions where the force vector is directed in the anterior to posterior direction in the sagittal plane. This force causes external rotation at one or both SI joints, resulting in open-book type injury. Injury may be unilateral or bilateral. An associated finding is broadening of the iliac wing on the AP view. A summary of the features of APC injuries by grade is presented in the table below.

Summary of features of APC injuries by grade

APC injury type	Pubic symphysis diastasis	Effect on SI joints	Rotational stability	Vertical stability
APC 1	< 2.5 cm	None	Preserved	Preserved
APC 2	> 2.5 cm	Anterior joint widening	Compromised	Preserved
APC 3	Complete disruption	Complete disruption of SI ligaments with dissociation of the iliac wing and sacrum	Compromised	Compromised

Clinical synopsis	The patient underwent closed reduction of his left posterior hip dislocation and open reduction internal fixation with symphyseal plating of his anterior pelvic ring injury.

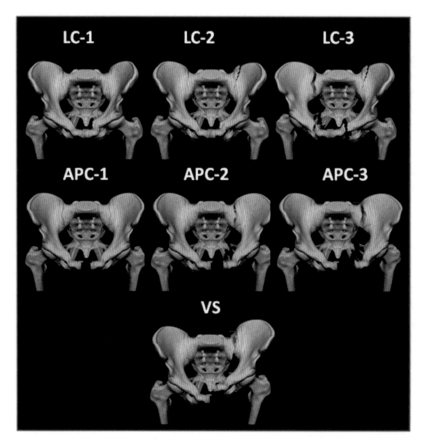

Young and Burgess classification system of pelvic ring injury. (LC: lateral compression; APC: anterior posterior compression; VS: vertical shear; combined type not shown)

(Reproduced with permission from *Radiographics*; see Further reading)

Self-assessment

- *What is the most common pelvic ring injury?*

- *What is the importance of L5 transverse process fracture in pelvic injury?*

- *Hemorrhage is most prevalent in which type of bony pelvic injury?*

- Lateral compression type injury.

- The L5 transverse process is the site of attachment of the iliolumbar ligament. An L5 transverse process fracture may be the only indication of posterior ring injury on radiographs, and is an independent predictor of instability.

- APC injury.

Spectrum of pelvic APC injury

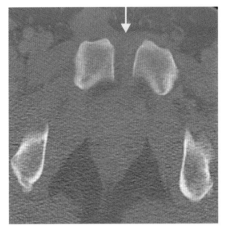

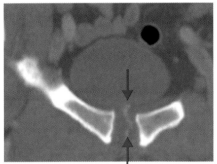

APC 1 injury

This patient presented after a motor vehicle accident. Axial (upper image) and coronal CT of the pelvis with IV contrast demonstrate widening of the pubic symphysis to 1.5 cm (yellow arrow). Subtle contrast extravasation in the region of the pubic symphysis (red arrows) denotes active hemorrhage. The posterior ring was found to be intact at the time of surgery.

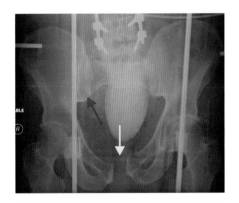

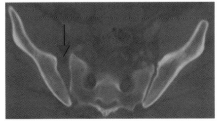

APC 3 injury

This 52-year-old male presented with pulseless cardiac arrest after a motorcycle accident. An AP radiograph of the pelvis demonstrates gross pubic diastasis (yellow arrow) and widening of the right SI joint (red arrow). Axial CT image confirms external rotation of the right hemipelvis and widening of the right SI joint (red arrow), more prominent anteriorly, although both the anterior and posterior aspects of the right SI joint are disrupted. Preoperative placement of a pelvic binder or sheet may reduce or lessen the degree of widening and deformity, making it difficult to detect at imaging, especially in absence of fractures. The patient underwent open reduction and internal fixation.

Differential diagnosis of pelvic APC injury

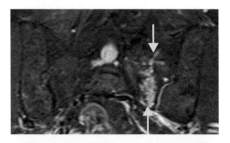

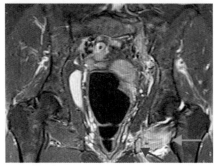

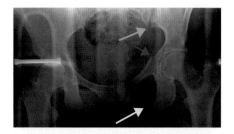

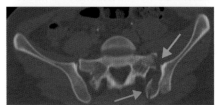

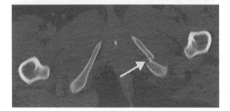

Lateral compression (LC) 1 fracture

LC injuries are the most common form of pelvic injury, usually occurring in side-impact motor vehicle accidents and resulting in internal rotation of the hemipelvis. In LC 1 fracture, laterally directed forces result in sacral crush injury with ipsilateral horizontal pubic ramus fractures. These injuries are considered stable and usually do not require surgery. This elderly patient presented after a fall from standing. Coronal STIR MRI demonstrates a linear vertical fracture through the left sacral wing (yellow arrows), fracture of the left inferior pubic ramus (red arrow), and edema within the obturator externus muscle consistent with muscle strain (blue arrow). There were also non-displaced fractures of the left superior pubic ramus and parasymphyseal region (not shown).

Lateral compression (LC) 2 fracture

In LC2 injury, lateral compression forces result in anterior sacral injury and posterior SI joint disruption or fracture through the ipsilateral iliac wing. LC2 fractures are considered rotationally unstable. This 18-year-old female presented after a motor vehicle accident. AP radiograph and axial CT of the pelvis demonstrate minimally overlapping fractures of the left inferior pubic ramus (yellow arrows) and acetabulum (red arrow) with widening of the left SI joint (blue arrows). The CT also demonstrates a displaced crescent-shaped fracture of the left iliac bone (green arrow) at the attachment site of the posterior SI ligament.

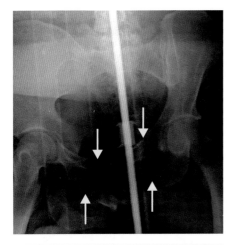

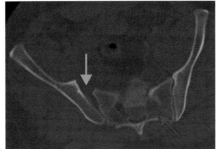

Lateral compression (LC) 3, "windswept pelvis" injury

LC 3 injury, also known as "windswept pelvis," is usually the consequence of high-velocity lateral compression forces causing ipsilateral internal rotation and contralateral external rotation. LC 3 injuries are both rotationally and vertically unstable. This 28-year-old male presented with hemodynamic instability after being struck by a motor vehicle from the left. Frontal radiograph of the pelvis demonstrates bilateral displaced superior and inferior pubic ramus fractures (yellow arrows). Axial CT demonstrates a minimally displaced sacral fracture on the side of impact (red arrow), with widening of the right SI joint and external rotation of the right ilium. (Images reproduced with permission from *Radiographics*; see Further reading.)

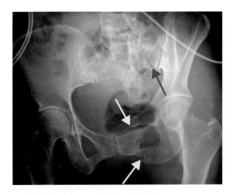

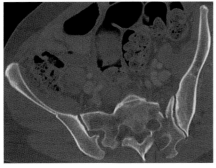

Vertical shear (VS) injury

In VS injury, inferior–superior directed forces cause a vertically oriented fracture of the pubic ramus with fracture of the sacrum. The SI ligaments are disrupted, and there is resultant cranial displacement of the hemipelvis on the side of impact. VS injuries are usually both vertically and rotationally unstable and are frequently associated with pelvic visceral injuries. This 53-year-old female presented after a motor vehicle accident. A frontal radiograph of the pelvis demonstrates minimal cranial displacement of the left hemipelvis with left-sided superior and inferior pubic ramus fractures (yellow arrows) and disruption of the left sacral arches (red arrow). Axial CT confirms the displaced left sacral fracture (red arrow) and demonstrates preservation of the SI joints.

Further reading

Campbell SE. Radiography of the hip: lines, signs, and patterns of disease. *Semin Roentgenol* 2005;40(3):290–319.

Kellam JF, Mayo KA. *Pelvic Ring Disruption: Skeletal Trauma* 3rd edn. Philadelphia, PA: Saunders, pp. 1052–1108.

Khurana B, Sheehan SE, Sodickson AD, Weaver MJ. Pelvic ring fractures: what the orthopedic surgeon wants to know. *Radiographics* 2014;34(5):1317-1333.

Stambaugh LE, Blackmore CC. Pelvic ring disruptions in emergency radiology. *European Journal of Radiology* 2003;48(1):71–87.

White CE, Hsu JR, Holcomb JB. Haemodynamically unstable pelvic fractures. *Injury* 2009;40(10):1023–1030.

Khurana B *et al.* Abbreviated MRI for patients presenting to the emergency department with hip pain. *AJR* 2012;198(6):W581–588.

Case 69   58-year-old male complains of thumb pain after punching a wall

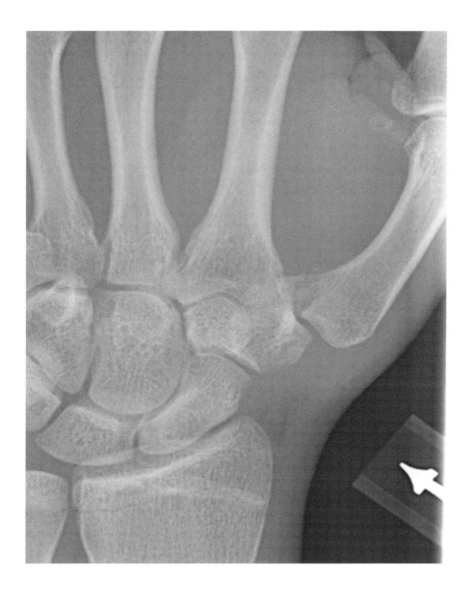

Diagnosis: **Bennett fracture-dislocation of the first metacarpal base**

PA radiograph of the hand demonstrates an intra-articular fracture through the thumb metacarpal base (arrow), with mild radial subluxation of the dominant radial metacarpal fracture fragment.

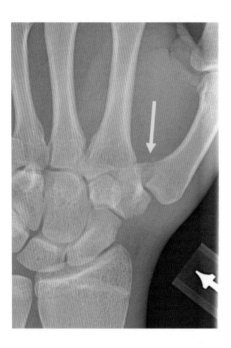

Discussion

Overview and mechanism of Bennett fracture

- A Bennett fracture is an intra-articular fracture through the ulnar articular margin of the volar beak of the base (arrow) of the thumb metacarpal, with varying degrees of associated subluxation or dislocation of the radial metacarpal fragment by traction from the abductor pollicis longus tendon. The smaller ulnar fragment remains in place due to anchoring by the attached anterior oblique ligament.
- The mechanism most commonly involves axial compression on a partially flexed thumb.

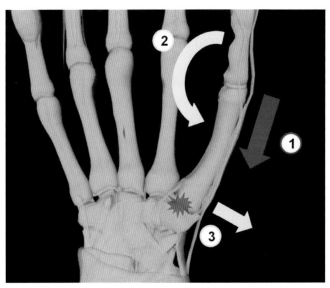

Axial compression along the shaft of the thumb (1), combined with flexion at the thumb metacarpophalangeal (MCP) joint (2), produces a fracture of the ulnar metacarpal base with lateral subluxation of the first metacarpal (3).

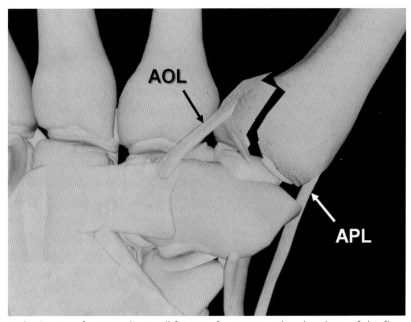

In the Bennett fracture, the small fracture fragment at the ulnar base of the first metacarpal is held in place by the anterior oblique ligament (AOL), and the radial component of the first metacarpal subluxes laterally under tension from the abductor pollicis longus tendon (APL).

Imaging of Bennett fracture

- Dedicated PA radiographs of the thumb base with the forearm in slight pronation are often required to adequately characterize the fracture fragment size.
- CT can be used to better characterize the degree of articular involvement in cases with ambiguous plain radiograph findings.

Treatment of Bennett fracture

- Closed reduction can be attempted if there is <3 mm of fragment displacement, although percutaneous pin fixation may be ultimately required.
- Open reduction and internal fixation (ORIF) is often required with fracture fragment displacement >3 mm. Other indications for ORIF include significant impaction of the central articular surface seen on CT, clinical findings of neurovascular injury, or failure of closed reduction.

Clinical synopsis   The patient underwent closed reduction with percutaneous pinning.

Differential diagnosis of Bennett fracture

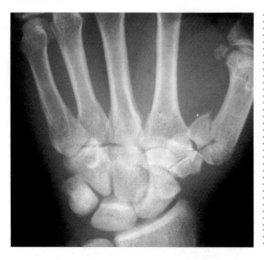

Rolando fracture

Rolando fracture is a $\geq$3-part fracture of the thumb metacarpal base, which can be described as Y-shaped, T-shaped, or comminuted. These injuries typically require open reduction and internal fixation, with generally worse post-treatment functional outcomes in contrast to Bennett fractures, which are non-comminuted (hence the mnemonic "Bennett is better"). Radiograph of the hand demonstrates a three-part, intra-articular (arrow) fracture of the thumb metacarpal base with a Y-shaped configuration.

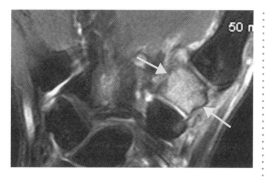

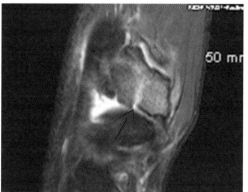

Trapezium fracture

Trapezium fractures are uncommon and may be associated with a fracture of the first metacarpal base. Nondisplaced fractures can be occult and cross-sectional imaging may be needed for diagnosis of these fractures. Displaced fractures often require ORIF. Coronal and sagittal T2-weighted MR images of the wrist with fat suppression demonstrate diffuse bone marrow edema within the trapezium (yellow arrows), with a fracture line most evident on the sagittal image (red arrow).

Further reading

Bennett, E. H. (1886). "On fracture of the metacarpal bone of the thumb." *Br Med J* 2(1331): 12–13.

Breen, T. F., R. H. Gelberman, *et al.* (1988). "Intra-articular fractures of the basilar joint of the thumb." *Hand Clin* 4(3): 491–501.

Cannon, S. R., G. S. Dowd, *et al.* (1986). "A long-term study following Bennett's fracture." *J Hand Surg Br* 11(3): 426–431.

Freeland, A. E., W. B. Geissler, *et al.* (2002). "Surgical treatment of common displaced and unstable fractures of the hand." *Instr Course Lect* 51: 185–201.

Jupiter, J. B., H. Hastings, II, *et al.* (2010). "The treatment of complex fractures and fracture-dislocations of the hand." *Instr Course Lect* 59: 333–341.

Kjaer-Petersen, K., O. Langhoff, *et al.* (1990). "Bennett's fracture." *J Hand Surg Br* 15(1): 58–61.

Langhoff, O., K. Andersen, *et al.* (1991). "Rolando's fracture." *J Hand Surg Br* 16(4): 454–459.

Pollen, A. G. (1968). "The conservative treatment of Bennett's fracture-subluxation of the thumb metacarpal." *J Bone Joint Surg Br* 50(1): 91–101.

Rockwood, C. A., D. P. Green, *et al.* (2006). *Rockwood and Green's fractures in adults*. Philadelphia: Lippincott Williams & Wilkins.

Case 70   23-year-old female with visible deformity of the forearm following a direct blow to the hyperextended forearm

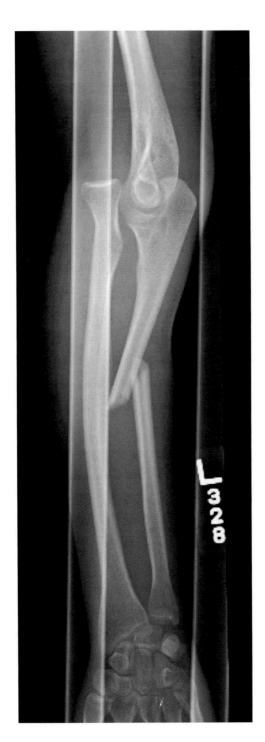

Diagnosis:
Monteggia
fracture–
dislocation

Frontal radiograph of the forearm demonstrates a displaced mid ulnar diaphyseal fracture (yellow arrow), with anterior dislocation of the radial head (red arrow). The radius is partially obscured by overlying trauma board.

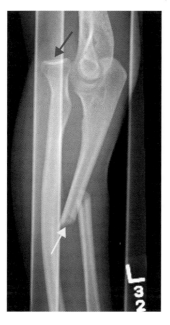

Discussion

Overview and mechanism of Monteggia fracture–dislocation

- A Monteggia fracture–dislocation is the combination of an ulnar fracture with radiocapitellar dislocation, commonly due to posterolateral direct impact onto a hyperextended forearm.

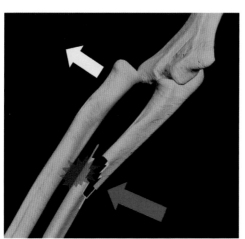

Impact on the proximal ulna (red arrow) with the arm in hyperextension causes fracture of the ulnar diaphysis and anterior dislocation of the radial head (yellow arrow), consistent with a Monteggia fracture–dislocation, Bado type I.

Classification of Monteggia fracture–dislocation

- Monteggia fracture–dislocations are classified according to the Bado system, which distinguishes injuries based on direction of dislocation, angulation of fracture fragments, and the presence of an associated radius fracture.
  - **Type I**: fracture of the proximal or middle third of the ulna with apex anterior angulation and anterior dislocation of the radial head.
  - **Type II**: fracture of the proximal or middle third of the ulna with apex posterior angulation and posterior dislocation of the radial head.
  - **Type III**: fracture of the proximal ulna with apex medial angulation and lateral dislocation of the radial head.
  - **Type IV**: Monteggia fracture–dislocation with a fracture of the radial shaft. Anterior direction of radial head dislocation is typical.

Imaging of Monteggia fracture–dislocation

- Radiographs are usually sufficient, though radiocapitellar dislocation can often be overlooked in the presence of a displaced ulnar fracture.
- CT is recommended to evaluate for additional fractures when Monteggia-type mechanism is suspected.

Treatment of Monteggia fracture–dislocation

- While these injuries have been treated conservatively in the past, recent improvements in surgical technique have shown improved functional outcomes with surgery. Early surgical repair is now the most common treatment strategy for all Monteggia-type lesions.

Clinical synopsis

The physical examination revealed gross deformity of the left forearm with tenting of the skin by the radial head and impending skin disruption. Additionally, there was complete loss of sensation in the radial sensory nerve distribution and complete motor loss of posterior interosseous nerve innervated muscles (forearm extensors). The patient underwent urgent open reduction and internal fixation of the ulna fracture and open reduction of the radial head with annular ligament repair.

Self-assessment

- *True or false: anterior dislocation of the radial head and proximal ulnar fracture are the two necessary components of Monteggia lesion.*

- *True or false: most Monteggia lesions are treated conservatively in adults.*

- False: the Monteggia lesion is defined as any ulna fracture with radiocapitellar dislocation. The radial head may be dislocated anteriorly, posteriorly, or laterally.

- False: early surgical repair is now the most common treatment strategy for all Monteggia-type lesions due to better functional outcomes.

Differential diagnosis of Monteggia fracture–dislocation

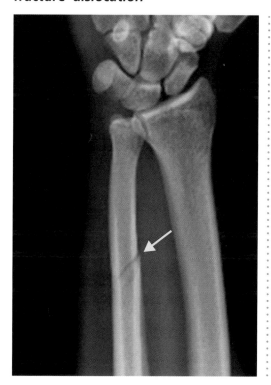

Nightstick fracture

A nightstick fracture is an isolated fracture of the distal ulna due to a direct impact (classically from a nightstick with the victim's hand raised in self-defense). Frontal radiograph of the forearm demonstrates a minimally displaced transverse fracture of the distal ulnar diaphysis (arrow).

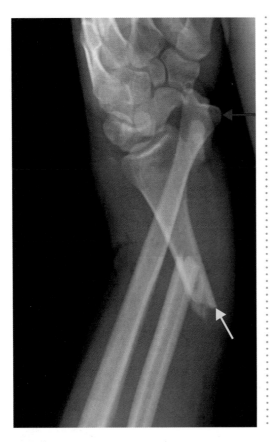

Galeazzi fracture

A Galeazzi fracture is a fracture of the distal radius with dislocation of the distal radioulnar joint. Oblique forearm radiograph demonstrates a displaced fracture of the distal radius with apex volar angulation (yellow arrow), with dislocation of the distal radioulnar joint (red arrow).

Further reading

Bado, J. L. (1967). "The Monteggia lesion." *Clin Orthop Relat Res* 50: 71–86.

Beutel, B. G. (2012). "Monteggia fractures in pediatric and adult populations." *Orthopedics* 35(2): 138–144.

Dymond, I. W. (1984). "The treatment of isolated fractures of the distal ulna." *J Bone Joint Surg Br* 66(3): 408–410.

Nicolaidis, S. C., D. H. Hildreth, *et al.* (2000). "Acute injuries of the distal radioulnar joint." *Hand Clin* 16(3): 449–459.

Ring, D., J. B. Jupiter, *et al.* (1998). "Monteggia fractures in adults." *J Bone Joint Surg Am* 80(12): 1733–1744.

Rockwood, C. A., D. P. Green, *et al.* (2006). *Rockwood and Green's fractures in adults*. Philadelphia: Lippincott Williams & Wilkins.

Case 71   22-year-old male with elbow pain after a fall onto outstretched hand

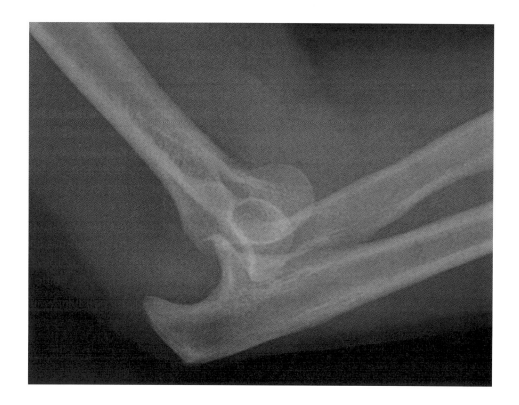

Diagnosis: Lateral radiograph demonstrates a posterior elbow dislocation, with the distal
Posterior humerus positioned anterior to the coronoid process and ulna dislocating
elbow posteriorly. There is cortical irregularity of the coronoid process (arrow), sus-
dislocation picious for fracture.

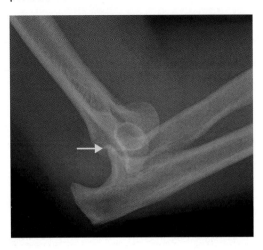

Discussion

Overview of elbow dislocation

- Elbow dislocation is defined by the relative position of the proximal ulna and
  radius relative to the distal humerus. Posterior dislocations are more common
  and typically occur after a fall onto outstretched hand (FOOSH). The specific
  mechanism of injury most commonly involves a combination of axial
  compression, supination, and valgus stress.

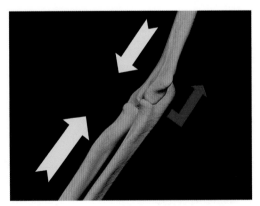

Fall onto outstretched hand with the arm in
slight supination and valgus angulation at
the elbow produces axial compression
forces at the elbow (yellow arrows), which
can cause posterior dislocation of the ulna
relative to the humerus (red arrow).

Classification of elbow dislocation

- **Simple**: no associated fractures.
- **Complex**: associated fractures, such as radial head and coronoid process fractures (the terrible triad is the combination of posterior dislocation with both of these fractures). Additional fractures of the capitellum or olecranon may be seen.
- **Posterolateral rotatory instability (PLRI)** is a progression of (predominantly) lateral ligamentous injuries caused by external rotation and posterior subluxation of the ulna with respect to the distal humerus. The most severe form of PLRI is a frank posterior dislocation, in which case there is also medial ligamentous injury. PLRI can clinically present with painful clicking, snapping, or locking, often associated with the subjective feeling of apprehension with activities such as pushing to rise from a chair. PLRI is thought to occur in a progressive sequence:
    1. Stage 1: lateral ulnar collateral ligament (LUCL, an important lateral stabilizer that connects the lateral epicondyle of the humerus to the ulna) injury only.
    2. Stage 2: radial collateral ligament (RCL, a secondary radial/lateral stabilizer that connects the lateral epicondyle to the annular ligament) and LUCL injury. Stage 2 PLRI presents as near-complete dislocation with perching of the humerus on the coronoid process.
    3. Stage 3: anterior bundle of the medial collateral ligament (the most important medial/ulnar stabilizer that connects the medial epicondyle to the sublime tubercle of the proximal ulna) injury, in addition to LUCL and RCL injury. Once the medial-sided ligaments are injured, it is possible to have a dislocation even without a fracture.

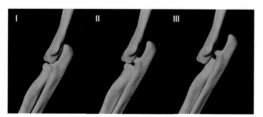

Posterolateral elbow instability can be described in stages ranging from mild instability (I) to perching of the humerus on the coronoid process (II) to frank dislocation (III).

Associated injuries

- **"Terrible triad"**: the previously discussed "terrible triad" is a posterior dislocation with associated radial head and coronoid process fractures. Surgery is almost always indicated for best management. Note that a posterior dislocation that has spontaneously reduced may be radiographically occult if there is no associated fracture. Posterior dislocations should be suspected if a coronoid process fracture is detected.

- **Coronoid process fracture:** CT can be used to better characterize coronoid process fracture morphology. Fractures of the anteromedial facet of the coronoid process and sublime tubercle of the proximal ulna can predispose to posteromedial rotary instability (PMRI) since the sublime tubercle serves the attachment site of the anterior band of medial collateral ligament, a primary radial/medial-sided stabilizer of the elbow. Note that PMRI is always associated with a coronoid process fracture and is due to varus stress.

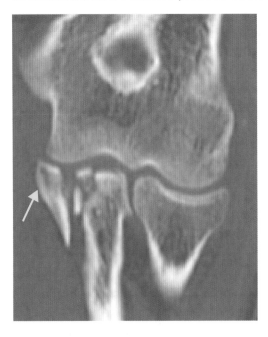

Coronal CT reformation showing a comminuted intra-articular fracture of the proximal ulna involving the ulnohumeral articulation and the sublime tubercle (arrow).

- **Ligamentous injury:** MR is often helpful after posterior dislocation to better evaluate the medial and lateral ligaments and for associated bony contusions.

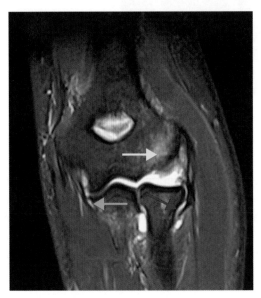

Coronal STIR MR shows marrow edema in the capitellum / lateral epicondyle (yellow arrow) and apposing radial head following recent elbow dislocation. There is a full-thickness tear of the LUCL (red arrow). The RCL (not visualized on this image) was also injured. There is a partial-thickness tear of the deep surface of the medial collateral ligament (MCL), manifested by fluid interposed between the MCL and the sublime tubercle, also known as the "T-sign" (blue arrow). MCL injury in the setting of posterior dislocation is consistent with stage 3 PLRI.

- **Osborne–Cotterill** lesion: the Osborne–Cotterill lesion is a fracture of the posterolateral capitellum at the attachment site of the LUCL secondary to impaction of the radial head with the capitellum. Similar to a coronoid process fracture, the Osborne–Cotterill lesion may be the only radiographic sign of significant ligamentous trauma or a spontaneously reduced dislocation.

Treatment of posterior elbow dislocation

- Simple dislocations can be treated conservatively with early post-reduction mobilization, provided there is no significant post-reduction instability.
- Complex dislocations most often require surgery.

Clinical synopsis

The post-reduction radiograph demonstrated radial head (yellow arrow) and coronoid process (red arrow) fractures (the terrible triad), with persistent widening of the ulnohumeral joint. The patient underwent surgical repair.

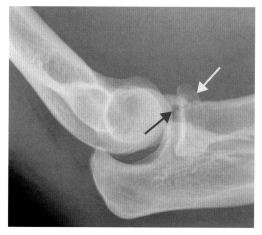

Self-assessment

- *What is the terrible triad of the elbow?*

- The combination of posterior elbow dislocation with radial head and coronoid process fractures has been described as the terrible triad (as seen in the index case). It is associated with extensive ligament damage that could result in chronic instability and secondary arthritis if inadequately treated.

- *What are the primary stabilizers of the elbow?*

- The anterior band of medial collateral ligament (medially), the LUCL (laterally), and ulnohumeral articulation constitute primary stabilizers of the elbow. Disruption of any of these structures will result in elbow instability.

Differential diagnosis of posterior elbow dislocation

Anterior dislocation

Most commonly seen in children, most often due to rebound after a posterior dislocation.

Monteggia fracture-dislocation

Fracture of proximal ulna in association with radiocapitellar dislocation. Please see Case 70 for images and further discussion.

Chronic valgus stress

Chronic valgus overload syndromes are seen in throwing athletes. The medial ligaments are typically involved, with intact lateral ligaments. There may be impaction injuries to the lateral osseous structures (radial head and capitellum). In contrast, in a posterior dislocation, the lateral ligaments are disrupted first.

Further reading

Cheung, E. V. (2008). "Chronic lateral elbow instability." *Orthop Clin North Am* 39(2): 221–228.

Chung, C. B., and L. S. Steinbach (2010). *MRI of the upper extremity : shoulder, elbow, wrist and hand.* Philadelphia, PA; Wolters Kluwer Health / Lippincott Williams & Wilkins.

Coonrad, R. W., T. F. Roush, *et al.* (2005). "The drop sign, a radiographic warning sign of elbow instability." *J Shoulder Elbow Surg* 14(3): 312–317.

Cotten, A., J. Jacobson, *et al.* (1997). "Collateral ligaments of the elbow: conventional MR imaging and MR arthrography with coronal oblique plane and elbow flexion." *Radiology* 204(3): 806–812.

Morrey, B. F., and J. Sanchez-Sotelo (2009). *The elbow and its disorders.* Philadelphia, PA: Saunders/Elsevier.

O'Driscoll, S. W., J. B. Jupiter, *et al.* (2003). "Difficult elbow fractures: pearls and pitfalls." *Instr Course Lect* 52: 113–134.

O'Driscoll, S. W., J. B. Jupiter, *et al.* (2001). "The unstable elbow." *Instr Course Lect* 50: 89–102.

Ring, D., J. B. Jupiter, *et al.* (2002). "Posterior dislocation of the elbow with fractures of the radial head and coronoid." *J Bone Joint Surg Am* 84-(A4): 547–551.

Rockwood, C. A., D. P. Green, *et al.* (2006). *Rockwood and Green's fractures in adults.* Philadelphia, PA: Lippincott Williams & Wilkins.

Rodriguez-Martin, J., J. Pretell-Mazzini, *et al.* (2011). "Outcomes after terrible triads of the elbow treated with the current surgical protocols: a review." *Int Orthop* 35(6): 851–860.

Rosas, H. G., and K. S. Lee (2010). "Imaging acute trauma of the elbow." *Semin Musculoskelet Radiol* 14(4): 394–411.

Sheehan S. E., G. S. Dyer, *et al.* (2013). "Traumatic elbow injuries: what the orthopedic surgeon wants to know." *Radiographics* 33: 869–888

Whiting, W. C., and R. F. Zernicke (2008). *Biomechanics of musculoskeletal injury*. Champaign, IL: Human Kinetics.

Case 72 67-year-old female with shoulder pain and limited range of motion following a fall onto an outstretched hand

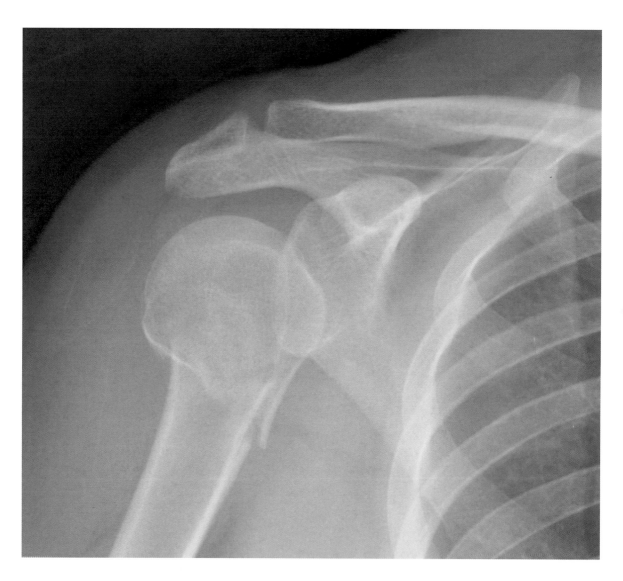

***Diagnosis:*
**Fracture
through the
surgical neck
of the humerus**

AP radiograph of the right shoulder demonstrates a slightly displaced transverse fracture (arrow) below the greater and lesser tuberosities (the surgical neck) of the proximal humerus.

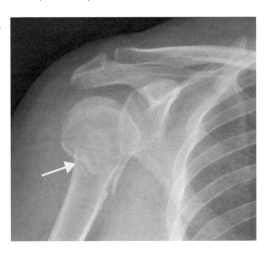

Discussion

- Proximal humerus fractures most commonly occur as a result of a fall onto an outstretched hand, with the humeral head impacting the hard-packed bone of the glenoid, but can occur with a number of mechanisms.
- Proximal humeral fractures can occur in several characteristic locations. The surgical neck (a nearly transverse line below the tuberosities) is much more commonly fractured than the anatomic neck (an oblique line above the tuberosities), which is rarely fractured in isolation.

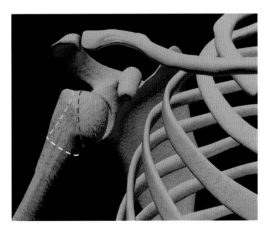

Typical proximal humerus fractures include the surgical neck (yellow dashed line), anatomic neck (red dashed line), and greater tuberosity (orange dashed line).

Classification of proximal humerus fractures

- Imaging of proximal humerus fractures.
- Proximal humeral fractures are most commonly classified according to the Neer classification system (discussed below), or alternately the Association for Osteosynthesis / Association for the Study of Internal Fixation (AO/ASIF) system (beyond the scope of this discussion). Differences in local institutional preferences may favor one system over the other.
- The Neer classification is based on the number and location of large fracture fragments or displaced "parts." Humeral head fractures are classified as having up to four parts, with the four parts being the humeral head, greater tuberosity, lesser tuberosity, and humeral shaft. A part is considered separate if it is displaced by 1 cm or more or is angulated 45 degrees or more. For instance, a four-part fracture must have at least 1 cm of displacement or 45 degrees of angulation of *each* part. Conversely, it is possible to have a comminuted fracture that is classified as one-part if no individual fragment meets these criteria.

Imaging of proximal humerus fractures

- Radiographs are sufficient for diagnosis in the majority of cases, with CT providing an adjunct role in classification of complex injuries and pre-surgical planning.
- CT and/or CT angiogram may be required in cases of neurovascular compromise.
- Fractures of the anatomic neck are associated with increased risk of avascular necrosis. The risk of avascular necrosis is increased with disruption of the medial periosteum of the proximal humeral metaphysis. Imaging findings suggestive of medial periosteal disruption include a short spur attached to the anatomic head measuring less than 8 mm or displaced by more than 2 mm.

Treatment issues

- Determination of overall treatment strategy is complex, with clinical factors such as ultimate functional outcome, surgical risk, and comorbid medical conditions playing a significant role.
- Early reduction is most beneficial, with failure of closed reduction often indicating open reduction in patients amenable to surgery.
- One-part and minimally displaced two-part fractures with post-reduction stability may undergo conservative treatment.
- Unstable or significantly displaced two-, three-, or four-part injuries will most often undergo surgical treatment.
- Anatomic neck fractures and fracture or fragmentation of the humeral head are associated with poor outcomes relating to humeral head ischemia.

Spectrum of proximal humerus fractures

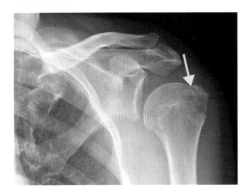

Greater tuberosity fracture

Isolated greater tuberosity fractures account for 20% of proximal humerus fractures and are associated with anterior glenohumeral dislocation. Up to two-thirds of fractures can be missed on initial radiographs. Nondisplaced or slightly displaced fractures are typically treated conservatively. Grashey radiograph of the left shoulder demonstrates a minimally displaced fracture of the greater tuberosity (arrow).

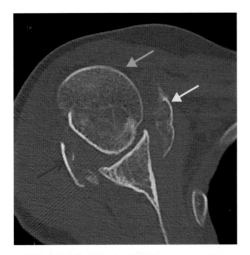

Four-part proximal humerus fracture

Four-part proximal humerus fractures are severe injuries with prognosis and treatment strategies depending on the degree of displacement of the fragments. Axial (upper image) and sagittal CT images of the right shoulder demonstrate a four-part proximal humerus fracture consisting of lesser tuberosity (yellow arrows), greater tuberosity (red arrows), humeral head (blue arrows), and humeral shaft (green arrow; seen on the sagittal only). This patient was treated with a hemiarthroplasty.

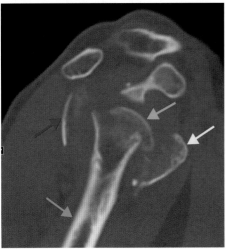

Differential diagnosis of proximal humerus fractures

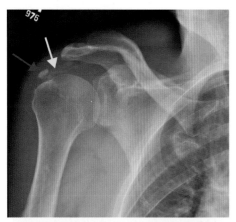

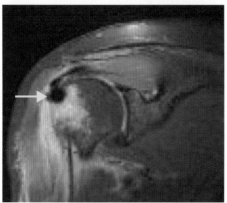

Calcific tendinitis/bursitis

Deposition of calcium hydroxyapatite within the rotator cuff tendons may cause acute pain when the deposits erupt from the tendon into the joint space, adjacent subacromial/subdeltoid bursa, or even the bone. The acute clinical presentation may mimic fracture; however, radiographs demonstrate globular/amorphous mineralization projecting over the course of the rotator cuff tendons or adjacent bursa and no fracture is evident. AP radiograph of the shoulder demonstrates globular, ill-defined mineralization along the expected course of the supraspinatus tendon (yellow arrow), with slightly more dense mineralization projecting over the subacromial/subdeltoid bursa (red arrow). Coronal proton density (PD) weighted MR with fat suppression demonstrates globular low signal at the supraspinatus insertion (yellow arrow) with marked reactive edema of the humeral head and adjacent soft tissues.

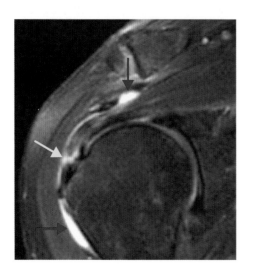

Acute rotator cuff tear

Although rotator cuff tears are most commonly secondary to degeneration, acute rotator cuff tear may be caused by trauma. Radiographs are typically negative. Coronal PD-weighted MR with fat suppression demonstrates a full-thickness defect (yellow arrow) of the critical zone of the supraspinatus, just proximal to the footprint. There is mild subacromial/subdeltoid bursal fluid (red arrows).

Further reading

Davies, A. M., and J. Hodler (2006). *Imaging of the shoulder: techniques and applications*. Berlin, New York: Springer.

Flatow, E. L., F. Cuomo, *et al.* (1991). "Open reduction and internal fixation of two-part displaced fractures of the greater tuberosity of the proximal part of the humerus." *J Bone Joint Surg Am* 73(8): 1213–1218.

Kilcoyne, R. F., W. P. Shuman, *et al.* (1990). "The Neer classification of displaced proximal humeral fractures: spectrum of findings on plain radiographs and CT scans." *AJR Am J Roentgenol* 154(5): 1029–1033.

Mattyasovszky, S. G., K. J. Burkhart *et al.* (Dec. 2011) "Isolated fractures of the greater tuberosity of the proximal humerus." *Acta Orthop* 82(6): 714–720.

Mirzayan, R. (2004). *Shoulder and elbow trauma*. New York: Thieme.

Müller, M. E., S. M. Perren, *et al.* (1991). *Manual of internal fixation: techniques recommended by the AO–ASIF Group*. Berlin, New York: Springer-Verlag.

Neer, C. S., II (1970). "Displaced proximal humeral fractures. I. Classification and evaluation." *J Bone Joint Surg Am* 52(6): 1077–1089.

Rasmussen, S., I. Hvass, *et al.* (1992). "Displaced proximal humeral fractures: results of conservative treatment." *Injury* 23(1): 41–43.

Rockwood, C. A. (2009). *The shoulder*. Philadelphia, PA: Saunders/Elsevier.

Rockwood, C. A., D. P. Green, *et al.* (2006). *Rockwood and Green's fractures in adults*. Philadelphia: Lippincott Williams & Wilkins.

Sandstrom, C. K., Kennedy, S. A., Gross, J. A., (2015). Acute Shoulder Trauma: What the Surgeon Wants to Know. *Radiographics* 2015; 35: 475–492.

Siebenrock, K. A., and C. Gerber (1993). "The reproducibility of classification of fractures of the proximal end of the humerus." *J Bone Joint Surg Am* 75(12): 1751–1755.

Whiting, W. C., and R. F. Zernicke (2008). *Biomechanics of musculoskeletal injury*. Champaign, IL: Human Kinetics.

Case 73

34-year-old female complains of elbow pain and limited range of motion after falling onto an outstretched hand

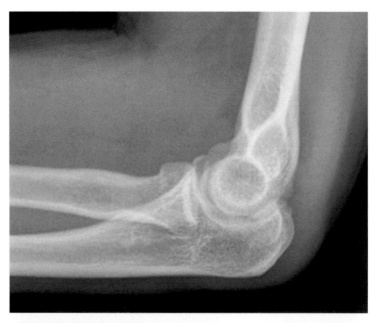

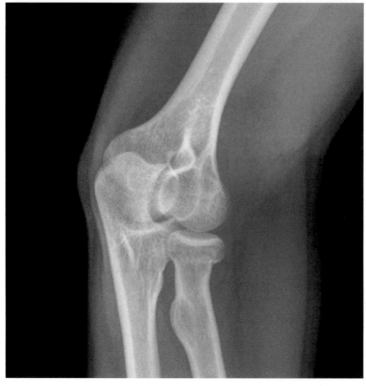

**Diagnosis:
Radial neck
fracture**

Lateral (left image) and AP radiographs of the elbow demonstrate elevated anterior and posterior fat pads (yellow arrows), indicative of an elbow joint effusion. There is a subtle depressed fracture of the radial neck (red arrows), best appreciated on the AP radiograph.

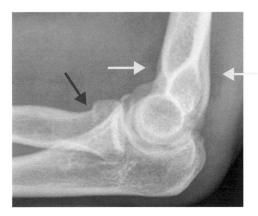 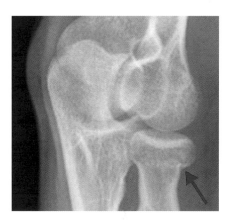

Discussion

Overview of radial head and neck fractures

- Often radiographically occult, fractures through the radial head or neck most commonly occur following a fall onto outstretched hand (FOOSH), with the radial head impacting upon the capitellum.
- Radial head or neck fractures can be seen with posterior elbow dislocations and as a component of complex injuries about the elbow.

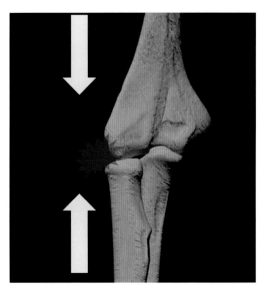

Axial loading at the elbow (yellow arrows), commonly seen in a fall on outstretched hand (FOOSH), causes impact of the radial head on the capitellum with potential for radial head fracture.

Radial head fractures are commonly classified according to the Mason classification system.

- **Type I:** Minimally displaced (<2 mm displacement) radial head or neck fracture.

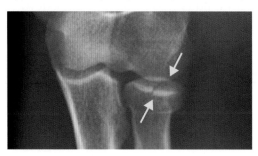

AP radiograph of the elbow demonstrates a minimally displaced radial head fracture (arrows), consistent with Mason I fracture.

- **Type II:** Displaced single fracture (>2 mm displacement) with <30% articular involvement.

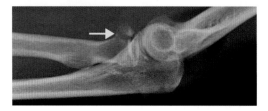

Lateral radiograph of the elbow demonstrates a displaced fracture of the radial head (arrow) with associated posterior dislocation of the radius at the radiocapitellar articulation. There is also posterior subluxation of the ulna, with perching of the distal humerus on the coronoid process tip.

- **Type III:** Comminuted radial head fracture.

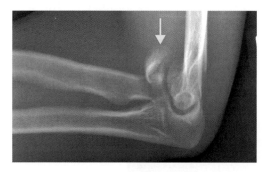

Lateral radiograph of the elbow demonstrates a comminuted radial head fracture (arrow).

- **Type IV:** Radial head fracture with associated dislocation of the radial head from the radiocapitellar articulation.

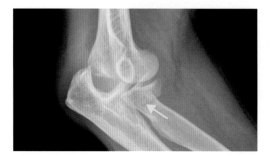

Lateral-oblique radiograph of the elbow demonstrates a radial head fracture (arrow) and dislocation of both the radiocapitellar and ulnohumeral articulations.

Imaging of radial head fractures

- Proximal radius fractures can be radiographically occult on initial imaging. The presence of an effusion (as indicated by elevation of the posterior or anterior fat pads) can suggest occult fracture.
- CT can be used for further evaluation in cases of high clinical suspicion.
- MRI can demonstrate edema or a low signal intensity fracture line.

Treatment issues

- Nondisplaced (Type I) fractures are most commonly treated conservatively.
- Minimally displaced fractures (Type II) can undergo a trial of conservative therapy if functional range of motion is preserved, but significant displacement, comminution (Type III), and dislocation (Type IV) most often require surgical treatment.

Differential diagnosis of radial head/ neck fractures

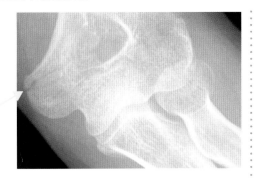

Supracondylar humerus fracture

Supracondylar fractures are typically seen in children, and are rare in adults. Oblique radiograph of elbow demonstrates a transverse, minimally displaced supracondylar fracture (arrow).

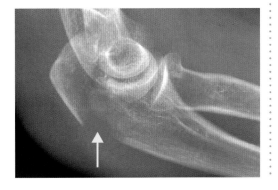

Olecranon fracture

Fractures of the olecranon can be due to direct impact on a flexed elbow or triceps avulsion injury. These fractures are considered intra-articular. Lateral radiograph of the elbow demonstrates a displaced, slightly comminuted olecranon fracture (arrow).

Further reading

Johnston, G. W. (1962). "A follow-up of one hundred cases of fracture of the head of the radius with a review of the literature." *Ulster Med J* 31: 51–56.

Major, N. M., and S. T. Crawford (2002). "Elbow effusions in trauma in adults and children: is there an occult fracture?" *AJR Am J Roentgenol* 178(2): 413–418.

Mason, M. L. (1954). "Some observations on fractures of the head of the radius with a review of one hundred cases." *Br J Surg* 42(172): 123–132.

Miller, M. D. (2000). *Review of orthopedics*. Philadelphia, PA: Saunders.

Morrey, B. F., and J. Sanchez-Sotelo (2009). *The elbow and its disorders*. Philadelphia, PA: Saunders/Elsevier.

Rockwood, C. A., et al. (2006). *Rockwood and Green's fractures in adults*. Philadelphia, PA: Lippincott Williams & Wilkins.

Sheehan, S. E., S. G. Dyer *et al.* (2013). "Traumatic elbow injuries: what the orthopedic surgeon wants to know." *Radiographics* 33: 869–888.

Case 74   45-year-old female with chest pain after a motor vehicle accident

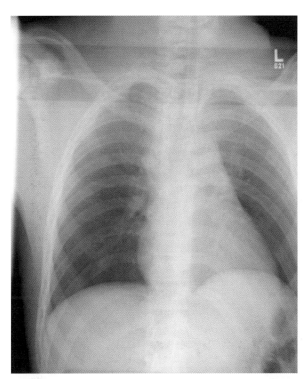

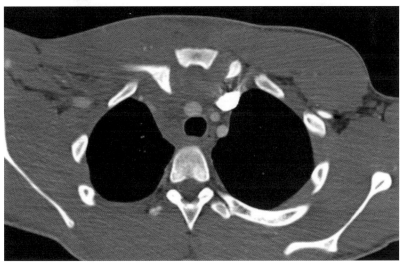

Diagnosis:
Right
sternoclavicular
joint
dislocation

Chest radiograph demonstrates subtle asymmetry in the position of the medial clavicles in this intubated patient. Axial contrast-enhanced CT through the upper chest reveals right posterior sternoclavicular dislocation (yellow arrow) with an anterior mediastinal hematoma (red arrows). The left sterno-clavicular joint is normal.

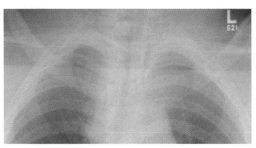 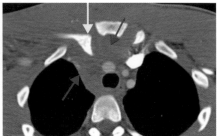

Discussion

Overview of sternoclavicular dislocation

- Sternoclavicular dislocation is most often due to high-energy injuries, and can be seen as a result of direct and indirect forces about the joint. Indirect mechanisms are more common, caused by lateral compression of the shoulder girdle.

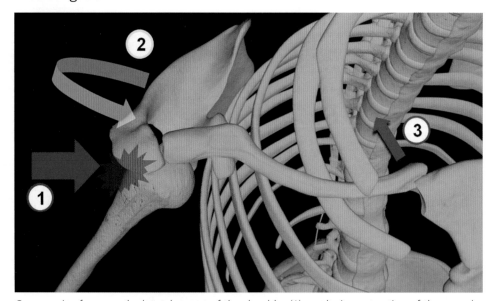

Compressive force on the lateral aspect of the shoulder (1) results in protraction of the scapula (2), with compressive force transmitted along the shaft of the clavicle to produce posterior dislocation at the sternoclavicular joint (3). Alternately, if the compressive force vector causes retraction (rather than protraction) of the scapula, then anterior dislocation of the clavicle at the sternoclavicular joint can result.

- The classification of sternoclavicular dislocation primarily depends on the direction of dislocation at the sternoclavicular joint, with anterior dislocations occurring much more commonly.
- Posterior dislocations have an increased risk of associated soft tissue injuries, including injuries to the great vessels or the trachea.
- Patients under 25 years old may have injury to the proximal clavicle physis.

Imaging of sternoclavicular dislocation

- Sternoclavicular dislocations are usually occult or very difficult to see on standard chest radiographs. Sometimes slight asymmetry in the alignment of the sternoclavicular joints can be seen, although this finding can be difficult to distinguish from positional variation.
- Serendipity views (frontal radiograph with 40 degree cephalic tilt) can better show the anterior and posterior displacement.
- CT is recommended for full characterization of extent of injuries, particularly vascular, tracheal, or lung injuries in the setting of posterior dislocations. Dyspnea or dysphagia can result from compression of the trachea and esophagus in posterior dislocations.

Treatment issues

- Early closed reduction can be attempted, though surgical reduction is often required.
- Posterior dislocations should undergo urgent reduction in an operative setting due to the high risk of associated soft tissue injuries.
- Over-reduction of anterior dislocation can cause injury to underlying chest structures, including the great vessels, trachea, and lungs. Closed reduction of anterior dislocations should therefore be performed only with close coordination with thoracic surgery.

Clinical synopsis
The patient underwent successful closed reduction of the right sternoclavicular joint under fluoroscopy. An outpatient follow-up chest CT showed interval decrease in mediastinal hematoma and satisfactory alignment of both sternoclavicular joints.

Self-assessment

- *What type of sternoclavicular dislocation can be fatal?*
- The mediastinal vascular structures including the aorta are at risk with posterior sternoclavicular dislocation. CT is the modality of choice to characterize associated injuries.

Differential diagnosis of sternoclavicular dislocation

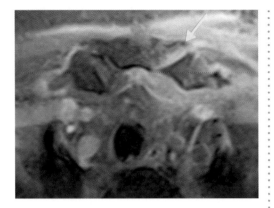

Sternoclavicular septic arthritis

Septic arthritis of the sternoclavicular joint is an uncommon form of infection seen predominantly in patients with predisposing risk factors, such as immunosuppression or history of intravenous drug abuse. Axial post contrast T1-weighted MR image with fat suppression in a 44-year-old intravenous drug abuser shows diffuse capsular enhancement and cortical irregularity of the left margin of the sternum (arrow), in keeping with septic arthritis and osteomyelitis. The alignment is intact.

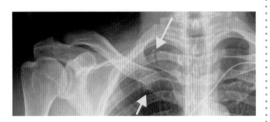

Medial clavicle fracture

Clavicle fractures are typically caused by a direct blow to the lateral shoulder or fall on an outstretched arm. Middle third of clavicle fractures comprise the majority of clavicle fractures, and operative management is generally performed if there is greater than one shaft's-width displacement. The pectoralis major muscle and weight of the arm displace the lateral segment of the clavicle inferiorly. Fractures involving the medial clavicle are rare and may result in compression of mediastinal structures with posterior displacement. These injuries therefore require rapid diagnosis, and CT is the examination of choice to assess the displacement and integrity of mediastinal structures. Frontal radiograph demon-strates a comminuted fracture of the medial right clavicle with greater than one shaft's-width inferior displacement of the distal fracture fragment (arrows).

Further reading

Kennedy, P. T., and H. J. Mawhinney (1995). "Retrosternal dislocation of the sternoclavicular joint." *J R Coll Surg Edinb* 40(3): 208–209.

Nettles, J. L., and R. L. Linscheid (1968). "Sternoclavicular dislocations." *J Trauma* 8(2): 158–164.

Robinson, C. M., P. J. Jenkins, *et al.* (2008). "Disorders of the sternoclavicular joint." *J Bone Joint Surg Br* 90(6): 685–696.

Rockwood, C. A., D. P. Green, *et al.* (2006). *Rockwood and Green's fractures in adults.* Philadelphia: Lippincott Williams & Wilkins.

Whiting, W. C., and R. F. Zernicke (2008). *Biomechanics of musculoskeletal injury.* Champaign, IL: Human Kinetics.

Wirth, M. A., and C. A. Rockwood, Jr. (1996). "Acute and chronic traumatic injuries of the sternoclavicular joint." *J Am Acad Orthop Surg* 4(5): 268–278.

Case 75   18-year-old male with finger pain after jamming his finger attempting to catch a baseball

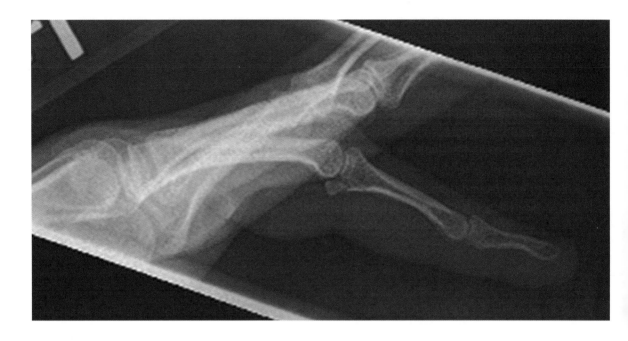

Diagnosis:
Volar plate
avulsion
fracture

Lateral radiograph of the second digit demonstrates a volar plate avulsion fracture (arrow) at the proximal interphalangeal (PIP) joint, without dislocation.

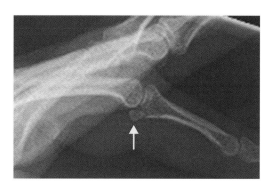

Discussion

Overview of volar plate injury

- The volar plate is a ligamentous structure of the PIP joint that prevents hyperextension.
- A volar plate injury may involve the ligament only, or may involve an osseous avulsion fracture. A volar plate avulsion is a fracture of the volar aspect of the articular base of the middle phalanx, and is commonly caused by a hyperextension injury with axial pressure applied to the fingertip.
- Volar plate fractures are often associated with dorsal subluxation or dislocation at the PIP joint.

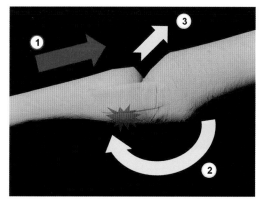

Axial loading along the shaft of the middle phalanx (1) and hyperextension at the PIP joint (2) can cause avulsion injuries at the base of the middle phalanx with dorsal subluxation at the PIP joint (3).

Classification of volar plate fractures

- Volar plate fractures are classified according to the stability of the joint after reduction. The volar plate may remain inserted on an avulsed distal fracture fragment, but collateral ligaments may be disrupted, or can remain inserted on either the volar or dorsal fragments.
  - **Stable fractures** are generally small fractures with <40% articular surface involvement, as the proper collateral ligaments are not functionally disrupted. This type of stable fracture is often referred to as a volar plate avulsion "chip" injury.
  - **Unstable fractures** most often involve >40% of the articular surface, commonly with frank dorsal dislocation. Significant dislocation implies complete functional disruption of the volar plate, with associated collateral ligament disruption or proper collateral ligament insertion on the small volar fracture fragment.

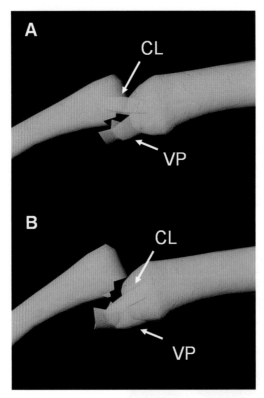

Illustration of the PIP joint in a lateral projection with volar plate (VP) fractures and dorsal phalanx dislocation. Stability is maintained when the fracture fragment is small and the proper collateral ligament (CL) maintains its insertion on the larger dorsal fracture component (A). When the fracture fragment is large, the proper collateral ligament either inserts onto the fracture fragment (as diagrammed in B), or the ligament is frankly disrupted and the fracture is unstable.

Imaging of volar plate injuries

- PA and true lateral finger radiographs are essential to diagnosis, though the presence or size of the fracture fragment may not reflect the degree of functional instability. The "V" sign represents divergence of the proximal and middle phalanges at the dorsal aspect of the PIP articulation, as seen on the lateral radiograph. The presence of a "V" sign indicates dorsal subluxation and probable instability.

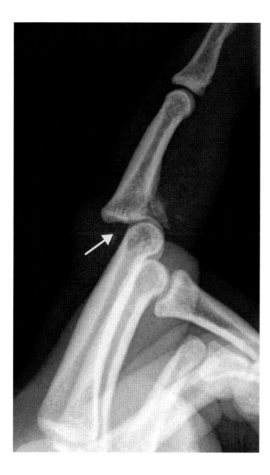

Lateral radiograph of the index finger demonstrates a "V" sign (arrow), with dorsal subluxation of the middle phalanx and a volar plate fracture.

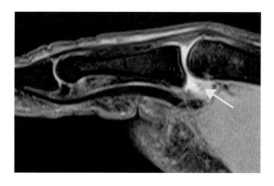

MRI can be obtained to directly evaluate the degree of ligamentous and soft tissue injuries, particularly injuries to the collateral ligaments. Sagittal proton density MRI with fat suppression demonstrates complete disruption of the volar plate (arrow) at the PIP joint of the 2nd digit.

Treatment issues

- Nonoperative treatment is usually considered for small fractures (<40% articular surface involvement), provided post-reduction functional stability is maintained. There is increased risk of an unstable injury with larger avulsion fragments, which will likely require surgical screw fixation or volar plate arthroplasty with repair of collateral ligament injury.
- Failed reduction due to soft tissue interposition usually requires open reduction and internal fixation.

Clinical synopsis

The patient was managed conservatively, with buddy taping and early mobilization with hand therapy.

Self-assessment

- *What is the most common mechanism of volar plate injury?*

- Hyperextension mechanism is the most common cause of volar plate injury.

Differential diagnosis of volar plate injury

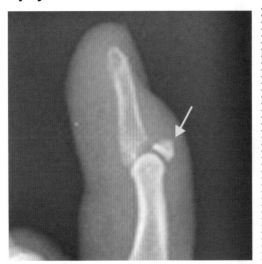

Mallet fracture

A mallet fracture is an avulsion injury of the extensor digitorum longus tendon at its insertion into the dorsal aspect of the distal phalanx. Significant displacement of the avulsion fragment or >50% articular surface involvement usually requires surgical treatment. In contrast to a volar plate fracture, the mallet avulsion occurs at the dorsal aspect of the finger and at the distal interphalangeal (DIP) joint rather than the PIP joint. Lateral radiograph demonstrates an avulsion fracture (arrow) of the dorsal aspect of the DIP.

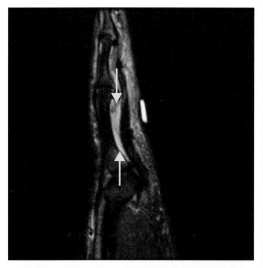

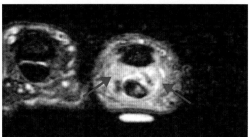

A2 pulley injury

Each finger flexor tendon passes through a fibro-osseous tunnel extending from the head of the metacarpals to the DIP joints. Each component of this tunnel is an alphanumeric-designated pulley. A2 and A4 are the largest pulleys and the primary preventers of flexor tendon bowstringing when the finger is flexed. The A2 pulley is located at the proximal-to-mid aspect of the proximal phalanx and the A4 is at the proximal-to-mid aspect of the middle phalanx. The typical mechanism for pulley injury is finger flexion under extreme loads, as may be experienced by rock climbers. Sagittal PD-weighted MRI with fat suppression demonstrates edema (yellow arrows) interposed between the proximal phalanx and the volarly displaced flexor tendon. Axial PD-weighted MR with fat suppression confirms separation of the flexor tendon from the phalanx with surrounding edema and full-thickness tears of the radial and ulnar aspects of the A2 pulley (red arrows).

Further reading

Bailie, D. S., L. S. Benson, et al. (1996). "Proximal interphalangeal joint injuries of the hand. Part I: anatomy and diagnosis." Am J Orthop (Belle Mead NJ) 25(7): 474–477.

Benson, L. S., and D. S. Bailie (1996). "Proximal interphalangeal joint injuries of the hand. Part II: Treatment and complications." Am J Orthop (Belle Mead NJ) 25 (8): 527–530.

Clavero, J. A., X. Alomar, et al. (2002). "MR imaging of ligament and tendon injuries of the fingers." Radiographics 22(2): 237–256.

Combs, J. A. (2000). "It's not 'just a finger.'" J Athl Train 35(2): 168–178.

Dionysian, E., and R. G. Eaton (2000). "The long-term outcome of volar plate arthroplasty of the proximal interphalangeal joint." J Hand Surg Am 25(3): 429–437.

Eaton, R. G., and M. M. Malerich (1980). "Volar plate arthroplasty of the proximal interphalangeal joint: a review of ten years' experience." J Hand Surg Am 5(3): 260–268.

Miller, M. D. (2000). Review of Orthopedics. Philadelphia, PA: Saunders.

Rockwood, C. A., D. P. Green, et al. (2006). Rockwood and Green's fractures in adults. Philadelphia, PA: Lippincott Williams & Wilkins.

Case 76   32-year-old male with shoulder pain status post motor vehicle accident

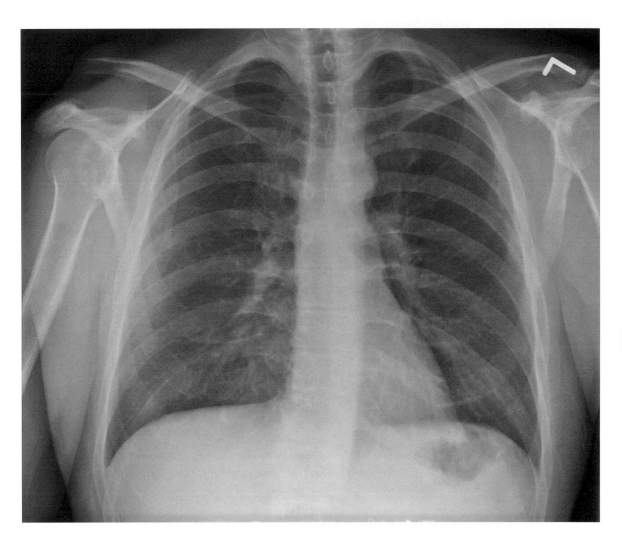

Diagnosis:
Type III
acromiocla-
vicular joint
separation
with coraco-
clavicular
ligament
avulsion

Magnified view of an AP chest radiograph demonstrates elevation of the distal clavicle (yellow arrow) relative to the acromion (red arrow) with widening of the coracoclavicular space. There is osseous irregularity at the superior aspect of the coracoid (blue arrow), consistent with coracoclavicular ligament avulsion.

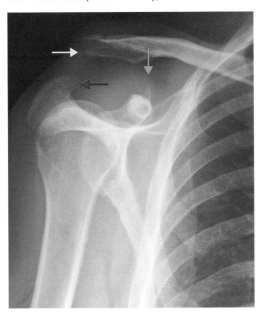

Discussion

Overview of acromioclavicular (AC) joint separation

- AC joint separation, generically referred to as "shoulder separation," describes a spectrum of injuries that most commonly occur as a result of a fall onto the lateral aspect of the shoulder with the arm in flexion and adduction.

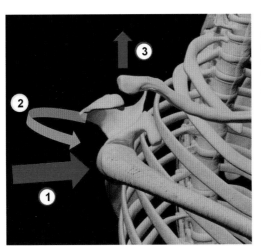

Impact onto the lateral aspect of the shoulder (1), as seen with a fall onto the shoulder, produces protraction of the scapula (2), with compressive force transmitted to the AC joint, causing superior displacement of the distal clavicle (3) with respect to the acromion.

Classification of acromioclavicular injuries

- Acromioclavicular injuries are most commonly classified according to the Rockwood classification system.
  - **Type I:** AC ligament sprain.
  - **Type II:** AC ligament tear with intact coracoclavicular (CC) ligament.
  - **Type III:** AC and CC ligament tears with widening of the coracoclavicular distance up to 100% compared to the contralateral side.
  - **Type IV:** AC and CC ligament tears with posterior displacement of clavicle.
  - **Type V:** AC and CC ligament tears with superior displacement of clavicle of greater than 100% compared to the contralateral side.
  - **Type VI:** AC and CC ligament tears with inferior/subacromial displacement of clavicle.

Imaging of acromioclavicular injuries

- Measurement thresholds of 6 mm and 7 mm have been suggested as upper limits of normal for acromioclavicular joint space on frontal radiographs for women and men, respectively. Similarly, a coracoclavicular space of 13 mm has been shown to be the upper limit of normal. Some authors have indicated that measurements exceeding these values suggest AC or CC ligament injury. However, the orthopedic surgery literature favors comparison with the (presumed normal) contralateral side. Greater than a 25–50% measurement discrepancy with the normal side has been suggested to correlate with ligament injury. This method is problematic in cases of bilateral injury, or when contralateral imaging is unavailable.
- Type I injuries are radiographically occult or may show soft tissue swelling at the AC joint, with the diagnosis dependent on the patient's symptoms and clinical suspicion.
- Type II injuries can be ambiguous, showing only minimal widening of the AC space.
- Weight-bearing radiographs (with weights held in hands) have been suggested to aid in detection of occult Type III injuries; however, studies have shown mixed results regarding efficacy.
- Type III, IV, and VI injuries may be difficult to distinguish clearly on radiographs, as differentiation depends on the relative three-dimensional displacement of the clavicle. In type IV injuries, the clavicle is displaced posteriorly, while in type VI injuries the distal clavicle is dislocated inferiorly, underneath the coracoid process. CT may be required to discriminate between these types. CT angiography should be considered if a type IV injury (posterior clavicular displacement) with vascular compromise is suspected.
- Type V injuries can be diagnosed with a 100–300% increase in the CC interspace on frontal radiographs.
- MRI has been shown to demonstrate ligamentous and associated soft tissue injury, and can be useful in resolving diagnostic ambiguity between type II

(intact coracoclavicular ligament) and type III (torn coracoclavicular ligament) injuries, particularly if surgical intervention is being contemplated. MRI is not indicated for uncomplicated injuries.

Treatment issues

- AC joint injury types I and II are almost always treated conservatively.
- Type III injuries may undergo a trial of conservative treatment versus early surgical intervention, depending on institutional and patient preferences and functional goals. Optimal treatment of these injuries is highly controversial.
- Type IV–VI injuries most commonly require surgical treatment.

Clinical synopsis   The patient was treated conservatively and made a full recovery.

Self-assessment

- *When is the AC joint width considered pathologic?*

- An AC joint width of greater than 7 mm in men and 6 mm in women may be pathologic if there is a history of trauma.

- *What are the two parts of the coracoclavicular ligament?*

- The coracoclavicular ligament consists of the conoid (triangular-shaped) ligament medially and trapezoid (quadrilateral-shaped) ligament laterally.

Spectrum of acromioclavicular injury

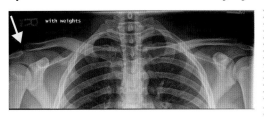

Type I/II AC injury

Frontal radiograph of the AC joints with weights in both hands demonstrates minimal asymmetric widening of the right AC joint (arrow). Non-weighted view was normal.

Type II AC injury

Frontal radiograph demonstrates widening of the AC joint (arrow). The coracoclavicular distance is normal.

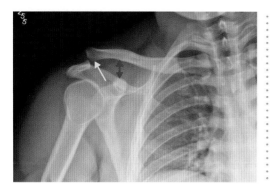

Type III AC injury

Frontal radiograph demonstrates disruption of the AC joint with superior displacement of the clavicle (yellow arrow) and widened coracoclavicular distance (red arrows), indicative of tears of the AC and CC ligaments. In contrast to the index case, the coracoid is intact.

Differential diagnosis of acromioclavicular injury

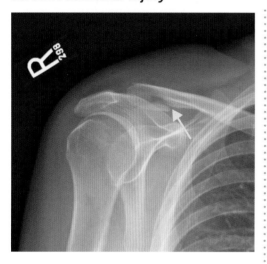

Distal clavicle fracture

AP radiograph of the right shoulder demonstrates mild widening of the acromioclavicular distance. The widening is due to a mildly displaced fracture of the distal 1/3 of the clavicle (arrow).

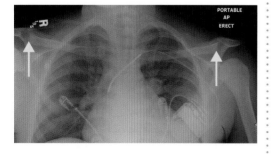

Subperiosteal resorption of the distal clavicles

Frontal chest radiograph in a patient with hyperparathyroidism demonstrates subperiosteal resorption of the distal clavicles (arrows). Although the imaging appearance may be similar to traumatic osteolysis seen in weightlifters (discussed below), resorption of the distal clavicles is seen in older patients with chronic hyperparathyroidism or chronic renal disease.

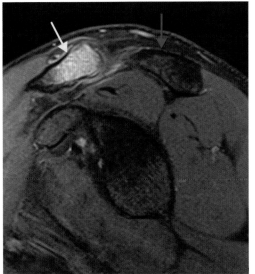

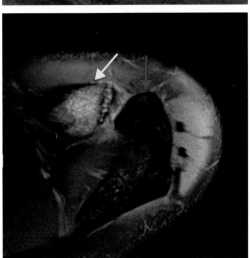

Traumatic osteolysis of the distal clavicle

Traumatic osteolysis of the distal clavicle is a painful condition seen in otherwise healthy weightlifters. Sagittal (upper image) and axial PD-weighted MR images with fat suppression in a weightlifter without history of acute trauma demonstrate marked edema of the distal clavicle (yellow arrows). This imaging finding is not specific and can also be seen with focal contusion and acromioclavicular arthropathy, but the lack of trauma and weightlifting history suggest traumatic osteolysis. The anterior acromion (red arrows) is intact.

Further reading

Alyas, F., M. Curtis, *et al.* (2008). "MR imaging appearances of acromioclavicular joint dislocation." *Radiographics* 28(2): 463–479; quiz 619.

Bearden, J. M., J. C. Hughston, *et al.* (1973). "Acromioclavicular dislocation: method of treatment." *J Sports Med* 1(4): 5–17.

Gstettner, C., M. Tauber, *et al.* (2008). "Rockwood type III acromioclavicular dislocation: surgical versus conservative treatment." *J Shoulder Elbow Surg* 17(2): 220–225.

Mulier, T., J. Stuyck, *et al.* (1993). "Conservative treatment of acromioclavicular dislocation: evaluation of functional and radiological results after six years follow-up." *Acta Orthop Belg* 59(3): 255–262.

Petersson, C. J., and I. Redlund-Johnell (1983). "Radiographic joint space in normal acromioclavicular joints." *Acta Orthop Scand* 54(3): 431–433.

Rockwood, C. A., D. P. Green, *et al.* (2006). *Rockwood and Green's fractures in adults*. Philadelphia: Lippincott Williams & Wilkins.

Schlegel, T. F., R. T. Burks, *et al.* (2001). "A prospective evaluation of untreated acute grade III acromioclavicular separations." *Am J Sports Med* 29(6): 699–703.

Spencer, E. E., Jr. (2007). "Treatment of grade III acromioclavicular joint injuries: a systematic review." *Clin Orthop Relat Res* 455: 38–44.

Whiting, W. C., and R. F. Zernicke (2008). *Biomechanics of musculoskeletal injury*. Champaign, IL: Human Kinetics.

Case 77   48-year-old male complains of shoulder pain and limited range
of motion after a fall with arm flexed and abducted

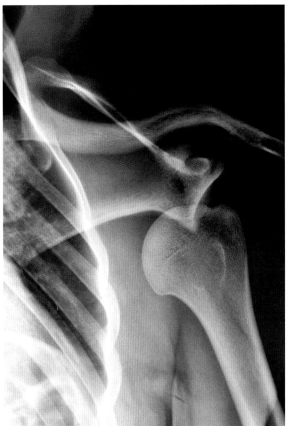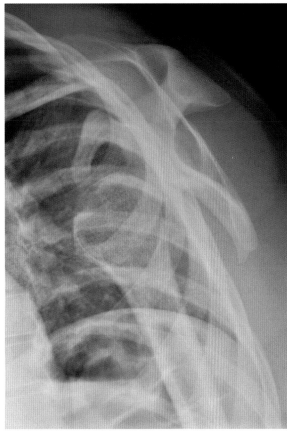

Diagnosis:
Anterior
shoulder
dislocation

AP radiograph of the shoulder (left image) demonstrates an anterior subcoracoid shoulder dislocation with the humeral head (yellow arrow) inferiorly displaced relative to the glenoid. Scapular-Y radiograph of the shoulder confirms that the humeral head (yellow arrow) is dislocated anterior to the glenoid and inferior to the coracoid process (red arrow).

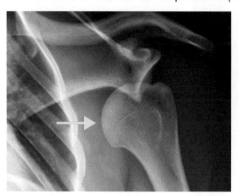 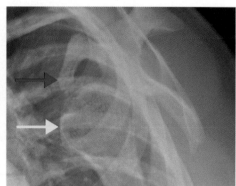

Discussion

Overview of glenohumeral dislocation

- Glenohumeral dislocation is defined as complete loss of glenohumeral articulation. In contrast, subluxation is characterized by partial articulation of the humeral head with the glenoid. Shoulder dislocation is classified based on direction, humeral head location, and presence of associated injuries.
- The vast majority of shoulder dislocations are anterior in direction (~95%), and are further subclassified as subcoracoid (A), subglenoid (B), or subclavicular (C) based on resting pre-reduction position of the humeral head.

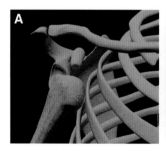 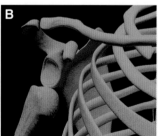 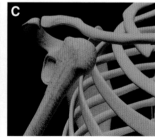

- Anterior dislocations are most commonly the result of hyperflexion with the arm in abduction and external rotation, often in association with an anteriorly directed force onto the posterior aspect of the shoulder.

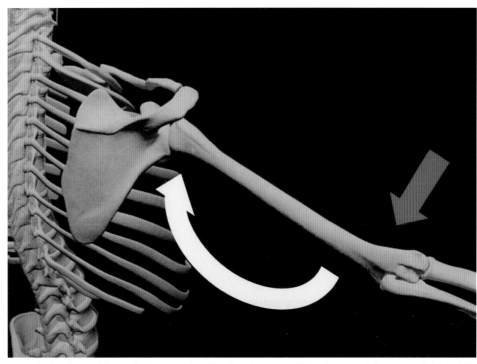

Posteriorly directed force (red arrow) on the distal aspect of the flexed, abducted and externally rotated arm produces an anteriorly directed force at the glenohumeral joint (yellow arrow), which can cause anterior shoulder dislocation.

Injuries associated with anterior shoulder dislocation

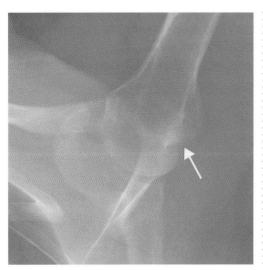

Hill–Sachs lesion

The Hill–Sachs lesion is an impaction fracture of the posterolateral humeral head, caused by contact of the humeral head upon the anterior-inferior glenoid after dislocation. Stryker notch radiograph of the shoulder (upper image) demonstrates a depression in the posterolateral humeral head (arrow), consistent with a Hill–Sachs lesion. AP radiograph in a different patient (lower image) demonstrates a Hill–Sachs lesion as linear sclerosis of the superolateral humeral head (arrow).

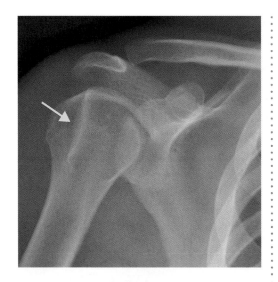

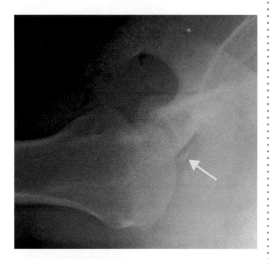

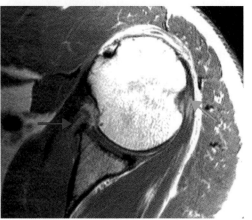

Anterior-inferior glenolabral complex injury

A Bankart lesion is an injury to the anterior-inferior glenoid labrum caused by impaction of the humeral head after dislocation. The glenoid is intact with a soft tissue Bankart injury, while a bony Bankart includes an avulsion fracture of the anterior-inferior glenoid rim. West Point radiograph of the shoulder (upper image) demonstrates a slightly displaced fracture of the anterior glenoid rim (yellow arrow), suggestive of a Bankart fracture due to prior anterior shoulder dislocation. Axial T1-weighted MR image of the shoulder in a different patient demonstrates an anterior-inferior labral tear consistent with a Bankart lesion (red arrow), and a partially imaged Hill–Sachs lesion (blue arrow).

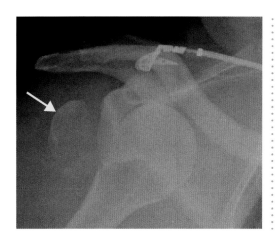

Greater tuberosity fracture

Greater tuberosity fractures are often associated with anterior dislocation and are relatively uncommon in isolation. There may be limitation in functional ability if there is significant displacement of the fracture. Treatment is typically operative, with repair of the often-concomitant rotator cuff tear. AP radiograph demonstrates anteromedial shoulder dislocation with a displaced greater tuberosity fracture (arrow).

Imaging of glenohumeral dislocation

- Initial pre-reduction radiographs should be obtained to verify diagnosis and to evaluate for the presence of any abnormality that may complicate reduction, such as a large loose bone fragment or comminuted glenoid fracture.
- Stryker notch and West Point views can be obtained for optimal radiographic evaluation of Hill–Sachs and osseus Bankart injuries, respectively.
- MRI can be obtained in suspected massive rotator cuff tear, or if there is concern for significant soft tissue interposition complicating reduction.
- Suspected vascular injuries may require emergent CT angiography.

Treatment of glenohumeral dislocation

- Early reduction is critical and should not be delayed to obtain advanced imaging for uncomplicated dislocations.
- Surgical reduction may be required for failure of closed reduction.
- Surgical treatment may ultimately be required, especially in younger patients who are at risk for recurrent dislocations or shoulder instability.

Clinical synopsis   A closed reduction of the shoulder was performed in the Emergency Department and the patient was managed conservatively without surgery.

Self-assessment

- *What is the most common site of glenoid fracture in anterior dislocation?*

- The anteroinferior glenoid fracture (osseous Bankart lesion) is the most common glenoid fracture seen with anterior dislocation.

- *In which age group is there a high incidence of rotator cuff failure with anterior dislocation?*

- There is an 80% incidence of associated rotator cuff tear in patients over 60 years of age, compared to only 30% in patients under 40 years of age. Recurrent instability, however, is more common in younger patients and usually requires surgery.

Differential diagnosis of anterior dislocation

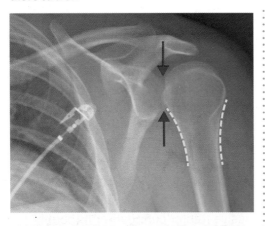

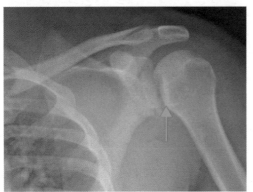

Posterior dislocation

Posterior dislocations are typically caused by sudden global muscle contraction in electric shock or seizures. Posterior dislocations are much less common than anterior dislocations but are more difficult to diagnose on the AP radiograph. Signs of posterior dislocation on the AP radiograph include the "light bulb" sign (due to fixed internal rotation) and loss of the normal "half-moon overlap" sign (caused by lateral displacement of the humerus and absence of the normal overlap of the medial humeral head with the glenoid). A reverse Hill–Sachs lesion is known as the "trough" sign, and appears as linear sclerosis of the humeral head. An injury of the posteroinferior glenoid known as a "reverse Bankart" lesion may also be present. Specific signs of posterior dislocation on the Grashey radiograph have not been named but there is generally loss of glenohumeral congruence. AP radiograph (upper image) shows both the lightbulb sign (dashed yellow lines) and loss of the half-moon overlap sign (red arrows). AP radiograph of a different patient (bottom image) shows linear sclerosis (blue arrow) of the humeral head indicating the "trough" sign.

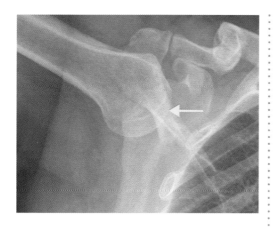

Inferior dislocation

Inferior dislocations are the least common type of dislocation, and are thought to be the result of hyperabduction of the arm with leverage of the humeral metaphysis about the acromion. There is an increased incidence of associated rotator cuff tear and neurologic injury. Luxatio erecta is inferior dislocation of the humeral head with the arm locked pointing upwards. Frontal shoulder radiograph demonstrates luxatio erecta with inferior displacement of the humeral head (arrow) with respect to the glenoid.

Further reading

Arciero, R. A., J. H. Wheeler, et al. (1994). "Arthroscopic Bankart repair versus nonoperative treatment for acute, initial anterior shoulder dislocations." Am J Sports Med 22(5): 589–594.

Burgess, B., and B. J. Sennett (2003). "Traumatic shoulder instability: nonsurgical management versus surgical intervention." Orthop Nurs 22(5): 345–350; quiz 351–352.

Chung, C. B., and L. S. Steinbach (2010). MRI of the upper extremity: shoulder, elbow, wrist and hand. Philadelphia: Wolters Kluwer Health / Lippincott Williams & Wilkins.

Freundlich, B. D. (1983). "Luxatio erecta." J Trauma 23(5): 434–436.

Mallon, W. J., F. H. Bassett, III, et al. (1990). "Luxatio erecta: the inferior glenohumeral dislocation." J Orthop Trauma 4(1): 19–24.

Miller, M. D. (2000). Philadelphia, PA: Saunders.

Netto, N. A., M. J. Tamaoki, et al. (July 2012). "Treatment of Bankart lesions in traumatic anterior instability of the shoulder: a randomized controlled trial comparing arthroscopy and open techniques." Arthroscopy 28(7): 900-908.

Provencher, M. T., R. M. Frank, et al. (2012). "The Hill–Sachs lesion: diagnosis, classification, and management." J Am Acad Orthop Surg 20(4): 242–252.

Rockwood, C. A., D. P. Green, et al. (2006). Rockwood and Green's fractures in adults. Philadelphia: Lippincott Williams & Wilkins.

Wang, R. Y., R. A. Arciero, et al. (2009). "The recognition and treatment of first-time shoulder dislocation in active individuals." J Orthop Sports Phys Ther 39(2): 118–123.

Whiting, W. C., and R. F. Zernicke (2008). Biomechanics of musculoskeletal injury. Champaign, IL: Human Kinetics.

Case 78   68-year-old female with wrist pain and deformity following a fall onto an outstretched hand

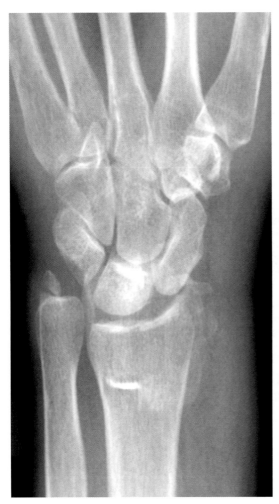
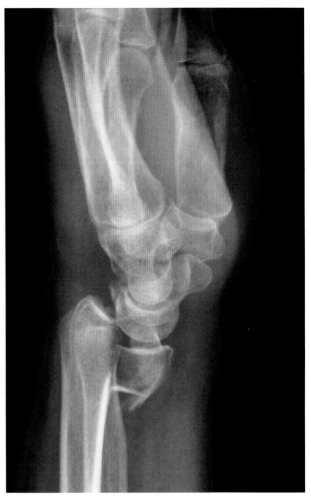

Diagnosis: **Volar shear fracture of the distal radius (Volar Barton fracture)**

Frontal and lateral radiographs of the wrist show a comminuted fracture of the distal radius with intra-articular extension to the radiocarpal articulation (yellow arrow) and volar displacement of the distal fragment (red arrow). There is also a fracture of the ulnar styloid (blue arrow).

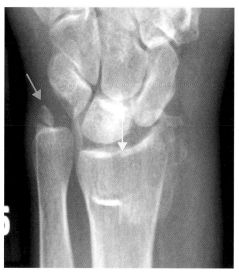
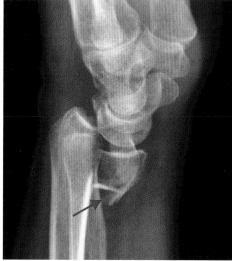

Discussion

Overview of Barton fracture

- Barton fracture is a shear-type fracture of the distal articular surface of the radius with translation of the distal radius fragment with the carpus. The volar and dorsal subtypes are distinguished by the direction of displacement of the radius fragment that articulates with the carpus.
- Barton fractures are most commonly due to axial compression from a fall onto an outstretched hand (FOOSH), with the force vector transmitted through the distal radius. Affected patients are usually over 50 years of age.

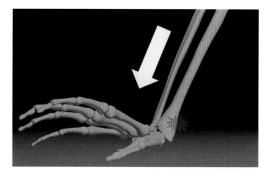

Axial loading at the wrist (arrow), commonly seen in a fall on an outstretched hand (FOOSH), causes the force vector to be transmitted to the distal radius with potential for distal radius fracture.

Classification of distal radius fractures

- Multiple systems have been developed for classification of distal radius fractures. The Fernandez and Jupiter system (further discussed on the following pages) is the most commonly used classification among orthopedic surgeons since it addresses the mechanism of injury and accurately reflects prognosis.

Common named distal radius fractures

- Several eponyms for distal radius fractures remain in common use, often described in conjunction with the Fernandez and Jupiter classification (indicated in parentheses).
- **Colles** (type I) fracture is the most common wrist fracture of older adults, and is a bending-type fracture characterized by dorsal angulation of the distal fragment. **Smith** fracture is a reverse Colles, characterized by volar angulation of the distal fragment.
- **Barton** (type II) fracture, as illustrated in the index case, is a shear-type intra-articular fracture of the distal radius. The carpus may be displaced in a volar or dorsal direction with respect to the distal radius.
- **Die-punch** (type III) fracture is an impaction fracture of the lunate fossa of the distal radius.
- **Hutchinson** (type IV) fracture, also known as **chauffeur** fracture, is an intra-articular radial styloid fracture. These are high-energy injuries often associated with radiocarpal dislocations and ligamentous injuries.

Imaging of distal radius fractures

- PA and lateral wrist radiographs are most commonly obtained for initial evaluation, though additional external oblique view and PA view with the wrist in ulnar deviation may be necessary to evaluate the fracture morphology fully.
- CT is helpful in characterizing fragment displacement and degree of articular surface involvement.

Treatment issues

- Nonoperative management can be considered for minimally displaced or angulated Colles fractures.
- Risk factors for instability include high degree of dorsal angulation, significant dorsal metaphyseal comminution, intra-articular extension, associated ulnar fracture, and age >60.
- Closed reduction is attempted in all distal radial fractures, even those requiring immediate operative management. Operative fixation is recommended for Colles fractures with radial shortening >3 mm, dorsal

angulation >10 degrees, or an intra-articular displacement or step off of >2 mm. It is therefore important to mention these findings if evident on radiographs.

- It is critical for the clinician to evaluate for acute median nerve injuries or vascular compromise both pre- and post-reduction. Surgery is often required if neurovascular injury is suspected.

Self-assessment

- *True or false: Barton fractures are often stable.*

- • False: Barton fractures reflect shear forces and are often unstable.

- *True or false: Colles fractures represent compression type injuries.*

- • False: Colles fractures are bending type fractures.

Clinical synopsis	This patient, a 68-year-old female with an unstable volar shear (Barton) fracture of the distal radius, underwent open reduction and internal fixation.

Spectrum of distal radius fractures (Fernandez and Jupiter classification)

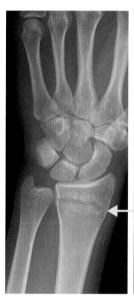 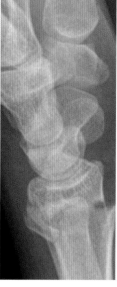

Type I distal radius fracture

Bending type fractures occur when opposing cortical surfaces undergo simultaneous tensile and compressive forces. A Colles fracture is a transverse fracture of the distal radial metaphysis with dorsal angulation and displacement of the distal fragment. Smith fracture is a reversed Colles fracture in which there is volar angulation of the distal fracture fragment. Frontal (left image) and lateral wrist radiographs demonstrate a transverse distal radius fracture (arrow) with minimal dorsal angulation of the distal fragment, consistent with a Colles fracture.

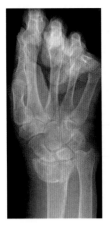
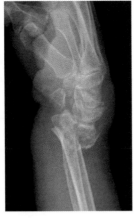

Type II distal radius fracture

A **Barton** fracture, as in the index case, results from shear type injury. In contrast to the index case, however, this case demonstrates dorsal displacement of the carpus with respect to the distal radius.

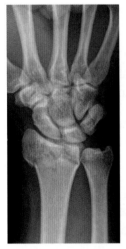
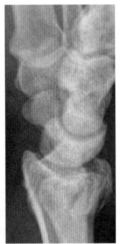

Type III distal radius fracture

Compression type fractures result from impaction of the carpus upon the distal radius. A **die-punch** fracture typically occurs from impaction of the lunate upon the lunate fossa of the distal radius articular surface, leading to fracture and subchondral collapse. Frontal (left image) and lateral radiographs demonstrate an intra-articular compression-type distal radius fracture with cortical depression of the distal radius apposing the scaphoid.

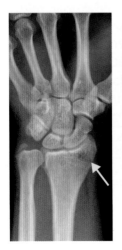
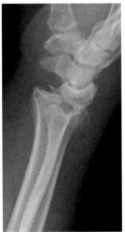

Type IV distal radius fracture

These are avulsion injuries involving the radial or ulnar styloid process. Although osseous injury of the radial or ulnar styloid does not cause significant morbidity in and of itself, these injuries are caused by a high-energy mechanism and there are often associated radiocarpal fracture-dislocations and ligamentous injuries. A type IV distal radius fracture involving the radial styloid is also known as a **chauffeur** or **Hutchinson** fracture. Frontal (left image) and lateral wrist radiographs demonstrate an obliquely oriented radial styloid fracture (chauffeur/Hutchinson fracture; arrow) with intra-articular extension. There is dorsal displacement of the carpus.

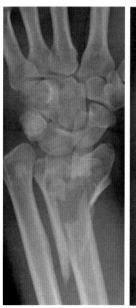 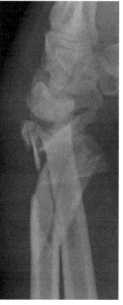

Type V distal radius fracture

Combined-type injuries result from combinations of the aforementioned mechanisms. Frontal (left image) and lateral wrist radiographs demonstrate a highly comminuted distal radius fracture with extensive intra-articular involvement and dorsal angulation of the distal fragment.

Further reading

Goldfarb, C. A., Y. Yin, *et al.* (2001). "Wrist fractures: what the clinician wants to know." *Radiology* 219(1): 11-28.

Lafontaine, M., D. Hardy, *et al.* (1989). "Stability assessment of distal radius fractures." *Injury* 20(4): 208-210.

Lichtman, D. M., R. R. Bindra, *et al.* (2010). "Treatment of distal radius fractures." *J Am Acad Orthop Surg* 18(3): 180-189.

Ilyas A. M., and J. B. Jupiter (Apr. 2007). "Distal radial fractures – classification of treatment and indications for surgery." *Orthop Clin North Am*; 38(2):167-173.

Miller, M. D. (2000). *Review of Orthopedics*. Philadelphia, PA: Saunders.

Rockwood, C. A., D. P. Green, *et al.* (2006). *Rockwood and Green's fractures in adults*. Philadelphia: Lippincott Williams & Wilkins.

Whiting, W. C., and R. F. Zernicke (2008). *Biomechanics of musculoskeletal injury*. Champaign, IL: Human Kinetics.

Section 9.3 Lower Extremity Trauma

Case 79 71-year-old female with a history of breast cancer presented with right hip and thigh pain

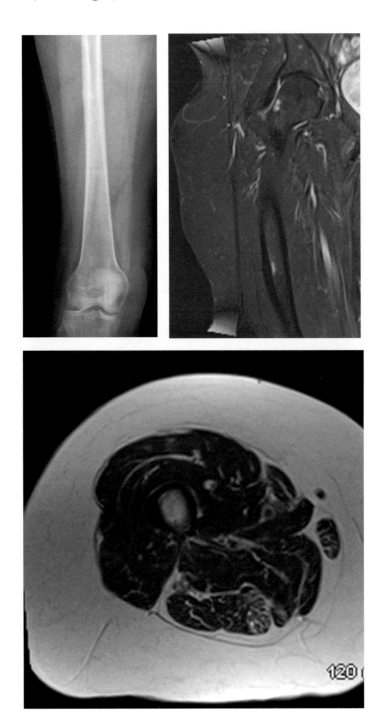

Diagnosis:
Atypical femoral insufficiency fracture in a patient on bisphosphonate therapy

Frontal radiograph of the right femur demonstrates focal cortical thickening along the lateral aspect of the proximal femoral diaphysis (arrow). Coronal STIR MR (middle image) demonstrates focal increased fluid signal along the lateral diaphyseal cortex (arrow). Axial T1-weighted image demonstrates focal cortical thickening laterally (arrow). *Case courtesy Ketan I. Patel, MD.*

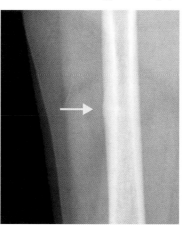 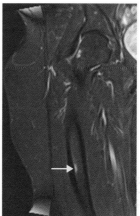 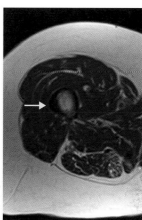

Discussion

Patients with fractures associated with long-term bisphosphonate use often report vague thigh pain with minimal or no trauma history.

- The proximal femur is exposed to substantial impact from normal activity on a daily basis; fracture of this normally strong bone in the absence of high-energy trauma is due to an underlying bone abnormality (insufficiency fracture, defined by normal stress on an abnormal bone).
- Abnormal bone remodeling from prolonged osteoclast suppression is the theorized cause of bisphosphonate-associated fractures.

Imaging of bisphosphonate-associated insufficiency fracture may be subtle.

- Radiographic findings include focal cortical thickening and transverse lucency through the lateral cortex (up to 98% specific). Findings may be very subtle, as in the index case. Fractures are usually close to the lesser trochanter. When complete, there may be a sharp medial projection or "medial spike", usually associated with the distal fragment, where the fracture line transitions steeply from horizontal to vertical. Comminution is unusual.

- In contrast to insufficiency fractures, fatigue fractures occur with abnormal stress on normal bone. These fractures tend to affect younger athletes rather than elderly patients with osteoporosis, and usually involve the medial rather than lateral cortex.

Clinical management of bisphosphonate-associated insufficiency fracture varies depending on clinical and radiographic findings.

- Bisphosphonate-associated fractures are often bilateral, and therefore, it is advisable to obtain radiographs of the contralateral femur to assess for clinically silent fractures when one is diagnosed.
- Management options include discontinuation of bisphosphonates, trial of non-weight bearing, and prophylactic placement of an intramedullary fixation rod. Many orthopedic surgeons recommend prophylactic fixation of nondisplaced bisphosphonate-associated fractures, as progression to displacement is common and generally results in increased pain, morbidity, and cost to the patient.
- Specific findings such as thickening of the lateral cortex, predominantly transverse orientation of the fracture line, and medial spike should be sought in all cases of subtrochanteric fracture in susceptible populations (elderly patients, patients with malignancy, etc.).

Clinical synopsis   The patient underwent prophylactic intramedullary femoral rod placement and discontinuation of bisphosphonate therapy.

Self-assessment

- *How do the findings in fractures from high-impact trauma differ from bisphosphonate-associated fractures of the proximal femur?*

- Traumatic femoral fractures not associated with bisphosphonate use are often oblique or spiral and comminuted. Focal lateral cortical thickening with or without a transversely oriented fracture line suggests bisphosphonate-associated insufficiency fracture.

- *What are the MRI and Tc99m-MDP bone scan findings of bisphosphonate-associated fracture?*

- T1-weighted MRI demonstrates lateral cortical thickening with low-signal marrow changes and corresponding high signal on STIR images. Tc99m-MDP bone scan will show increased focal uptake.

Spectrum of bisphosphonate-associated insufficiency fracture

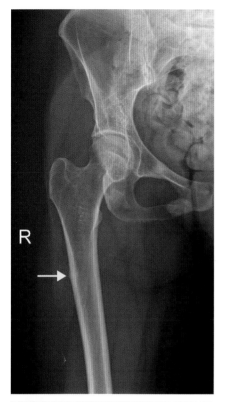

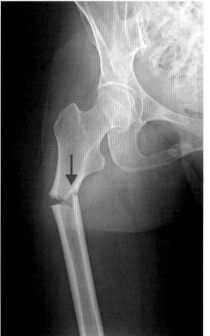

Progression from nondisplaced to complete fracture

In this case of bisphosphonate-associated insufficiency fracture, an initial radiograph (upper image) demonstrated subtle cortical thickening of the lateral cortex in the subtrochanteric femur (yellow arrow). Ongoing weight bearing ultimately resulted in complete transverse fracture at the same site, as seen on the follow-up image taken when the patient presented with acute pain. The distal fracture fragment has a medial spike (red arrow), which is characteristic of a bisphosphonate-associated insufficiency fracture.

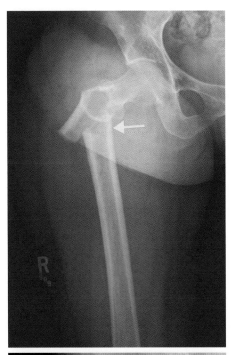

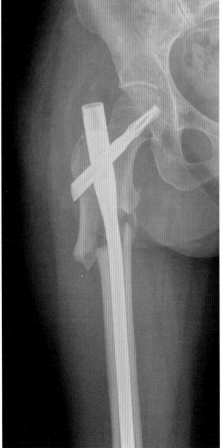

Displaced insufficiency fracture

AP radiograph of a 60-year-old female patient (upper image) shows a transverse, displaced fracture with cranial displacement of the distal fragment and varus angulation. Note the medial spike (arrow) and lack of comminution. The fracture was treated with cephalomedullary nail fixation (bottom image).

Differential diagnosis of atypical femoral fracture

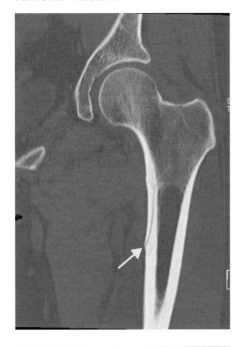

Typical subtrochanteric stress fracture

As opposed to bisphosphonate-associated fractures that tend to involve the lateral cortex, stress fractures most often involve the medial cortex and tend to occur in younger, active individuals. Stress fractures commonly occur in the pelvis (sacrum, pubic rami) or femur. Coronal CT of the left femur in a 53-year-old woman demonstrates a nondisplaced, longitudinal stress fracture (arrow) in the medial cortex.

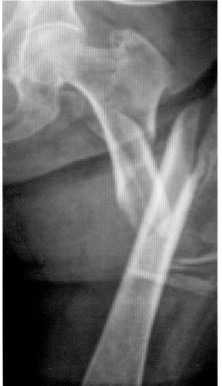

Typical subtrochanteric fracture

It can sometimes be difficult to distinguish between atypical femoral fracture due to bisphosphonate use and typical femoral fracture once the fracture is complete. Typical femoral fractures are usually oblique or spiral in orientation, in contrast to atypical femoral fractures, which are classically transverse. There is often more pronounced displacement and shortening with typical fractures due to oblique orientation of the fracture. Frontal radiograph demonstrates a displaced, obliquely oriented subtrochanteric fracture with foreshortening and varus (distal part pointing medial) angulation.

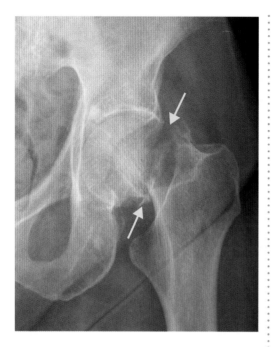

Subcapital fracture

Subcapital femur fracture is the most common intracapsular fracture of the hip. Transcervical (across the femoral neck) and basicervical (at the base of the femoral neck) fractures are slightly more distal but still intracapsular. In contrast, intertrochanteric and the previously discussed subtrochanteric fractures are extracapsular. Intra-capsular hip fractures have a greater risk of osteonecrosis in comparison to extracapsular fractures, due to disruption of the circumflex fem-oral arteries. Subcapital femoral neck fractures are classified with the Garden system from I (incomplete fracture) to IV (displaced fracture). Frontal radiograph of the left hip demonstrates a Garden IV displaced subcapital fracture (arrows).

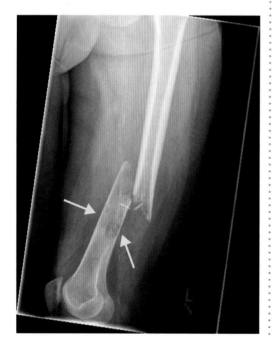

Pathologic fracture: multiple myeloma

Lateral radiograph of the left femur in a 74-year-old male patient with multiple myeloma demonstrates an oblique, displaced pathologic fracture of the mid-femoral shaft through a permeative, lytic, destructive lesion (arrows). Sites of fracture should always be investigated for underlying destructive lesions, especially in elderly patients and in the absence of substantial trauma.

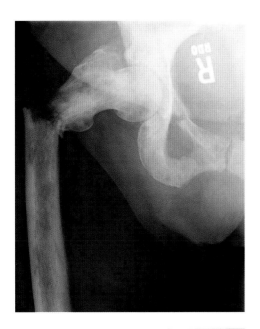

Pathologic fracture: metastatic breast cancer

AP radiograph of the right hip in a 57-year-old woman with metastatic breast cancer demonstrates diffuse sclerotic bone metastases in the femur and pelvis. There is a transverse, angulated, displaced pathologic fracture in the subtrochanteric region.

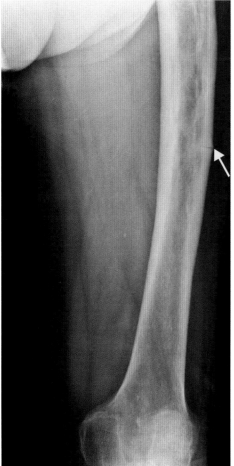

Looser zone: Paget's disease

Looser zones are focal collections of unmineralized osteoid that usually occur at the concave aspect of long bones in conditions such as Paget's disease, osteomalacia, rickets, and renal osteodystrophy. Looser zones typically occur at the medial aspect of the proximal femur, pubic bones, and dorsal aspect of the proximal ulna. This AP radiograph of the left femur in an 82-year-old male with known Paget's disease demonstrates trabecular coarsening, cortical thickening, and bone expansion. There is a linear cortical lucency (Looser zone; arrow) in the lateral cortex of the mid femur.

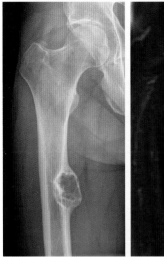
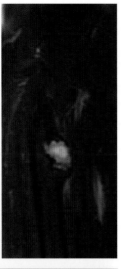

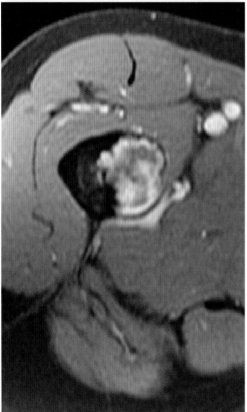

Benign bone lesion: chondromyxoid fibroma

A wide variety of benign and malignant primary bone neoplasms may occur in the proximal femoral diaphysis. Chondromyxoid fibroma is a benign primary bone tumor composed of chondromyxoid and fibrous elements. It is classically seen in young to middle-aged adults, and its typical radiographic appearance is an eccentric, lobulated lesion without aggressive-appearing periosteal reaction. Frontal radiograph of the right femur in a 52-year-old male with pain (upper left image) demonstrates a cortically based, expansile, lucent lesion at the medial aspect of the proximal femoral diaphysis with a narrow zone of transition and partially sclerotic margin. On MRI, the mass was found to be lobular in morphology, hyperintense on STIR (upper right image) and heterogeneously enhancing on post-contrast T1-weighted MR with fat suppression (lower image). The lesion demonstrates uptake on a Tc99m-MDP bone scan (not shown).

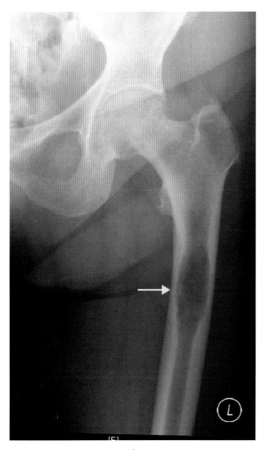

Bone metastasis with impending fracture: anaplastic cranial meningioma metastasis

This 87-year-old male with a history of anaplastic cranial meningioma presented with left thigh pain and weakness. A frontal radiograph of the left hip (upper image) demonstrates an aggressive, centrally located lytic lesion (yellow arrow) with endosteal scalloping, a wide zone of transition, and no internal matrix. A Tc99m-MDP bone scan (lower image) shows increased uptake in the same location (red arrows) and postsurgical uptake in the right frontal bone (blue arrow). The term "impending fracture" is variably defined, but generally describes situations in which a lesion erodes half to two-thirds of the cortical thickness (including the sum of the visible cortices), without frank fracture. With this finding, the referring clinician should be notified directly given the high risk of fracture.

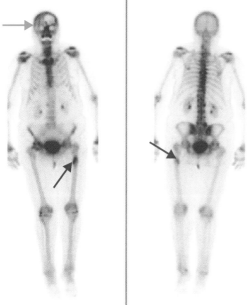

Further reading

Banffy MB *et al*. Nonoperative versus Prophylactic Treatment of Bisphosphonate-associated Femoral Stress Fractures. *Clin Orthop Relat Res* 469, 2028–2034 (2011).

Chew, FS *Skeletal Radiology: The Bare Bones*, 3rd edn. Philadelphia, PA: Lippincott Williams & Wilkins, 2010.

Porrino JA *et al*. Clinical Perspective: Diagnosis of Proximal Femoral Insufficiency Fractures in Patients Receiving Bisphosphonate Therapy. *AJR. American Journal of Roentgenology* 194, 1061–1064 (2010).

Venkatamarasimha N *et al*. Subtrochanteric Femoral Insufficiency Fractures Related to the Use of Long-term Bisphosphonates: A Pictorial Review. *Emerg Radiol* 17, 511–515 (2010).

Case 80   67-year-old male pedestrian who struck his left leg against a car

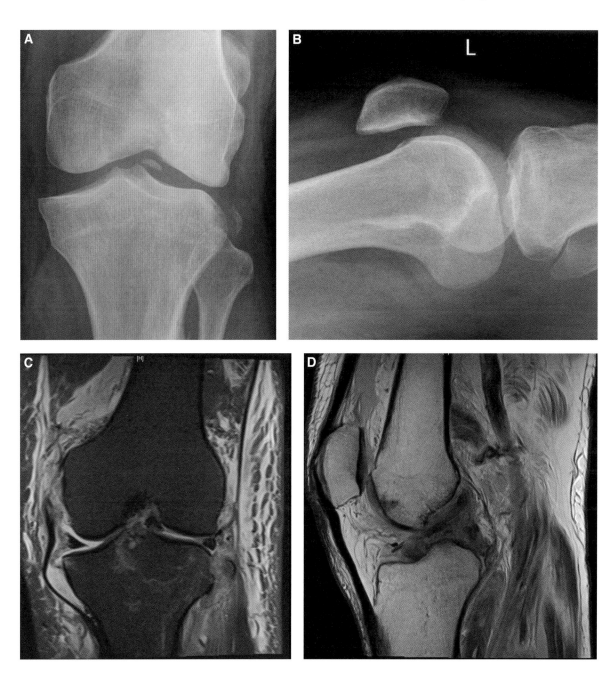

Diagnosis: **Segond fracture with complete tears of the anterior cruciate and medial collateral ligaments**

Frontal knee radiograph (A) demonstrates an avulsion fracture of the lateral tibial rim (Segond fracture; yellow arrow) and a fracture of the tibial eminence (red arrow). Cross-table lateral radiograph of the knee (B) shows a fat–fluid level, or lipohemarthrosis (blue arrow), indicating concomitant intra-articular fracture with leakage of marrow fat into the joint capsule. Coronal proton density fat-suppressed (C) and sagittal proton density (D) MR images show complete tears of the femoral attachment of the medial collateral ligament (green arrow) and anterior cruciate ligament (white arrow). The Segond fracture (yellow arrow) and avulsed tibial spine (red arrow) are also seen on the coronal image. There is focal bone narrow edema of the trochlea (black arrow).

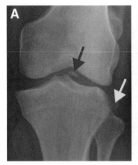 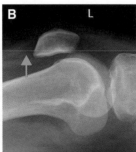 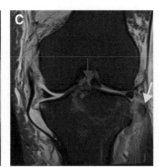 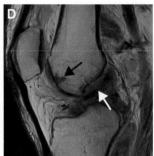

Discussion

A fracture of the non-articular surface of the lateral tibial rim is called a Segond fracture.

- The site of a Segond fracture is posterior and just proximal to Gerdy's tubercle, which is the tibial attachment of the iliotibial band.
- Opinion varies about the exact anatomic components involved in this injury. Paul Segond, who identified the injury in 1879 before the advent of x-rays, believed it was the result of avulsion of the central portion of the lateral capsular ligament. Since then, injury to the posterior fibers of the iliotibial band and the anterior oblique band of the fibular collateral ligament has been postulated, although the exact structures involved remain controversial.

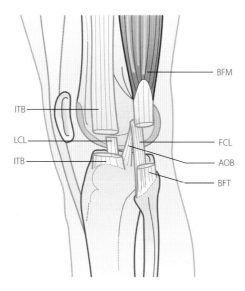

BFM: Biceps femoris muscle
BFT: Biceps femoris tendon
ITB: Iliotibial band
LCL: Lateral capsular ligament
FCL: Fibular collateral ligament
AOB: Anterior oblique band of fibular collateral ligament

- Segond fractures may be inconspicuous, but are essential to recognize, as the fracture is associated with extensive ligamentous injury and lateral knee instability. If the fracture is not initially identified and appropriately treated, chronic instability can occur.
- Radiographs are the initial imaging modality for detecting a Segond fracture. Once it has been identified by plain film, subsequent MRI is essential to evaluate for associated injuries, including:
  - anterior cruciate ligament (ACL) tears (most common, in 75–100% of cases)
  - medial or lateral meniscal tears (in 66–75% of cases)
  - other avulsion injuries including avulsion of the fibular head, tibial spine, and Gerdy's tubercle
  - posterolateral corner injuries

Clinical synopsis

The patient was discharged from the Emergency Department with a hinged knee brace and instructions for immobilization. He did well with conservative treatment.

Self-assessment

- *What is the "lateral capsular" sign?*

- *Is MR an optimal imaging modality for detection of a Segond fracture?*

- *How do Segond and arcuate complex avulsion fractures differ?*

- This term describes the Segond tibial rim avulsion fracture fragment.

- No. In most patients, the fracture fragment may not be apparent on MRI, even when it is seen on radiography. If there is lateral tibial plateau edema on MR, a Segond fracture should be suspected – the ligaments and menisci should be closely scrutinized. Often, Segond fracture is the only finding on radiographs in patients with ACL tear.

- Segond fractures involve the lateral tibial rim, while arcuate complex avulsion fractures involve the proximal fibula. On plain AP radiographs, Segond fracture fragments typically project parallel to the tibial shaft, while arcuate complex avulsion fracture fragments project perpendicular to the long axis of the tibia and fibula.

Spectrum of Segond fracture

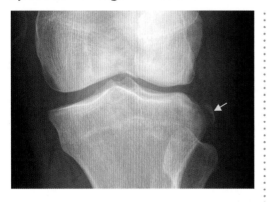

Typical Segond fracture

The cortical avulsion fracture is typically elliptical or curvilinear, and is oriented parallel to the tibial shaft, as best seen on the AP view. The fracture is located distal and lateral to the lateral tibial articular surface. Hemarthrosis may also be present. The mechanism of this injury is forceful internal rotation and varus stress on the knee, with tension on the lateral ligamentous structures. AP radiograph demonstrates a curvilinear avulsion of the lateral tibial rim (arrow).

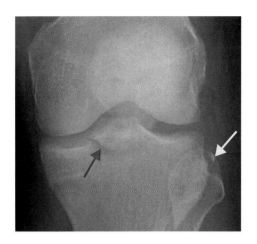

Segond fracture with ACL avulsion injury

Segond fractures often occur in conjunction with other injuries. The ACL attaches to the anterior tibial eminence, and avulsion of the ACL can result in a bone fragment projecting in the intercondylar notch on the AP view. AP knee radiograph demonstrates a small Segond fracture (yellow arrow), associated with avulsion of the tibial eminence (red arrow). MR should be obtained to determine the extent of ACL injury and evaluate for other injuries. MR imaging demonstrated a complete ACL tear in this case.

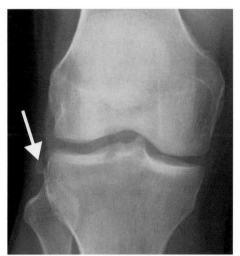

Chronic Segond fracture

A well-corticated bony protuberance can sometimes be identified, representing remote Segond fracture. If the bony protruberance is contiguous with the lateral tibia it is called a Bosch–Bock bump. In the presence of chronic instability, MR should be recommended to evaluate for internal derangement. Frontal radiograph demonstrates a rounded corticated mineralization (arrow) adjacent to the lateral tibial rim.

Differential diagnosis of Segond fracture

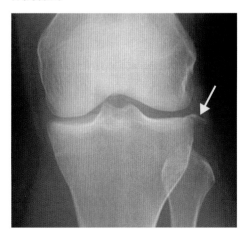

Arcuate complex avulsion fracture

The arcuate complex includes the arcuate, fabellofibular, and popliteofibular ligaments, which insert onto the fibular styloid process. The "arcuate" sign is the term given to an avulsion fracture of the arcuate complex. The fracture fragment is typically displaced superiorly and lies perpendicular to the long axis of the fibula. This is an important fracture to recognize; if left untreated, chronic posterolateral instability and failure of cruciate ligament repair can occur. If this fracture is

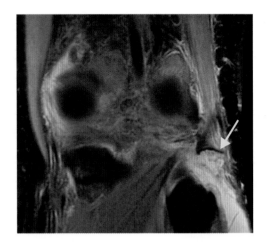

detected on radiographs, MRI should be obtained to assess for other injuries (most commonly to the PCL and MCL). Frontal radiograph demonstrates a curvilinear fracture fragment adjacent to the lateral tibia, oriented perpendicular to the fibular shaft (arrow), representing the arcuate sign. Coronal proton density-weighted MR with fat suppression demonstrates a moderately displaced avulsion of the arcuate complex (arrow) from the proximal fibula.

Iliotibial band avulsion fracture

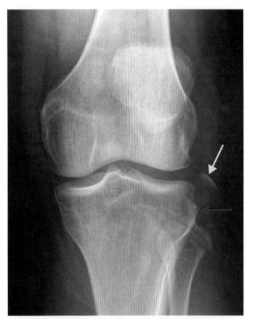

The iliotibial band inserts onto the anterolateral aspect of the tibial condyle at Gerdy's tubercle; hence, iliotibial band avulsion occurs more anteriorly and distally than a Segond fracture. MRI is usually able to identify the avulsed bony fragment and allows for identification of iliotibial band retraction as in this case. Frontal radiograph (upper image) demonstrates an avulsion fragment lateral to the proximal tibia (yellow arrow), with cortical irregularity of the lateral aspect of the proximal tibia (red arrow) that is slightly more distal than the donor site of a Segond fracture. Coronal proton density-weighted MR with fat suppression (lower image) demonstrates complete avulsion of Gerdy's tubercle (yellow arrow), with an undulating contour of the retracted iliotibial band (blue arrow).

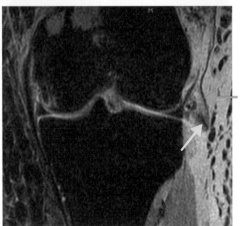

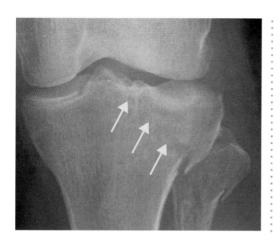

Fracture of the lateral tibial plateau

When cortical irregularity of the lateral tibia is identified, it is important to differentiate a Segond fracture from a fracture extending to the articular surface of the lateral tibial plateau. Frontal radiograph demonstrates a split-type (Schatzker type I) lateral tibial plateau fracture (arrows). Fracture of the proximal fibula is also present.

Further reading

Bolog, N., & Hodler, J. (2007). MR imaging of the posterolateral corner of the knee. *Skeletal radiology*, 36(8), 715–728.

Campos, J. C., Chung, C. B., Lektrakul, N., Pedowitz, R., Trudell, D., Yu, J., & Resnick, D. (2001). Pathogenesis of the Segond fracture: anatomic and MR imaging evidence of an iliotibial tract or anterior oblique band avulsion. *Radiology*, 219(2), 381–386. Retrieved from www.ncbi.nlm.nih.gov/pubmed/11323461

Gottsegen, C. J., Eyer, B. A, White, E. A, Learch, T. J., & Forrester, D. (2008). Avulsion fractures of the knee: imaging findings and clinical significance. *Radiographics: a review publication of the Radiological Society of North America, Inc,* 28(6), 1755–1770.

Huang, G. S., Yu, J. S., Munshi, M., *et al.* (2003). Avulsion fracture of the head of the fibula (the "arcuate" sign): MR imaging findings predictive of injuries to the posterolateral ligaments and posterior cruciate ligament. *AJR Am J Roentgenol*, 180(2), 381–387.

Strub, W. M. (2007). The arcuate sign. *Radiology*, 244(2), 620–621.

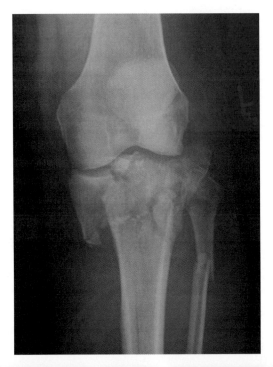

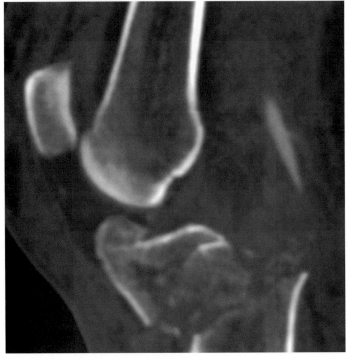

Diagnosis:
**Schatzker
type VI tibial
plateau
fracture,
proximal
fibular fracture,
and traumatic
popliteal
arterial
dissection**

AP radiograph of the knee demonstrates a comminuted bicondylar fracture of the tibial plateau, transverse fracture of the tibial metaphysis, and a fracture of the proximal fibula. Sagittal CT angiogram demonstrates smooth short segment tapering with complete distal occlusion of the popliteal artery (arrow).

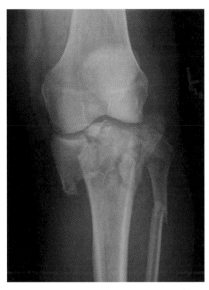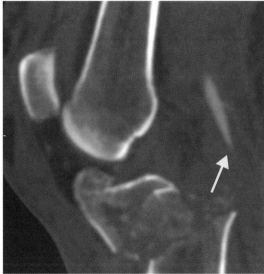

Discussion

Imaging of tibial plateau fractures

- Radiographs are the initial imaging evaluation of knee trauma. Some tibial plateau fractures can be missed or difficult to identify by radiography. The presence of a lipohemarthrosis on the cross-table lateral view should prompt further evaluation by CT to detect a radiographically occult fracture. A subtle band of sclerosis of the medial or lateral tibial plateau may indicate an impacted fracture.
- While plain radiographs are typically the initial imaging modality for assessing for fractures, these often underestimate fracture extent, depression, and grade. Cross-sectional imaging with MR or CT is the standard of care for assessing tibial plateau fractures seen on radiographs. MR can detect associated ligamentous and tendinous injuries. CT angiography is used to assess for vascular compromise or when there is clinical suspicion of compartment syndrome.

Grading of tibial plateau fractures

- The most widely used grading system for fractures of the articular surface of the tibial plateau is the Schatzker classification. Schatzker categories range from I to VI, with higher grades indicating increased severity and worse prognosis. As the grade increases, the likelihood of damage to menisci, ligaments, neurovascular structures, and soft tissues increases.
- Types I through III typically occur due to low-energy injury and management centers on repairing damaged articular cartilage and stabilizing the tibial plateau. Types IV through VI typically occur as a result of high-energy injury and management centers both on repairing soft tissue damage and bony stabilization.

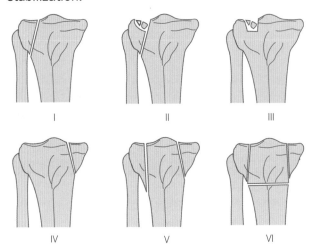

- Type I: lateral split fracture with little (less than 4 mm) or no depression
- Type II: lateral split fracture with depression
- Type III: compression fracture of the articular surface
- Type IV: medial split fracture with or without depression
- Type V: bicondylar split fracture
- Type VI: bicondylar split fracture with transverse fracture of metaphysis

---

Clinical synopsis

This patient, a 52-year-old male with a Schatzker grade VI fracture and popliteal artery dissection, was admitted and underwent fasciotomies, a popliteal bypass, external fixation, and multiple soft tissue debridements. A limb salvage and ORIF of the complex fracture was attempted; however, a transfemoral amputation was ultimately necessary.

Self-assessment

- *What neurovascular structures are at risk for compromise in fracture–dislocation type injuries of the tibial plateau?*

- *What other injuries may be associated with grade V and VI Schatzker fractures?*

- *How does fracture morphology differ based on the patient's age?*

- The popliteal vessels and peroneal nerve.

- Patients with grade V and VI Schatzker fractures are at risk for neurovascular injury, compartment syndrome, meniscal and ligamentous injury, and postoperative infection. The status of the soft tissues determines the timing and choice of surgical repair.

- Older patients with osteopenic bones tend to depress the tibial plateau in low-energy injuries, while younger patients tend to cleave the bone in high-energy injuries.

Spectrum of tibial plateau fractures

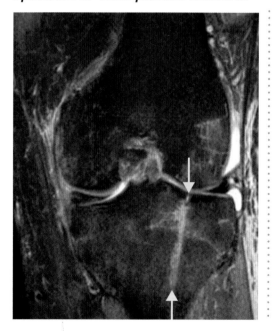

Schatzker type I

Schatzker type I fractures are characterized by a split fracture of the lateral tibial plateau without depression. This fracture type typically occurs in young patients and associated injuries include ACL, medial collateral ligament (MCL), and lateral meniscal tears. Meniscal tears can become entrapped in the fracture and management centers on repair of the articular cartilage and fixation of the lateral plateau. Coronal PD-weighted MR with fat suppression demonstrates a nondisplaced split fracture of the lateral tibial plateau (arrows). Bone marrow edema is seen in the apposing lateral femoral condyle, and fluid surrounds the medial and lateral collateral ligaments.

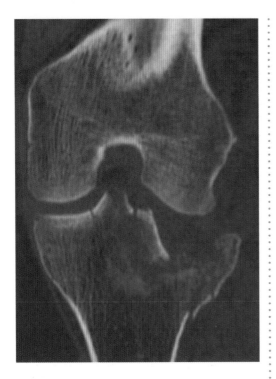

Schatzker type II

A Schatzker type II fracture is a split fracture of the lateral tibial plateau with depression, as seen on this coronal CT. Depression is measured as the distance between the depressed fragment and the intact medial plateau. Common associated injuries include meniscal and MCL tears. Treatment is lateral fixation and elevation of the plateau with bone graft.

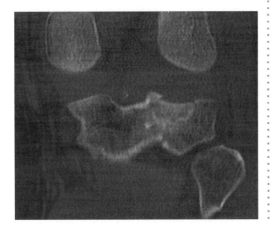

Schatzker type III

A Schatzker type III is a pure compression fracture of the lateral tibial plateau, as seen on this coronal CT. This fracture type tends to occur in older patients and is subdivided into IIIA (lateral depression) and IIIB (central depression). The finding may be subtle on plain radiographs, and should be suspected in the presence of a sclerotic line or lipohemarthrosis. Treatment depends on the presence of joint instability with fixation and elevation of the plateau.

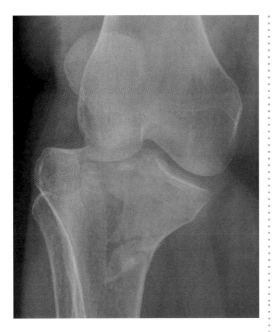

Schatzker type IV

Schatzker type IV is a split fracture of the medial tibial plateau with or without depression, often with concomitant dislocation or subluxation of the joint, as seen in this case demonstrating lateral subluxation of the tibia with respect to the femur. Fractures with associated dislocation carry a worsened prognosis, with injuries often involving the neurovascular structures, ACL, MCL, lateral collateral ligament (LCL), and the posterolateral corner. Treatment is medial plateau fixation and repair of soft tissue injury.

Schatzker type V

Schatzker type V is a bicondylar split fracture sparing the metaphysis. Associated injuries include fracture of the intercondylar eminence (suggesting ACL injury), meniscal tears, and neurovascular compromise. There is a high risk of postoperative infection in this type of fracture.

Schatzker type VI

Schatzker type VI is a transverse fracture through the metaphysis combined with fracture of either the medial, central, or lateral tibial plateau. There is a significant concomitant risk of neurovascular compromise, compartment syndrome, and meniscal, ACL, and collateral ligament injury. The status of the soft tissues often dictates surgical management.

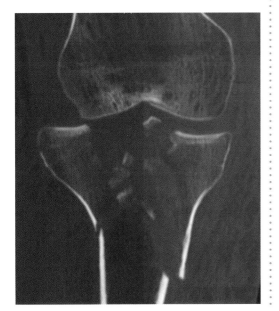

Differential diagnosis of tibial plateau fracture

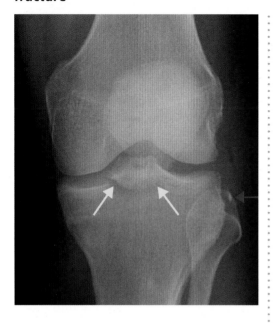

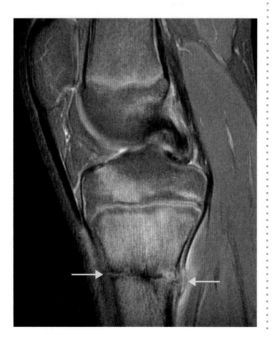

Fracture of the tibial eminence

Fracture of the tibial eminence can often be seen in conjunction with fractures of either the lateral or medial tibial plateau, although this fracture is not included in the Schatzker classification. The tibial attachment of the ACL is the anterior intercondylar area and this type of fracture should raise suspicion for ACL injury. Frontal radiograph demonstrates a mildly displaced fracture of the tibial eminence (yellow arrows). There is an additional fracture of the lateral tibial rim (with the fracture fragment superimposed upon the fibular head; red arrow), known as a Segond fracture. A Segond fracture is critical to recognize (especially in isolation), as this fracture almost always indicates serious internal derangement, typically an ACL injury.

Stress fracture of the tibia

The posteromedial proximal tibial metaphysis is a common site for this type of overuse injury. In contrast to tibial plateau fractures, stress fractures of the proximal tibia spare the articular surface and occur more distally. Plain radiographs may show a sclerotic band perpendicular to the cortex. The fracture is often better seen on MR. Sagittal proton density-weighted MR image with fat suppression in a 17-year-old female runner (upper image) shows a transverse metadiaphyseal junction stress fracture (arrows) with both cortical and trabecular disruption and some posterior callus formation. Frontal knee radiograph in a different skeletally immature patient shows sclerosis (arrow) of the medial tibial metaphysis, representing a healing stress fracture.

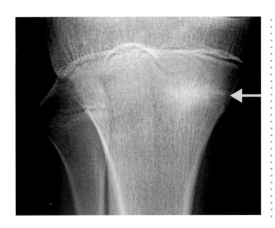

Further reading

Berquist, T. H. (2007). Osseous and myotendinous injuries about the knee. *Radiologic clinics of North America*, 45(6), 955–968, vi.

Markhardt, B. K., Gross, J. M., & Monu, J. (2009). Schatzker classification of tibial plateau fractures: use of CT and MR imaging improves assessment. *Radiographics*, 29(2), 585–598.

te Stroet, M. A. J., Holla, M., Biert, J., & van Kampen, A. (2011). The value of a CT scan compared to plain radiographs for the classification and treatment plan in tibial plateau fractures. *Emergency radiology*, 18(4), 279–283.

Case 82   78-year-old female presented with immediate pain, swelling, and
inability to bear weight after twisting injury to the left ankle

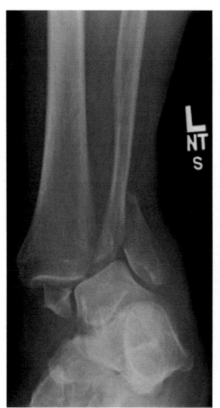
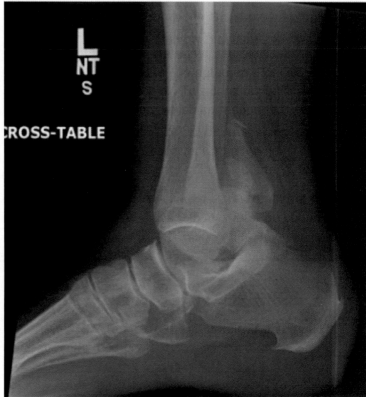

**Diagnosis:
Supination
external
rotation (SER)
stage 4 ankle
fracture**

Frontal and lateral radiographs of the left ankle demonstrate displaced fractures of the medial (yellow arrow), lateral (red arrow), and posterior (blue arrow) malleoli, widening of the tibiofibular space (green arrows), and anterior and medial displacement of the tibia, consistent with SER stage 4 injury.

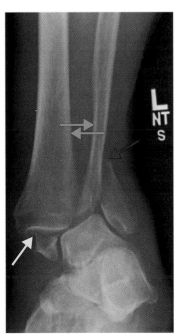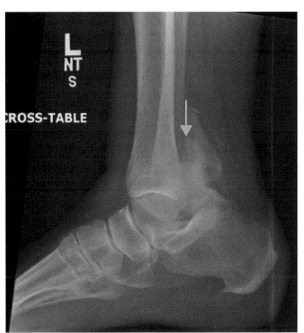

Discussion

The Lauge–Hansen classification system associates ankle injury types with mechanisms of injury, which allows consistent predictions of ligamentous injury patterns with each mechanism.

- The classification system is based on two parts: the position of the ankle at the time of injury and the direction that the talus is displaced or rotated relative to the mortise.
- The ankle may be in pronation (external rotation and eversion of the forefoot and abduction of the hindfoot) or in supination (internal rotation and inversion of the forefoot and adduction of the hindfoot) at the time of trauma. The three deforming forces are abduction, adduction, and external rotation. Therefore, the combined patterns of injury include supination adduction, supination external rotation (SER, as in the index case), pronation abduction, pronation external rotation, and pronation dorsiflexion.

The Danis–Weber classification is a much simpler classification of ankle fractures based on the location of the fibular fracture in relation to the tibiofibular syndesmosis.

- Type A is an infrasyndesmotic fibular fracture, type B is a transsyndesmotic fibular fracture, and type C is a suprasyndesmotic fibular fracture. This simplified system is most helpful with type A and type C fractures, since in type A the syndesmotic ligaments are intact, and in type C the syndesmotic ligaments are disrupted. The status of the syndesmotic ligaments is indeterminate in type B fractures.

Approximately 40–70% of all ankle fractures are secondary to SER, which is the most common mechanism of ankle fracture. When the foot is in supination, the deltoid ligament is relaxed and there is tension on the lateral ligamentous structures; hence, the sequential and stepwise patterns of injury first affect the lateral side. Injury due to SER force is sequentially graded as follows:

- SER stage 1: lateral rotation of the talus stresses and leads to the rupture of the anterior-inferior tibiofibular ligament (AITFL). It is considered a stable injury and is usually radiographically occult.
- SER stage 2: increased stress on the talus leads to spiral fracture of the fibular malleolus, in the direction of low anterior to high posterior, at the tibiofibular syndesmosis. It is considered a stable injury. Patients with isolated fibular fractures at the level of syndesmosis (SER 2) require a gravity stress view for assessment of the deltoid ligament. If there is widening of the medial clear space (> 4 mm), deltoid ligament disruption should be suspected (deltoid ligament disruption upgrades the injury to SER stage 4).
- SER stage 3: increased SER force causes injury to the posterior structures: rupture of the posterior-inferior tibiofibular ligament (PITFL) or fracture of the posterior malleolus of the tibia in addition to rupture of the AITFL and spiral fracture of the fibular malleolus (stage 1 and 2 injury).
- SER stage 4: stage 4 injury is characterized by injury to the deltoid ligament / medial collateral ligament (MCL) complex or medial malleolus in addition to the lateral and posterior structures (stage 1–3 injuries). It is considered an unstable injury and requires open reduction more often than any other fracture type. If unrecognized, it can lead to talar subluxation, malunion, and arthrosis. If the diagnosis is suspected, follow-up radiographs or a stress series should be obtained to identify deltoid complex injury.

Clinical synopsis   The patient underwent open reduction and internal fixation using locking and nonlocking screws.

Self-assessment

- *What is the most common mechanism of ankle fracture?*

- *What constitutes SER stage 4 injury?*

- *Why is knowledge of ankle fracture mechanism important?*

- *Name the components of the syndesmotic ligament complex.*

- Supination external rotation (SER).

- Injury to medial structures (disruption of the deltoid ligament complex or fracture through the medial malleolus) in addition to lateral and posterior structures.

- Knowledge of the mechanism allows inference of the fracture and soft tissue injury pattern, which is important for surgical planning.

- The anterior-inferior tibiofibular (AITFL), posterior-inferior tibiofibular (PITFL), transverse tibiofibular ligaments, and the interosseous ligament.

Spectrum of SER stage 4 injury

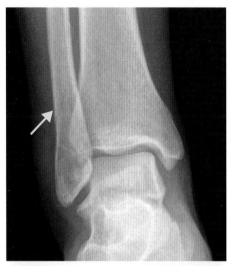

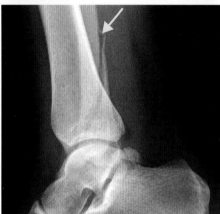

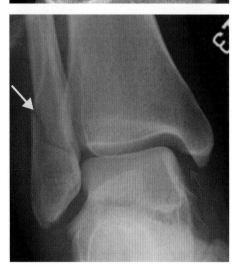

SER stage 4 injury

This 20-year-old patient presented with ankle pain after twisting injury. Frontal, lateral, and mortise radiographs of the ankle demonstrate a mildly comminuted spiral fracture of the distal fibula (yellow arrows) at the tibiofibular syndesmotic joint, with the fracture line oriented from low anterior to high posterior. Widening (8 mm) of the medial clear space (red arrow) denotes injury of the MCL complex. This pattern is consistent with SER stage 4 injury due to disruption of the MCL complex.

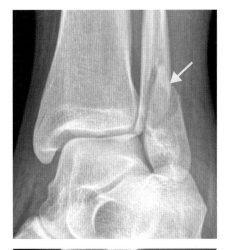

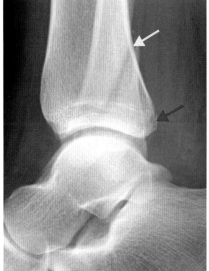

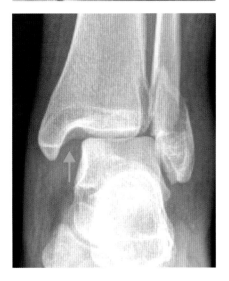

SER stage 4 injury evident on gravity stress view

This 22-year-old male presented with ankle pain and swelling after a fall. Mortise (upper image) and lateral (middle image) radiographs demonstrate a distal fibular fracture (yellow arrows) extending into the syndesmosis. Mild irregularity of the posterior malleolus represents a fracture (red arrow). Gravity stress view (lower image) reveals marked widening of the medial mortise, suggestive of MCL complex injury (blue arrow). Injury to the MCL complex makes this an SER 4 injury.

Differential diagnosis of SER injury

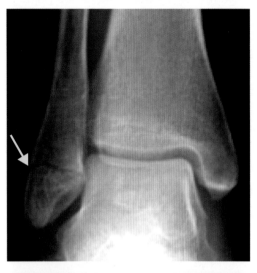

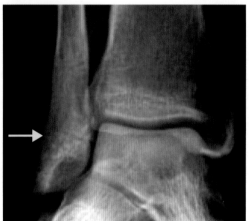

Supination adduction, stage 1

This 70-year-old female presented with right ankle pain after a fall. Frontal and mortise radiographs of the right ankle demonstrate a nondisplaced, transverse fracture of the lateral malleolus (arrows) just below the level of the tibial plafond. The joint spaces of the ankle mortise are maintained, and the medial malleolus is intact. Supination adduction (SA) injury is caused by adduction forces upon the talus, leading to stretching of the lateral structures. Stage 1 injury, as in this case, is a stable injury characterized by transverse fracture of the lateral malleolus at or below the tibial plafond, with injury to the anterior talofibular ligament or calcaneofibular ligament (indicated by lateral mortise widening). Stage 2 injury, which is usually unstable, occurs with more severe adduction of the talus, and produces a vertical fracture of the medial malleolus in addition to the findings seen in stage 1 injury.

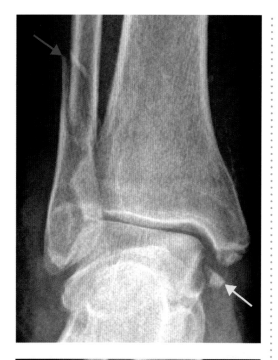

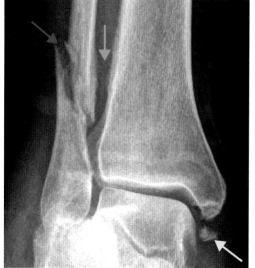

Pronation external rotation, stage 3

This 70-year-old female presented with right ankle pain after a twisting injury. Frontal and mortise views of the right ankle demonstrate a fracture of the medial malleolus (yellow arrows) and a mildly comminuted, minimally displaced oblique fracture of the distal fibula (red arrows). Mild widening of the distal tibiofibular joint indicates syndesmotic injury (blue arrow). In pronation external rotation (PER) injury, there is disruption of medial ankle structures, as the medial ligaments are under stress when the foot is pronated. Stage 1 injury is characterized by medial ligamentous injury, which may be occult or demonstrated by medial mortise widening or medial malleolar fracture. Stage 2 injury involves the AITFL along with the inter-osseous membrane. Progressive increases in force cause a spiral fracture of the fibula above the level of the tibiotalar joint (stage 3), and posterior malleolus fracture (stage 4).

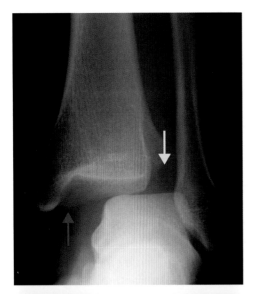

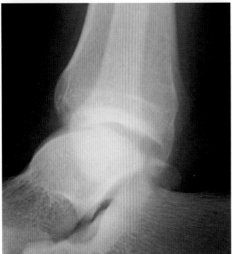

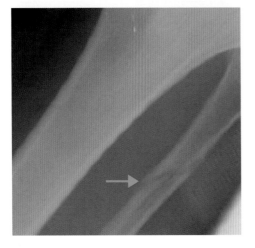

Pronation abduction, stage 1

This 20-year-old female presented with a 180-degree right ankle twisting injury. Mortise and lateral radiographs demonstrate gross disruption of the distal tibiofibular syndesmosis (yellow arrow), with severe widening of the medial ankle mortise (red arrow), and lateral/anterior subluxation of the talus relative to the tibia. There is an associated oblique, minimally displaced, proximal fibular diaphyseal Maisonneuve fracture (blue arrow). While the foot is pronated, abduction force on the talus leads to stress on the medial ligaments, which may cause ligamentous sprain or medial malleolus fracture. Isolated injury to the medial ligaments or medial malleolus is a pronation abduction (PA) stage 1 injury. In stage 2 injury, the posterior malleolus is fractured. With more severe forces, lateral ankle structures are involved, with the characteristic fibular fracture line crossing from high lateral to low medial (stage 3 injury).

Further reading

Clare MP. A rational approach to ankle fractures. *Foot Ankle Clin*. Dec. 2008;13(4): 593–610.

Okanobo H, Khurana B, Sheehan S, Duran-Mendicuti A, Arianjam A, Ledbetter S. Simplified diagnostic algorithm for Lauge–Hansen classification of ankle injuries. *Radiographics*. Mar.–Apr. 2012;32(2):E71–84.

Perrich KD, Goodwin DW, Hecht PJ, Cheung Y. Ankle ligaments on MRI: appearance of normal and injured ligaments. *AJR Am J Roentgenol*. Sept. 2009;193(3):687–695.

31-year-old female presented with right foot and ankle pain after falling on her inverted right ankle

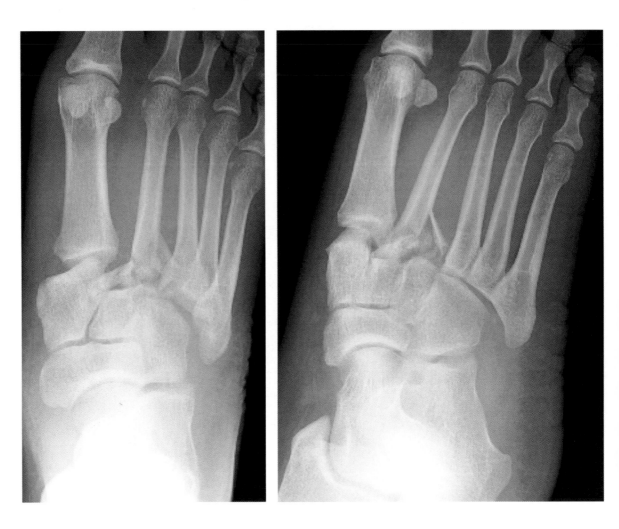

***Diagnosis:*
**Lisfranc
fracture–
dislocation,
homolateral
type**

Frontal and oblique radiographs of the right foot demonstrate a comminuted fracture through the base of the second proximal metatarsal (yellow arrows). There is widening and distortion of the Lisfranc joint (red arrow), with lateral displacement of all metatarsals including the first, consistent with homolateral injury.

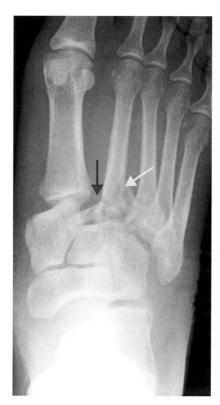
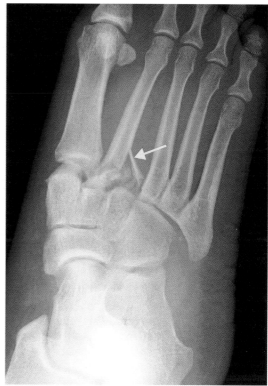

Discussion

The Lisfranc joint complex is comprised of tarsometatarsal (TMT), intermetatarsal, and intertarsal articulations, as well as ligaments including the Lisfranc, plantar tarsometatarsal, dorsal tarsometatarsal, and intermetatarsal ligaments, which are not routinely distinguished at MR imaging

- The Lisfranc ligament extends from the medial cuneiform to the base of the second metatarsal, and is divided into dorsal, interosseous, and plantar components, with the plantar component being the most important.

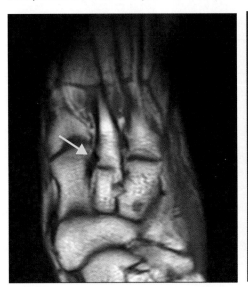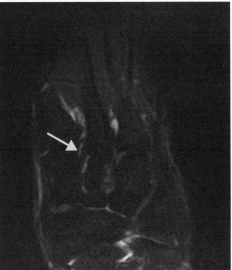

Normal Lisfranc ligament: Axial T1-weighted MR (left image) and T2-weighted MR with fat saturation depict the normal Lisfranc ligament connecting the medial cuneiform to the base of the second metatarsal (arrows). Note the normal very low signal of the ligament on both sequences without associated edema.

Lisfranc ligament sprains generally result from low-impact midfoot injury, while Lisfranc fracture–dislocations result from high-impact injury.

- These injuries account for 0.2% of all fractures and less than 1% of all dislocations.
- Delayed recognition leads to chronic pain, significant functional loss, and osteoarthritis.
- Common mechanisms of Lisfranc injury include direct trauma (such as crush injury) and indirect trauma (such as forced plantar flexion and forefoot abduction).
- Common clinical symptoms include pain at the TMT joint of the midfoot and inability to bear weight. Limited forefoot abduction or adduction, plantar ecchymosis, and shortening of the foot are less common presenting features.

There are two types of dislocation in Lisfranc injury.
- Homolateral dislocation is defined as lateral displacement of the first through fifth metatarsals.
- Divergent dislocation is defined as medial dislocation of the first metatarsal with lateral dislocation of the second through fifth metatarsals.

Most common fractures associated with Lisfranc injury involve the medial aspect of the second metatarsal base or the distal lateral aspect of the medial cuneiform.
- On radiography, more than 2 mm of separation between first and second metatarsal on weight-bearing views suggests Lisfranc ligament tear, while frank displacement of the second metatarsal and medial cuneiform is suggestive of complete tear.
- On radiography or MR, nonalignment of the lateral aspect of the first metatarsal and medial cuneiform and the medial aspect of the fourth metatarsal and cuboid suggest a Lisfranc injury.
- As many as 20% of Lisfranc joint injuries are estimated to be missed on conventional non-weight-bearing AP and lateral radiographs. CT is highly sensitive for identifying fractures not identified on plain radiographs or MR.
- MR findings of Lisfranc injury include abnormal signal (i.e., sprain) or frank disruption (i.e., tear) of the Lisfranc ligament, malalignment of the dorsal arch, TMT joint subchondral edema suggestive of avulsion fracture, and marrow edema within the metatarsals or medial and middle cuneiforms.

Clinical synopsis The patient underwent open reduction and internal fixation with arthrodesis of the first, second, and third TMT joints.

Self-assessment

- *Where is the Lisfranc ligament and what are its components?*
  - The Lisfranc ligament attaches the medial cuneiform to the base of the second metatarsal, and is divided into dorsal, interosseous, and plantar components.

- *Name the two types of Lisfranc fracture–dislocations.*
  - Homolateral (all metatarsals move laterally) and divergent (the first metatarsal moves medially and the second through fifth metatarsals move laterally).

- *What fractures indicate possible Lisfranc injury?*
  - Fracture of the medial aspect of the second metatarsal base or the distal lateral aspect of the medial cuneiform.

Spectrum of Lisfranc injuries

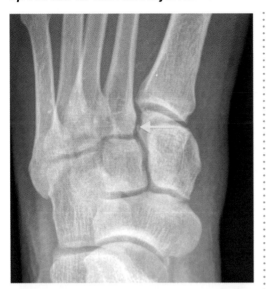

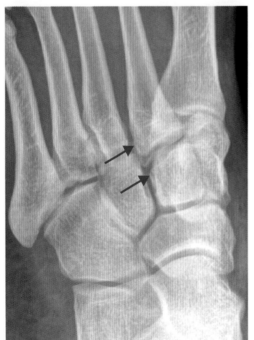

Lisfranc fracture–dislocation, homolateral type

Frontal and oblique radiographs demonstrate a tiny osseous fragment adjacent to the lateral aspect of the medial cuneiform (known as the "fleck sign"; yellow arrow), and offset at the second TMT joint (red arrows), best appreciated on the oblique view. Open reduction and plate and screw internal fixation was performed. Displacement of the second metatarsal and lateral shift of the base of the first metatarsal was noted during surgery, consistent with a homolateral type injury.

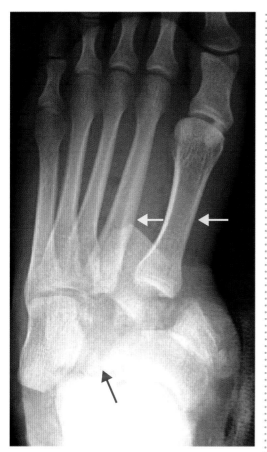

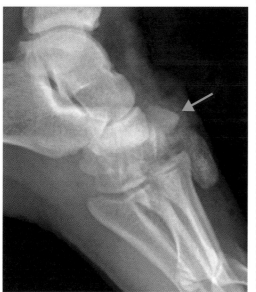

Lisfranc fracture–dislocation with additional midfoot fractures, homolateral type

A 19-year-old male presented after an industrial accident involving the left foot. Frontal radiograph shows lateral displacement of the first through fifth metatarsals (yellow arrows). An additional fracture involving the lateral aspect of the navicular bone (red arrow) is also seen. The lateral radiograph demonstrates dorsal displacement of the cuneiforms (blue arrow). These findings are consistent with a comminuted homolateral Lisfranc fracture–dislocation. The patient subsequently underwent open reduction and internal fixation at multiple forefoot and midfoot articulations.

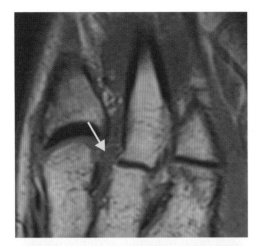

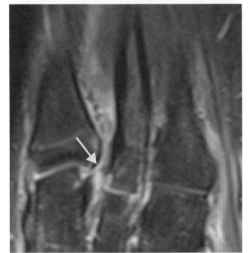

Full-thickness Lisfranc ligament tear

This patient presented with foot pain after a fall. Axial T1-weighted MR (upper image) and T2-weighted MR with fat saturation demonstrate a full-thickness tear of the Lisfranc ligament (arrows), with no intact fibers identified. There was no associated fracture or dislocation.

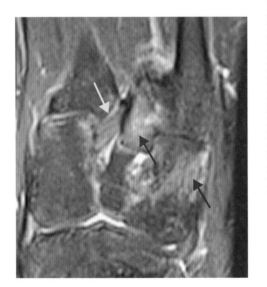

High-grade Lisfranc ligament sprain

This patient presented with foot pain after a twisting injury. Axial T2-weighted image with fat saturation demonstrates striated increased signal intensity of the Lisfranc ligament, consistent with sprain (yellow arrow). The ligament fibers are intact. Bone marrow edema within the lateral cuneiform and base of the second metatarsal (red arrows) is consistent with contusion.

Differential diagnosis of Lisfranc ligament injury

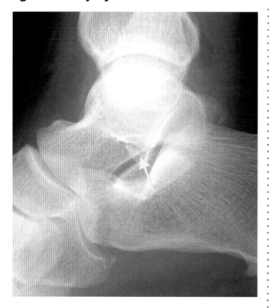

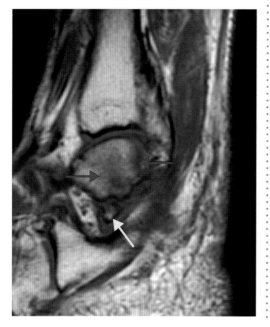

Lateral process of talus fracture

A lateral process of talus fracture occurs when the foot is dorsiflexed and inverted, causing shear stress to be transmitted from the calcaneus to the lateral process of the talus. Physical exam findings may show swelling and ecchymosis over the lateral talar process; however, because patients with this injury are frequently able to bear weight, they may be clinically misdiagnosed with an ankle sprain, especially since the imaging findings may be subtle. This patient presented with ankle pain after a snowboarding accident. Lateral radiograph and sagittal T1-weighted MR show a mildly displaced fracture of the lateral process of the talus (yellow arrows), which is associated with patchy edema of the talar body (red arrows).

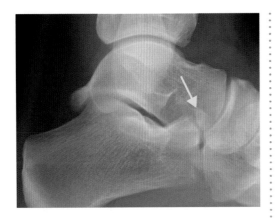

Avulsion fracture of anterior calcaneal process

There are two types of anterior calcaneal process injury: avulsion fracture (more common) and compression fracture. The avulsion fracture is caused by adduction with plantar flexion, which places tension on the bifurcate ligament that connects the anterior calcaneal process to the cuboid and navicular bones. Treatment is immobilization in a short leg cast for 4 weeks. Frequently, this fracture is overlooked due to overlap with the talus on radiographs. This patient presented with right ankle pain after twisting injury. A lateral radiograph of the right ankle demonstrates a mildly displaced avulsion fracture of anterior calcaneal process (arrow).

Second metatarsal base stress fracture

Stress fractures result from repetitive injury, and base of the second metatarsal stress fractures are characteristically seen in ballet dancers. Treatment is usually nonoperative. This patient presented with midfoot pain. A frontal radiograph of the foot demonstrates a subtle area of sclerosis (arrow) at the base of the second metatarsal, which suggests a healing stress fracture.

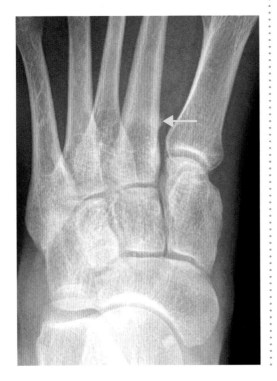

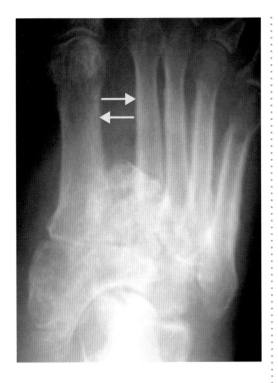

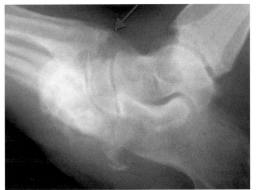

Charcot arthropathy

Charcot arthropathy, also known as neuropathic arthropathy, is a destructive joint disorder that is seen in patients with loss of sensation. In the ankle and foot, Charcot arthropathy is usually a sequela of uncontrolled diabetes. The typical clinical presentation is of swollen, painless joints, with normal systemic inflammatory markers and no fever. Radiographic features include bony sclerosis and degeneration with debris (intra-articular bodies), destruction of articular cartilage and subchondral bone, and dislocation/sublux-ations. Although Lisfranc dislocations can often be seen with Charcot arthropathy, the associated chronic-appearing destructive changes of the mid-foot should suggest a longstanding process rather than a traumatic fracture–dislocation. Frontal and lateral views of the foot in a patient with uncon-trolled diabetes demonstrate severe destruction of the midfoot with a widened first intermetatarsal interspace (yellow arrows) and dorsal subluxation (red arrow) of the TMT joint complex relative to the navicular bone.

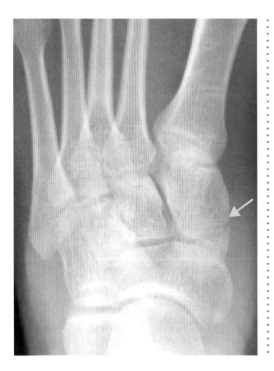

Isolated medial cuneiform fracture

This patient presented with foot pain after a twisting injury. Frontal radiograph of the foot demonstrates an isolated, nondisplaced fracture of the proximal aspect of the medial cuneiform (arrow). Intact alignment of the base of the second metatarsal and middle cuneiform is suggestive of an intact Lisfranc ligament, although a weight-bearing view can be obtained to confirm.

Further reading

Cheung Y, Rosenberg ZS. MR imaging of ligamentous abnormalities of the ankle and foot. *Magn Reson Imaging Clin N Am*. Aug. 2001;9(3):507–531.

Crim J. MR imaging evaluation of subtle Lisfranc injuries: the midfoot sprain. *Magn Reson Imaging Clin N Am*. Feb. 2008;16(1):19–27.

Dunfee WR, Dalinka MK, Kneeland JB. Imaging of athletic injuries to the ankle and foot. *Radiol Clin North Am*. Mar. 2002;40(2):289–312.

Macmahon PJ, Dheer S, Raikin SM, Elias I, Morrison WB, Kavanagh EC, Zoga A. MRI of injuries to the first interosseous cuneometatarsal (Lisfranc) ligament. *Skeletal Radiol*. Mar. 2009;38(3):255–260.

Nazarenko A, Beltran LS, Bencardino JT. Imaging evaluation of traumatic ligamentous injuries of the ankle and foot. *Radiol Clin North Am*. May 2013;51(3):455–478.

Stoller DW, Ferkel RD. The ankle and foot. (2-volume Set) In Stoller DW *et al*. (eds.) *Magnetic resonance imaging in orthopaedics and sports medicine*. Baltimore: Lippincott Williams & Wilkins, 2007, pp. 733–1050.

Haapamaki VV, Kiuru MJ, Koskinen SK. Ankle and foot injuries: analysis of MDCT findings. *Am J Roentgenol*. 2004:183:415–422.

Case 84   47-year-old female with foot pain after tripping on doormat

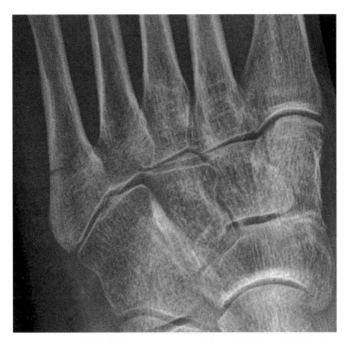

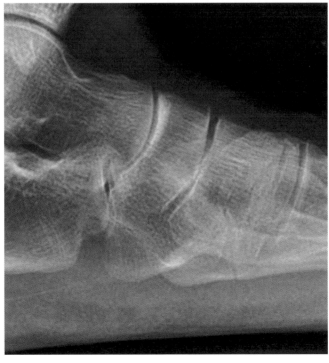

Diagnosis: Frontal and lateral radiographs of the left foot demonstrate a transversely
Acute proximal orientated, non-displaced, acute extra-articular fracture of the proximal fifth
fifth metatarsal metatarsal (zone 2; arrows).
fracture

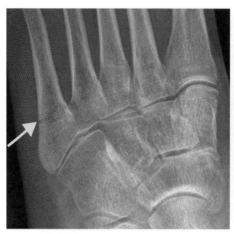
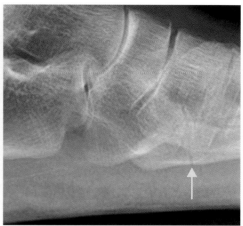

Discussion

Overview of fifth metatarsal fractures

- There are three types of proximal fifth metatarsal fractures, which are classified anatomically into zones. Zone 1 and 2 fractures tend to be caused by trauma, while Zone 3 fractures are seen in the setting of stress fracture.
- Zone 1 fracture, also known as an avulsion fracture, is the most proximal fracture type.
- Zone 2 fracture, commonly known as a Jones fracture, occurs at the fifth metatarsal metaphyseal–diaphyseal junction. Strictly speaking, a Jones fracture refers to a fracture at the metaphyseal–diaphyseal junction *without* intra-articular extension to the articulation of the fourth and fifth metatarsals; however, in common usage, the term "Zone 2 fracture" is often used synonymously with "Jones fracture".
- Zone 3 fracture is a diaphyseal fracture, typically occuring as a stress injury.

Anatomy at the base of the fifth metatarsal

- The peroneus brevis tendon attaches at the lateral base of the fifth metatarsal.
- The lateral aspect of the plantar aponeurosis attaches slightly more proximally at the plantar base of the fifth metatarsal.

- Avulsion fractures at the base of the fifth metatarsal are thought to be due to combined forces of the peroneus brevis tendon and lateral aspect of the plantar aponeurosis.

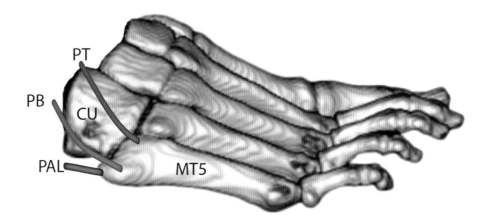

Illustration demonstrates the anatomy at the base of the fifth metatarsal. The peroneus brevis tendon (PB) attaches to the lateral base of the fifth metatarsal (MT5). The lateral aspect of the plantar aponeurosis (PAL) attaches to the plantar base of the fifth metatarsal. The peroneus tertius (PT) tendon attaches dorsally. The cuboid (CU) articulates with the base of the fifth metatarsal to form the fifth tarsometatarsal joint.

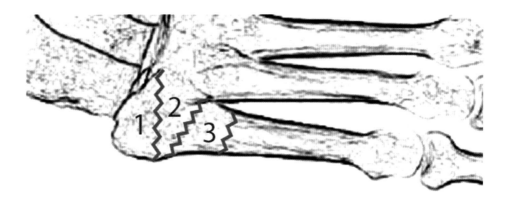

Illustration demonstrates the zonal anatomy at the base of the fifth metatarsal. Zone 1 fracture (most proximal) is an avulsion type. Zone 2 fracture (Jones fracture) occurs at the metaphyseal–diaphyseal junction. Zone 3 fracture is a proximal diaphyseal fracture.

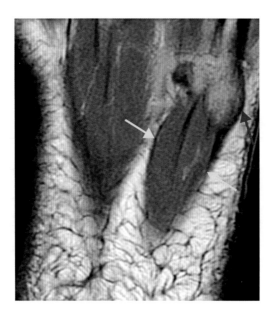

Axial PD-weighted MR of the base of the fifth metatarsal demonstrates normal anatomy of the lateral cord of the plantar aponeurosis (yellow arrows) inserting onto the base of the fifth metatarsal (red arrow)

Imaging of fifth metatarsal fractures

- Radiographs are the primary modality for imaging proximal fifth metatarsal fractures.
- Once the fracture has been identified on radiographs, attempts should be made to describe the zonal location, etiology (acute or stress fracture), degree of displacement, and the presence of intra-articular extension.

Treatment of fifth metatarsal fractures

- As a general principle, indications for surgical treatment include a more distal fracture, displacement of more than 2 mm, and intra-articular extension. Competitive athletes may also be treated surgically without these indications. Otherwise, most fractures are treated conservatively.
- The junction of the metatarsal metaphysis and diaphysis has a watershed vascular supply. With repetitive mechanical forces from weight-bearing, fractures in this tenuously vascularized region are susceptible to delayed healing.

Clinical synopsis

This patient, a 47-year-old female with a zone 2 acute fifth metatarsal fracture, was sent home from the Emergency Department with compression bandaging and crutches. A week later she was seen in the orthopedic clinic and underwent elective intramedullary screw fixation of the fifth metatarsal.

Self-assessment

- *What is the definition of a Jones fracture?*

- A Jones fracture is a transverse fracture at the junction of the diaphysis and metaphysis of the fifth metatarsal without intra-articular extension into the fourth and fifth intermetatarsal articulation.

- *What can you suggest if a fifth metatarsal fracture is not identified on routine views of the foot and an avulsion fracture is suspected?*

- Not all plain radiographs of the foot detect avulsion fractures. An AP view of the ankle to include the base of the fifth metatarsal can help identify these occult fractures.

- *Why is it important to review prior imaging of the foot?*

- Serial films may indicate signs of a developing stress fracture.

Spectrum of fifth metatarsal fractures

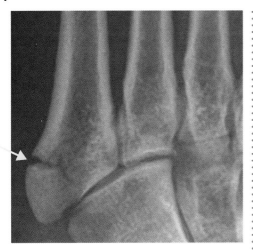

Tuberosity avulsion fractures (zone 1)

Tuberosity avulsion fractures are the most common proximal fifth metatarsal fractures, occuring during ankle inversion with the foot in plantar flexion. The exact mechanism of this injury is controversial, either involving contracture of the peroneus brevis muscle or the lateral band of the plantar fascia. Imaging findings include a transverse fracture through the tuberosity, usually without intra-articular extension into the cuboid-metatarsal joint. The majority of these fractures are treated conservatively, unless the patient is a high-level athlete. Oblique radiograph demonstrates a nondisplaced fifth metatarsal avulsion fracture (arrow) without definite intra-articular extension to the tarsometatarsal joint.

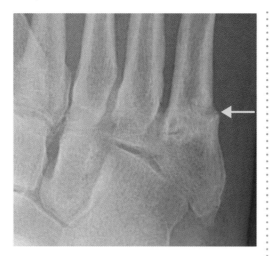

Fractures of the metaphysis–diaphysis junction (zone 2)

Fractures of the metaphysis–diaphysis junction are prone to poor healing. The mechanism of injury is a large adduction force to the forefoot with the ankle in plantar flexion. These fractures are typically transversely orientated at the junction of the metadiaphysis and diaphysis, with or without intra-articular extension into the fourth and fifth metatarsal articulation. Oblique radiograph demonstrates a healing zone 2 fracture (arrow) with blurring of the fracture margins and surrounding sclerosis.

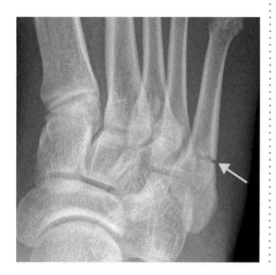

Fractures of the diaphysis (zone 3)

This is the rarest subtype of fracture and is prone to poor healing. It is usually a chronic stress injury in athletes. There is often an acute on chronic presentation of pain, and a review of serial imaging is important to detect subtle abnormalities prior to complete fracture. Frontal radiograph demonstrates a zone 3 fracture (arrow) with mild surrounding sclerosis, suggesting subacute chronicity.

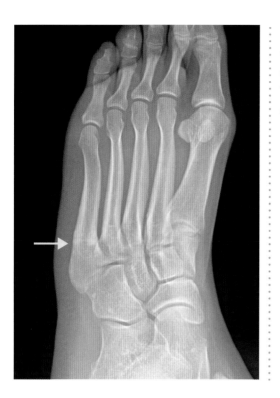

Healing stress fracture (zone 3)

Oblique radiograph demonstrates transversely oriented, linear sclerosis (arrow) of the proximal fifth metatarsal diaphysis, consistent with healing stress fracture.

Differential diagnosis of fifth metatarsal fracture

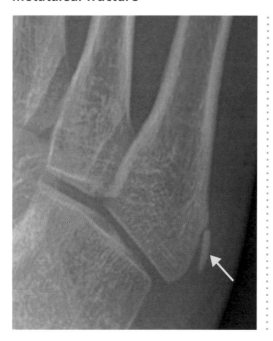

Apophysis

The normal apophysis is seen in girls between the ages of 9 and 11 and in boys between the ages of 11 and 14, and is not seen in patients over the age of 16. In contrast to a fracture, the apophysis is oriented parallel rather than perpendicular to the axis of the metatarsal shaft. Oblique radiograph in an adolescent demonstrates a smooth, well-corticated ossific density (arrow) along the lateral border of the metatarsal tuberosity, oriented parallel to the shaft.

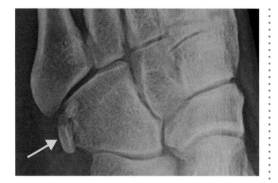

Os peroneum

An os peroneum is a sesamoid bone located within the peroneus longus tendon at the level of the cuboid tunnel. It is ossified in up to 20% of adults. It appears as a well-corticated ossification with rounded borders adjacent to the lateral border of the cuboid. It is most commonly an incidental finding; however, proximal retraction of an os peroneum may represent peroneus longus tendon tear. Painful os peroneus syndrome represents a spectrum of disorders, which may be related to fracture of the os peroneum or peroneus longus tendon pathology. Oblique radiograph demonstrates an ossified os peroneum (arrow) in its typical location lateral to the cuboid.

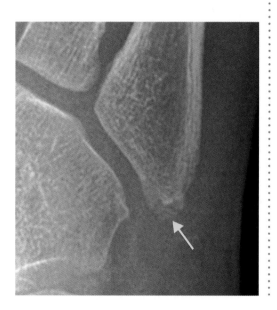

Os vesalianum

An os vesalianum is a very rare accessory bone of the foot (reportedly present in 0.1% of individuals) that is located within the peroneus brevis tendon, and is seen adjacent to the lateral border of the fifth metatarsal tuberosity. Coned-down oblique radiograph demonstrates a corticated mineralization (arrow) at the most proximal aspect of the fifth metatarsal.

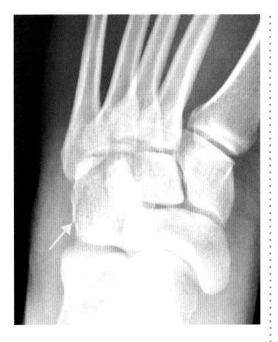

Cuboid fracture

Isolated fractures of the cuboid bone are rare; however, a lateral cuboid avulsion fracture may result from direct trauma. In contrast to an os peroneus, an acute cuboid fracture would typically not feature corticated margins. Indirect injury usually occurs through a torsional injury to the ankle and midfoot resulting in the cuboid being crushed between the calcaneus and metatarsals by forced plantar flexion and abduction, the so-called nutcracker fracture. Such fractures are most often associated with calcaneus, lateral metatarsal base, and navicular fractures. Frontal and lateral radiographs of the foot demonstrate a lucency through the lateral and plantar aspect of the cuboid bone (arrows), associated with mild overlying soft tissue swelling.

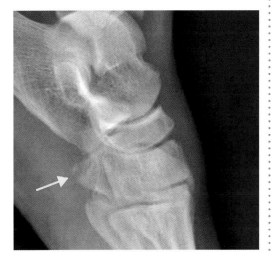

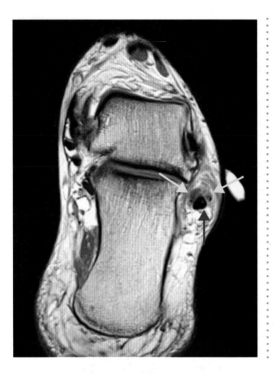

Peroneus brevis split tear

The peroneus brevis inserts on the base of the fifth metatarsal and is important for ankle eversion. Typically caused by lateral ankle inversion, injury of the peroneus brevis may clinically mimic base of fifth metatarsal fracture. Patients typically complain of lateral instability and pain localized posterior to the lateral malleolus. A split tear of peroneus brevis is the most common type of tear, typically demonstrating a "chevron" morphology. Axial-oblique PD-weighted MR demonstrates a split-tear of peroneus brevis with a chevron-shaped tendon (yellow arrows). Peroneus longus (red arrow) is intact.

Further reading

Fetzer, G. B., & Wright, R. W. (2006). Metatarsal shaft fractures and fractures of the proximal fifth metatarsal. *Clinics in sports medicine*, 25(1), 139–150, x.

Hatch, R. L., Alsobrook, J. A., & Clugston, J. R. (2007). Diagnosis and management of metatarsal fractures. *American family physician*, 76(6), 817–826.

Lawrence, S. J., & Botte, M. J. (1993). Jones' fractures and related fractures of the proximal fifth metatarsal. *Foot ankle*, 14(6), 358–365.

Pao, D. G., Keats, T. E., & Dussault, R. G. (Aug. 2000). Original report avulsion fracture of the base of the fifth metatarsal not seen on conventional radiography of the foot: the need for an additional projection. *Virginia Medical*, 549–552.

Theodorou, D. J., Theodorou, S. J., Kakitsubata, Y., Botte, M. J., & Resnick D. (Mar. 2003). Fractures of proximal portion of fifth metatarsal bone: anatomic and imaging evidence of a pathogenesis of avulsion of the plantar aponeurosis and the short peroneal muscle tendon. *Radiology*, 226(3), 857–865.

Zwitser, E. W., & Breederveld, R. S. (2010). Fractures of the fifth metatarsal: diagnosis and treatment. *Injury*, 41(6), 555–562.

Case 85   17-year-old male who caught his foot on the turf while playing football
and hyperextended his great toe

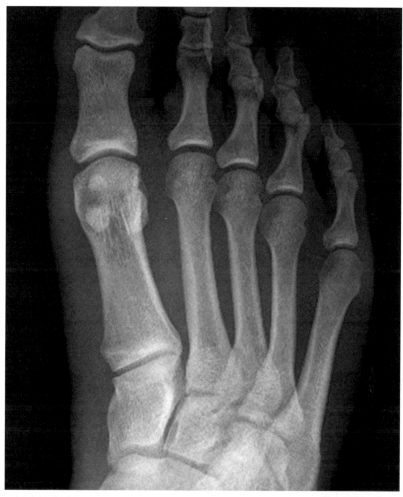

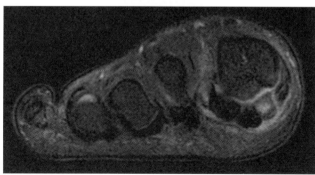

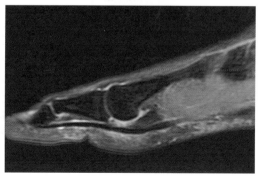

Diagnosis:
Medial (tibial) hallux sesamoid fracture and tear of the plantar plate and medial sesamoid-phalangeal ligament (turf toe)

Frontal radiograph of the right foot (upper image) demonstrates two distracted components of the fractured medial sesamoid (yellow arrows). Sharp margination of the apposing cortices suggests acute transverse fracture. Coronal T2-weighted MR with fat suppression (lower left image) reveals focal marrow edema in the fractured medial sesamoid (yellow arrow) with surrounding edema. There is linear increased signal (red arrow) at the attachment of the abductor hallucis to the medial sesamoid, consistent with tear. There is a tear of the medial sesamoid–phalangeal ligament (blue arrow). The lateral sesamoid (green arrow) and flexor hallucis longus tendon (white arrow) are intact. Sagittal STIR MR image demonstrates a torn plantar plate (orange arrow).

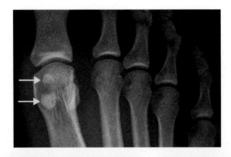

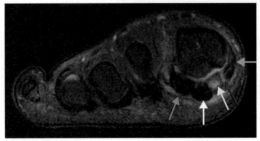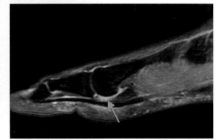

Discussion

Sesamoids are seed-like bones (the word "sesamoid" is derived from a Greek word meaning "resembling a sesame seed") that are embedded in tendons, typically spanning a joint.

- The sesamoids absorb shock, prevent tendon damage, and enhance joint gliding. Hallucal sesamoids associated with the great toe are prone to injury due to the large forces transmitted through them during gait.
- There are two hallucal sesamoids; the medial (tibial) sesamoid and the lateral (fibular) sesamoid. They are embedded in the flexor hallucis brevis tendon that spans the first metatarsophalangeal (MTP) joint in the plantar plate.

- Fractures usually relate to sudden loading of the forefoot as might occur from jumping or falling from height. Abnormal ossification can lead to a partite configuration that can be difficult to differentiate from fracture.
- Tenuous blood supply to sesamoids has been implicated in conditions such as avascular necrosis and delayed healing or nonunion of fractures.

Turf toe injuries are a spectrum of injuries of the plantar capsuloligamentous–sesamoid complex.

- The abductor hallucis tendon inserts on the medial sesamoid with fibers contributing to the medial capsule.
- The adductor hallucis muscle contributes fibers to the lateral sesamoid, capsule, and plantar plate.
- Flexor hallucis brevis inserts on the sesamoids, while flexor hallucis longus runs in between the plantar aspect of the sesamoids to continue to the distal phalanx.
- The medial and lateral sesamoid–phalangeal ligaments are stabilizing structures.

Imaging of sesamoid injury

- Standard weightbearing radiographs are typically the initial imaging modality to assess bone morphology and exclude other causes of first metatarsal pain.
- If an abnormality is suspected or if there is a high suspicion for sesamoid injury, then dedicated sesamoid axial and/or oblique stress radiographs can provide optimal visualization.
- Bone scan is a sensitive but nonspecific imaging modality. Both feet should be imaged to evaluate for abnormal asymmetric uptake. It is important to note that bone scan may show physiologically increased, symmetric uptake in asymptomatic patients.
- CT is useful to assess osseous detail in fractures and avascular necrosis, while the role of MRI is to detect marrow signal abnormality and evaluate the integrity of associated ligaments and tendons.

Clinical synopsis

Radiographs of the contralateral foot were obtained to exclude traumatic distraction of a bipartite medial sesamoid. The patient underwent open reduction and internal fixation of the medial sesamoid with reconstruction of the first MTP joint. In isolated sesamoid fracture, conservative therapy, such as non-weightbearing for several weeks, is commonly prescribed. Noncompliance can lead to complications such as avascular necrosis.

Self-assessment

- *Which sesamoid is more commonly injured and why?*

- The tibial (medial) sesamoid, because it is located under the metatarsal head and is more directly involved in weightbearing.

- *What is the role of radiographic imaging of the opposite, asymptomatic foot?*

- This is a useful troubleshooting tool to compare bone morphology in cases of suspected fracture. Partite sesamoids can be bilateral in 50 to 85% of individuals, while fractures are rarely bilateral. Acutely fractured sesamoids have sharper contours than those seen with displaced partition. Because fibular (lateral) sesamoids are less common, a "partite" lateral sesamoid is more likely to be fractured if the patient presents with pain in that area unless the margins are clearly corticated.

- *What is "turf toe?"*

- Turf toe is a hallux MTP joint injury involving the plantar joint capsule, ligaments, and plantar plate. The term describes a large spectrum of abnormalities with varying severities.

Spectrum of sesamoid fractures

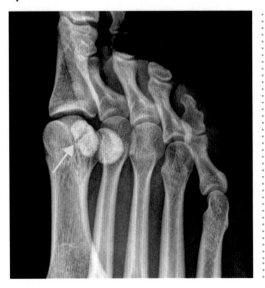

Sesamoid fracture: routine radiographs

Oblique radiograph of the foot demonstrates a non-displaced fracture of the medial hallux sesamoid (arrow). A sharp lucency without corticated edges favors fracture over a bipartite sesamoid.

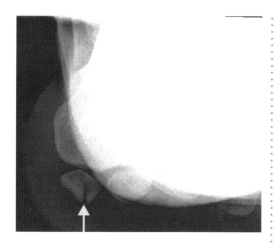

Sesamoid fracture: dedicated sesamoid view

A dedicated sesamoid view is obtained with the x-ray beam directed anterior–posterior through the sesamoids with the foot plantarflexed and the great toe dorsiflexed. Sesamoid view demonstrates a nondisplaced fracture of the medial sesamoid (arrow).

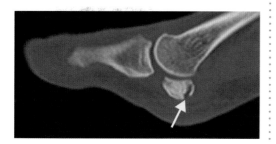

Sesamoid fracture: CT

CT is often helpful in detecting subtle acute fractures, as in this case. Sagittal CT demonstrates a nondisplaced medial sesamoid fracture (arrow).

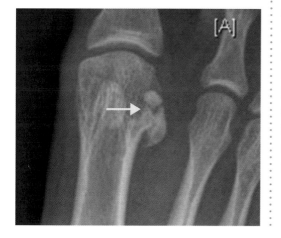

Chronic sesamoid fracture

Delayed union and nonunion are common complications of sesamoid fracture, as a single artery supplies each sesamoid. Non-united fractures have sclerotic margins, differentiating them from acute fractures. If symptomatic, marrow edema will be present on MR. Frontal radiograph demonstrates a chronic, non-united fracture of the lateral sesamoid (arrow), with sclerosis of the fragments.

Differential diagnosis of sesamoid fracture

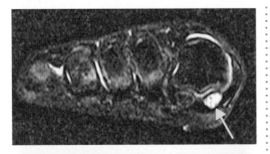

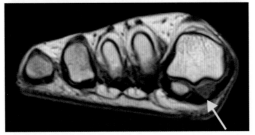

Sesamoiditis

Sesamoiditis is an inflammatory process that results from either direct repetitive trauma to the plantar aspect of the foot or other processes such as osteoarthritis, avascular necrosis, and infection. Radiographs are often normal. MR imaging detects diffuse marrow edema, which may be low signal on T1-weighted imaging when severe. Coronal STIR (upper image) and T1-weighted (lower image) images demonstrate high signal on STIR in the medial sesamoid (arrows), corresponding to low signal intensity on the T1-weighted image.

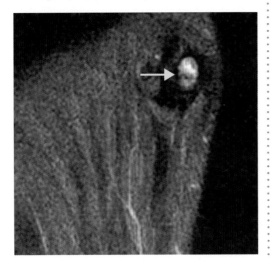

Sesamoid stress fracture

A stress (fatigue) fracture of the sesamoids is common in athletes and dancers who exert increased force across the first MTP joint. Radiographs are often normal. CT may demonstrate a lucent fracture line, with or without separation of fragments. Initial MR findings are nonspecific, with increased marrow edema, as seen in sesamoiditis. If physical activity continues, the fracture may become complete and displaced. Axial STIR image demonstrates diffuse edema in the medial sesamoid, with the suggestion of a low signal intensity fracture line (arrow).

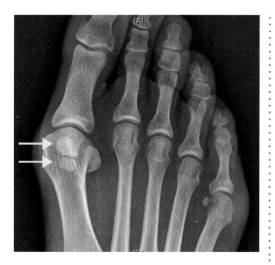

Asymptomatic bipartite sesamoid

Incomplete ossification during late childhood results in partitioned sesamoids. These are most commonly bipartite rather than multipartite. The lateral sesamoid is rarely partite. A partitioned sesamoid has well-corticated, rounded margins at the non-ossified cleft. Partitioned sesamoids are commonly bilateral, and imaging of the opposite foot is often useful to differentiate a bipartite sesamoid from an acute fracture. Frontal radiograph of the foot demonstrates a bipartite medial sesamoid, with well-corticated components (arrows).

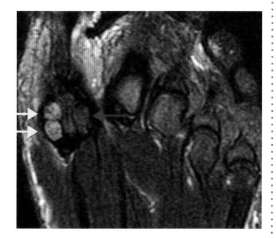

Symptomatic bipartite sesamoid

A bipartite sesamoid may be symptomatic – in such cases, the imaging findings can mimic trauma, with edema in the sesamoid components. One important clue to distinguishing a symptomatic bipartite sesamoid from a fractured sesamoid is that the sum of the bipartite components is often larger than a unipartite sesamoid. Axial proton density-weighted MR with fat suppression (in a different patient from above) demonstrates a bipartite medial sesamoid (yellow arrows) with marrow edema of both components – note that the sum of the bipartite medial components is larger than the normal lateral sesamoid (red arrow).

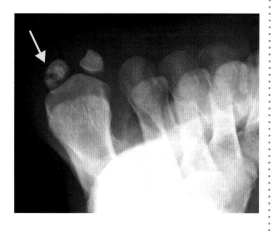

Avascular necrosis

Delicate, non-redundant blood supply predisposes the hallucal sesamoids to avascular necrosis in the setting of repetitive trauma. Radiographic appearance is often normal in the early stages, with MRI showing early marrow edema that later progresses to mixed signal with sclerosis. The hallmark imaging finding of later-stage avascular necrosis is bone fragmentation and sclerosis. Sesamoid view demonstrates irregularity, fragmentation, and sclerosis of the medial sesamoid (arrow).

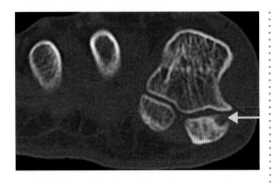

Arthritis

The first MTP joint is a common site of osteoarthritis, gout, and inflammatory arthritis. Imaging findings depend on the etiology of the arthritis, with osteoarthritic changes characterized by osteophyte production, cystic change, subchondral sclerosis, and cartilage space narrowing. Erosions can be seen in inflammatory causes. Coronal CT demonstrates subchondral cystic change of the medial sesamoid (yellow arrow) with a medially projecting osteophyte (red arrow) of the plantar aspect of the first metatarsal in a patient with osteoarthritis.

Further reading

Boike, A., Schnirring-Judge, M., & McMillin, S. (2011). Sesamoid disorders of the first metatarsophalangeal joint. *Clinics in Podiatric Medicine and Surgery*, 28(2), 269–285, vii.

Cohen, B. E. (2009). Hallux sesamoid disorders. *Foot and Ankle Clinics*, 14(1), 91–104.

Sanders, T. G., & Rathur, S. K. (2008). Imaging of painful conditions of the hallucal sesamoid complex and plantar capsular structures of the first metatarsophalangeal joint. *Radiologic Clinics of North America*, 46(6), 1079–1092, vii.

Index